Managerial Epidemiology for Health Care Organizations

MANAGERIAL EPIDEMIOLOGY FOR HEALTH CARE ORGANIZATIONS

SECOND EDITION

Peter J. Fos and David J. Fine

With contributions by
Brian W. Amy
Miguel A. Zúniga

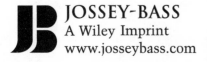

JOSSEY-BASS
A Wiley Imprint
www.josseybass.com

The previous edition of this book was published under the title *Designing Health Care for Populations: Applied Epidemiology in Health Care Administration*, ISBN 0-7879-5226-5.

Published by Jossey-Bass
A Wiley Imprint
989 Market Street, San Francisco, CA 94103-1741   www.josseybass.com

Jossey-Bass books and products are available through most bookstores. To contact Jossey-Bass directly call our Customer Care Department within the U.S. at 800-956-7739, outside the U.S. at 317-572-399386 or fax 317-572-4002.

Jossey-Bass also publishes its books in a variety of electronic formats. Some content that appears in print may not be available in electronic books.

Library of Congress Cataloging-in-Publication Data

Fos, Peter J.
 Managerial epidemiology for health care organizations / Peter J. Fos, David J. Fine.— 2nd ed.
    p. ; cm.
 Rev. ed. of: Designing health care for populations / Peter J. Fos, David J. Fine. 1st ed. c2000.
 Includes bibliographical references and index.
 ISBN-13 978-0-7879-7891-4
 ISBN-10 0-7879-7891-4 (alk. paper)
 1. Epidemiology. 2. Health services administration.
 [DNLM: 1. Epidemiologic Methods. 2. Health Services Administration. 3. Health Care Surveys. 4. Health Planning—methods. 5. Quality of Health Care.] I. Fine, David J. II. Zúñiga, Miguel A. III. Fos, Peter J. Designing health care for populations. IV. Title.
 RA652.F67 2005
 614.4—dc22
              2005003186

Printed in the United States of America
SECOND EDITION
HB Printing   10 9 8 7 6 5 4 3 2 1

CONTENTS

LIST OF TABLES, FIGURES, AND EXHIBITS

Tables

Figures

Exhibits

PREFACE

This book is intended to introduce the student and practitioner of health care management to the notion of health care for populations and the science of epidemiology. Outside the field, epidemiology may be viewed as a questionably relevant
but complicated set of terms, formulas, and statistics. In fact, epidemiology is a core
discipline pertinent to all branches of health care, including management. The mo-
tivating purpose of the text is to illustrate both the relevance and the benefit of epidemiology in the field of health care management and population health
management, and it has been jointly written by authors who bring both a managerial and an epidemiologic perspective to the work. Contemporary applications of epidemiology in health care management are found in monitoring the quality and
effectiveness of clinical services, strategic and program planning, marketing, and managing insurance and managed care. Traditional applications are found in such areas
as tumor registries, infection control programs, and public health programming. This
text is an updated version of the first edition of this book, published in 2000. This new
edition has been substantially rewritten to introduce epidemiologic principles, rein-
force the traditional uses of epidemiology, and illustrate its contemporary uses in planning, evaluating, and managing health care for populations.

   Teaching the practical application of epidemiology in health care management
is an important purpose of this text. Each chapter first presents epidemiologic principles, followed by examples and applications. Concepts, examples, and case studies

allow students and practitioners to understand epidemiology and its application in the design and management of health care for populations.

The text is organized in the following manner. Chapter One introduces the reader to the science of epidemiology. Definitions of epidemiology and an overview of its history in management are presented. Also, epidemiology's transition from its traditional role in health care management to its new role in population health care management is outlined. The chapter also features a historical perspective on the development of epidemiology into a scientific discipline. Chapter Two describes the health and needs of populations and their relevance to management. Included in this chapter is a discussion of the commonly available sources of data. Chapter Three presents epidemiologic measures used in health care, with an emphasis on measures of importance to managers. Chapter Four presents study designs and measures of the cause-and-effect relationship of health and disease across and among populations. Clinical trials, as an example of experimental study designs, are presented, along with the more commonplace observational designs. Chapter Five introduces the concept of confounding, the problem of misleading data interpretation, and methods to address this problem. It includes a discussion of the standardization of epidemiologic data and risk adjustment.

Chapter Six introduces clinical epidemiology as the core discipline of clinical outcomes research, clinical effectiveness, and medical management. Topics covered include validity and reliability, other measures of test performance, infectious disease epidemiology (including epidemiologic surveillance and monitoring infections), and the role of epidemiology in bioterrorism. Chapter Seven, which was written by Brian W. Amy, presents the relationship of epidemiology to planning health care for populations. Emphasis is placed on community health evaluation, performance improvement, and planning based on need. Chapter Eight, which is the result of the work of Miguel A. Zúniga, provides a discussion of health outcomes assessment and the relationships among traditional epidemiologic concepts; benchmarking, best practices, practice guidelines, and the measurement of quality of care are examined. Chapter Nine focuses on the use and benefit of epidemiology in planning and marketing. Chapter Ten describes the relationship between epidemiology and economic analysis, including the manner in which epidemiologic measures are used in the evaluation of health care delivery and the formulation of health care policy for populations. Burden of disease is discussed, with a focus on the economic impact of disease.

Chapters Eleven through Fourteen present case studies of the application of epidemiology to the planning for and management of health care for populations. Chapter Eleven presents a case study focusing on emergency care. The intent of this chapter is to apply general concepts presented throughout the text to establishing a plan for expansion of emergency health care services. The case study in Chapter Twelve focuses on quality of hospital care, and the one in Chapter Thirteen illustrates the application of epidemiology to the study of the pediatric inpatient services in a hospital network. Chapter Fourteen presents a case study focusing on community relations in a hospital service area, specific to both a pediatric and an adult population.

An appendix presents concepts not directly covered in the body of the text. These concepts are important for understanding the relevance of epidemiology to managing health care for populations. Topics included in the appendix are statistical power, hypothesis testing, categorical data analysis, sample size considerations, and the handling of outliers.

Each chapter is supplemented with study questions, intended to aid the reader in understanding and applying the epidemiologic concepts presented in a management context.

We anticipate that the primary users of this text will be health care management students and practitioners, for whom we have presented the material in a practical and applied manner. This book can serve as a classroom text as well as an on-the-job reference for practitioners. We expect that after reading and using this book, the student or practitioner will understand and appreciate the relevance of epidemiology and look forward to using it in everyday health care management practice.

This work has been the result of a multiyear collaboration. The special contributions of two of our former students, Miguel A. Zúniga, M.D., M.H.A., Dr.P.H., who is now the director of the Health Informatics program at the Medical College of Georgia, and Brian W. Amy, M.D., M.H.A., M.P.H., the State Health Officer in Mississippi, are gratefully acknowledged, particularly with respect to the chapter each contributed.

Finally, we would like to thank the students at Tulane University Medical Center School of Public Health and Tropical Medicine, the University of Wisconsin-Madison Medical School, the University of Indiana at South Bend, the University of St. Thomas Graduate School of Business, and the University of Alabama in Birmingham School of Health-Related Professions, whose comments on the first edition have been incorporated into this book. Their collective feedback has improved the book significantly.

P.J.F.
D.J.F.

For Lori Ann, Tammy, Tim, and Maggie
The loves of my life
PJF

For Jeffrey Fine
And his bright future
DJF

THE AUTHORS AND CONTRIBUTORS

Peter J. Fos is dean and professor of the College of Health at the University of Southern Mississippi. He earned his doctorate in health care decision analysis at Tulane University Graduate School following a career in clinical dentistry. Before he assumed the position of dean at the University of Southern Mississippi, he served as the chief science officer of the Mississippi State Department of Health, after spending almost twenty years at academic institutions, where he was active in curriculum development in the application of epidemiology to management, as well as the practice of managerial epidemiology, clinical effectiveness, and health outcomes research. He maintains adjunct faculty positions at Tulane University Health Sciences Center, the University of Mississippi Medical Center, the University of Alabama in Birmingham School of Health-Related Professions, and Dillard University.

David J. Fine is chief executive officer of the St. Luke's Episcopal Health System in Houston, Texas. Fine is a nationally and internationally known health care executive and consultant who has directed hospitals, hospital systems, multispecialty group practices, and managed care organizations. He has published extensively in leading journals and books. In 1985, Fine was the recipient of the prestigious Hudgens Medal from the American College of Healthcare Executives. He is a member of Delta Omega, the national public health honor society, and Omicron Delta Epsilon, the national economics honor society. Fine was recently named one of the one hundred most influential people in health care today by *Modern Healthcare*. He is professor of medicine at Baylor College of Medicine, professor of public health at the University of Texas Health Sciences Center, and professor of the practice of management at Rice University.

Contributors

Brian W. Amy is Mississippi State Health Officer and head of the Mississippi State Department of Health. He holds faculty positions at the College of Health, The University of Southern Mississippi, and the University of Mississippi Medical Center.

Miguel A. Zúniga is associate professor, Department of Health Informatics, School of Allied Health Sciences, Medical College of Georgia. He previously held faculty positions at Tulane University Health Sciences Center and Texas A&M University Health Science Center.

Managerial Epidemiology for Health Care Organizations

CHAPTER ONE

EPIDEMIOLOGY IN HEALTH CARE ADMINISTRATION

Chapter Outline

Introduction
Philosophic Framework
Focus and Uses of Epidemiology
Current Issues in Health Care Administration
The Concept of Populations and Communities
Managing Health Care for Populations and Communities
The Role of Epidemiology
Summary
Study Questions

Learning Objectives

Upon completing this chapter, the reader will be able to do all of the following:

- Define epidemiology
- Discuss the history of epidemiology
- Define managerial epidemiology
- Discuss the distinction between observational and experimental epidemiology
- Describe the uses of epidemiology
- Describe the field of social epidemiology
- Discuss the concept of populations and population health care management

Introduction

Epidemiology is recognized as a core discipline within the field of public health. It is a unique discipline that formally began as a result of the sanitary reform movement in seventeenth- and eighteenth-century England. Epidemiology is formally defined in a number of ways. First, epidemiology is the study of the distribution and determinants of diseases and injuries in human populations (Mausner and Kramer, 1985). A second definition emphasizes the study of all factors that affect the occurrence of health and disease in populations and their interdependence. Finally, epidemiology is the study of the distribution and determinants of health-related states and events in defined populations and the application of this study to the control of health problems (Last, 1995).

Common to all of these definitions is the concept of populations. Individuals are not the focus of epidemiology; *groups* of individuals are. Populations may represent large groups, such as the total population of the United States, or small groups, such as the employees of a factory, store, or government agency. Central to the concept of populations is that groups of individuals exhibit certain commonalities. For example, a group of individuals who are related geographically, such as those living in the same city, represent a population. A group of individuals who work in the same setting are a population. And a group of individuals who live and work together are a population, as in the case of military personnel. Groups of individuals of the same race or ethnic group are also considered populations.

Historically, epidemiology is a discipline that has experienced long and distinct development stages. It is reasonable to think that epidemiology began when humans first walked on earth. Darwin's theory of the "survival of the fittest" can be extended to assume that early humans acquired, over time, an understanding of the relationship between environment and health. One simple example is the use of animal hides and furs as protective clothing.

The relationship between the environment and health and disease is mentioned in the Old Testament. However, it wasn't until the Greek civilization was established that epidemiology began to emerge as a scientific discipline. Hippocrates (460–377 B.C.) wrote the classic work "On Airs, Waters, and Places," the first known treatise on what is referred to today as environmental epidemiology. His writing discussed the link between the environment and human health. Hippocrates provided accurate descriptions of the diseases tetanus, typhus, and phthisis (Singer and Underwood, 1962). His contribution, which is also the first documented use of observational techniques, earned Hippocrates the title of "father of epidemiology" and the designation as the first epidemiologist (Newcomb and Marshall, 1990).

In the 1600s, John Graunt developed the demographic approach to health and disease investigations. Graunt used quantitative methods to study sex differences in deaths and diseases, geographic differences in death rates (rates were found to be higher in cities), and age differences in death rates (infant mortality rates were high). His work represents a significant advancement in epidemiology from an observational to a quantitative discipline, and Graunt is considered the founder of the discipline known as demography (Dupaquier and Dupaquier, 1985). His work is referred to as the starting point of modern epidemiology (Newcomb and Marshall, 1990).

Another seventeenth-century epidemiologist was Thomas Sydenham, who is called the English Hippocrates (Meynell, 1988). Sydenham reemphasized and expanded the theories of Hippocrates. He was the first to describe the clinical manifestations of the condition known as Bell's palsy. He reinitiated scientific observations of health, Hippocrates' contribution, into the core fabric of modern epidemiology.

Medical registration of deaths began in Great Britain in 1801. William Farr (1807–1883), a statistical abstracter in the General Registry Office in London, established a national system of recording causes of death (Eyler, 1980). This standard classification system was the precursor to the International Classification of Diseases and Related Conditions (ICD). Farr's other contributions included involvement in the first modern census, use of the census to collect specific information on diseases and conditions (blindness and deafness), and invention of the standardized mortality rate (Newcomb and Marshall, 1990).

A colleague of William Farr, John Snow, used epidemiologic principles to study outbreaks of cholera in London in the 1850s (Lilienfeld, 2000). Snow demonstrated how scientific evidence can be used to support hypotheses and analytic investigations. He identified the source of the infectious agent, contaminated water, and the etiology of the cholera outbreak (Collins, 2003). His work has been described as a brilliant use of descriptive and quantitative epidemiologic principles (Winkelstein, 1995).

The years leading up to World War II marked the beginning of another important period in the development of epidemiology as a scientific discipline. Epidemiologic methods continued to evolve, with a focus on individual diseases and conditions. The case-control study design was developed during the 1930s. Cohort studies were pursued to observe the relationship of tobacco use and disease. Case-control studies became very popular in hospital-based studies, beginning around 1950 (Levin and others, 1950; Wynder and Graham, 1950; Doll and Hill, 1950). Since then, epidemiology has continued to develop as cohort studies and clinical trials have gained popularity. Well-known cohort studies include the Framingham Heart Study (Gordon and others, 1977) and the Bogalusa Heart Study (Voors and others, 1976).

At the dawn of the twenty-first century, epidemiology has begun to expand its focus to health status, health-related quality of life, and burden of disease. As a result of the terrorist attacks on the United States on September 11, 2001, epidemiology has taken on new roles in bioterrorism preparedness and management of health care services. With the significant number of emerging infectious diseases (including AIDS and SARS), epidemiology's initial role in the study of epidemics will regain prominence.

Philosophic Framework

Our population-based perspective on epidemiology lends itself quite well to the objectives of health care management in the twenty-first century. These new objectives—focused on populations, not individual patient care—have forced a modification in the focal point of the science of epidemiology, which calls for the specialized concentration known as managerial epidemiology. Managerial epidemiology is one result of the contemporary demands of epidemiology and has become the core discipline for planning and managing health care for populations. A functional definition of managerial epidemiology—the use of epidemiology for designing and managing the health care of populations—is the study of the distribution and determinants of health and disease, including injuries and accidents, in specified populations and the application of this study to the promotion of health, prevention, and control of disease, the design of health care services to meet population needs, and the elaboration of health policy.

This adaptation of epidemiology to a managerial focus has been nurtured by many different external forces. One set of forces is the transition from a traditional role of the health care executive to a population orientation. The traditional role of the health care executive has been in a facility context, encompassing such general management functions as planning, organization, leadership, and control. These functions all emphasize the management of facilities and personnel that provide health care services. Planning involves many activities, but in general, it is the determination of courses of action for individuals and organizations. Organization is essential for the coordination of activities and resources, both human and physical. Leadership is centered on the ability or skill to motivate and manage people. Control involves monitoring and periodically evaluating these activities.

The discipline of health care management continues to evolve from the individual patient perspective toward a managed population perspective. The current stage of evolution is highlighted by management of a network of services, management across traditional organizational boundaries, and management of the continuous improvement of quality of care (Shortell and Kaluzny, 1997).

The primary evolutionary pressures on the discipline of managerial epidemiology are cost containment and an underlying desire to maintain and improve the quality of health care. Epidemiology has emerged as a primary discipline in achievement of the population-oriented objectives of health care management.

Focus and Uses of Epidemiology

Epidemiology initially centered on observations and descriptions of health and disease and factors associated with health and disease. During its maturation into a science, experimental considerations were added to the discipline in the twentieth century. Over time, epidemiology developed a specificity for individual diseases, etiologic constellations (injury, chronic disease, and infectious disease epidemiology, for example), and situational uses (including environmental, occupational, molecular, and managerial epidemiology). Both observational and experimental aspects are characteristic in all of the uses of epidemiology.

Observational Epidemiology

Observational epidemiology involves the observation of health and disease in a population and the analysis of these observations. Observational study activities are the most common in epidemiology. Observational study methods include descriptive studies, historically the first type of epidemiologic study, and analytic epidemiologic study designs (cross-sectional, cohort, and case-control designs). Cross-sectional studies measure the prevalence of health and disease in a population. Cohort and case-control studies measure the incidence and risk of health and disease in a population. Chapter Four presents a thorough discussion of these concepts.

Experimental Epidemiology

Experimental epidemiology is concerned with planned studies in which the exposure to potential health and disease risk factors is controlled. The objective of this method is to improve the validity, or accuracy, of epidemiologic studies. Exposure to potential risk factors is accomplished by random assignment. This randomization is used to avoid bias in the study and to ensure validity. Clinical trials are the most commonly used experimental study design. Chapter Four discusses experimental epidemiology in greater detail.

Preventive Medicine

Epidemiology and medicine have always been linked as scientific disciplines. Epidemiology is an important tool of community health and preventive medicine. Specific uses of epidemiology have included determining etiologic or causal factors of diseases; describing factors that are associated with adverse conditions; community diagnosis of the distribution of disease; predicting disease occurrence, impact, and distribution; estimating the individual risk of suffering from diseases; evaluating preventive therapeutic and intervention activities; measuring the efficacy of health measures; studying historical disease trends; identifying disease syndromes; planning for current health needs; and predicting future needs.

Epidemiology plays a major role in controlling the distribution, frequency, and severity of disease in populations. This is accomplished through prevention of new cases (known as primary prevention), as well as by eliminating existing disease profiles

About linky article + risk + health promotion

and improving the health status and survival of individuals with those diseases (known as secondary and tertiary prevention). Primary prevention involves the removal or modification of intrinsic and extrinsic factors that effect a change in health status from absence of disease to preclinical disease. Primary preventive measures include health promotion and specific preventive measures. Health promotion involves health education and the provision of conditions that influence health (adequate food, housing, clothing, and so on). Specific preventive measures target diseases and groups of individuals, often based on the risk of acquiring a disease. These measures include purification of water supplies, immunization, protection from occupational hazards (for example, proper clothing and protective equipment), and protection from accidents (seat belts, for example).

Secondary prevention, which involves screening, early disease detection, and early treatment, often allows for the reversal or delay of the progression from preclinical to clinical disease. This is particularly beneficial in diseases for which control measures exist, such as hypertension. Tertiary prevention involves arresting the progression from clinical disease to disability and reversal of progression from disability to death, with restoration of function through rehabilitation.

Current Issues in Health Care Administration

The health policy experiments of various states, and the periodic policy debates at the federal level, focus on the evaluation and reformation of the manner in which health is promoted and disease and associated disability are controlled in the United States. The notions of improved or even universal access to more comprehensive and cost-effective health care services and the reduction of unnecessary or unproven services are central to such health system reform discussions. Understanding the health status and needs of populations is essential to the proper planning and organization of the health care system.

Contemporary reform of the U.S. health care delivery system from a federal standpoint began in 1965, when Title XVIII of the Social Security Act Amendments created Medicare and Title XIX created Medicaid. Medicare provided financing of health care services for citizens over the age of 65 and for the disabled. Medicaid provided financing of health care services for the medically indigent. These programs were driven by the concept of social equity and represent the first time that the federal government became involved with the financing and delivery of health care services for the general population.

In 1973, Congress passed the Health Maintenance Organization Act, which encouraged the formation and proliferation of health maintenance organizations (HMOs). The intent of this legislation was cost containment. The federal government began to recognize that the HMO model, when successful, reduces the cost of providing health care services and can motivate secondary and even primary prevention activities. This reform movement emphasized the federal government's concern with the cost of health care. A major change in the Medicare program occurred in 1982 with the creation of the prospective payment system (PPS). PPS was created by an act of Congress and focused on in-hospital Medicare charges (often known as "Part A"). A result of PPS was the establishment of diagnosis-related groups (DRGs) to permit the comparison of like admissions and the regulation of their cost. In 1990, Medicare was further reformed with the establishment of the resource-based relative value scale (RBRVS) for reimbursement of physician services (often known as "Part B"). RBRVS is an extension of PPS, and its intent is also cost containment. In 2000, additional PPS efforts were implemented by Medicare's mandate to use the ambulatory patient classification (APC). Payment for services under the outpatient PPS system is based on combining outpatient services into APC groups.

Current initiatives in health policy have centered on the provision of prescription medications and access to care for the uninsured. Medicare coverage has not included a benefit for outpatient prescription medication. The result has been that a significant proportion of elderly Americans must purchase medications using out-of-pocket resources. The latest information suggests that 86% of Medicare beneficiaries use prescription medications (Davis and others, 1999). In addition, about 35% of Medicare beneficiaries have no prescription medication insurance coverage. The Medicare Prescription Drug, Improvement, and Modernization Act of 2003 (Public Law 108-173) is intended to provide access to prescription drug coverage for seniors and individuals with disabilities for the first time in the history of the Medicare program.

Another segment of the population that has been targeted by health policy is children. In spite of Medicaid coverage, a significant number of children are uninsured. Congress passed the Balanced Budget Act of 1997, which created the State Children's Health Insurance Program, referred to as SCHIP. This program is intended to cover children of families who earn too much to be eligible for Medicaid benefits. It is similar to Medicaid in that each state administers its own unique program. Common services covered are physician office visits, immunizations, hospitalizations, and emergency room visits. That same year, Congress passed legislation that allows states to provide health insurance to more children in working families. These programs build on the Medicaid program that started covering children and adults in the mid-1960s. The Children's Health Insurance Program (CHIP) provides health insurance to children free or at low cost through state-sponsored programs. The costs vary by state and by family income, but when there are charges, they are minimal. Depending on income level and the specific state program, it may be possible for an entire family to receive health insurance.

Because health care reform activities will continue, understanding the health status of populations is a crucial success factor for health care executives. The health status of the population is dependent on the environmental conditions, socioeconomic factors, and the structure of the health care system. Future health policy efforts should focus on recognition of the health care needs of the population, with emphasis on services and programs associated with disease prevention, chronic disease, and long-term care, as well as acute care. This can occur by refocusing efforts and objectives of the health care system to promote quality of care, quality of life, and quality of physical function of individuals in the population.

Health care reform efforts inevitably result in a deviation from the traditional public health disease prevention and intervention model, which focuses on communicable and infectious diseases. Public health has begun to direct some of its efforts to behavioral interventions that are designed to reduce smoking, substance abuse, violence, risky sexual behaviors, and obesity. Disease screening, prenatal and child care, health education, and immunization have garnered increased attention. Planning and implementation of such services does not focus on the individual but is centered at the community or larger population levels.

The Concept of Populations and Communities

The concept of populations was first documented in the seventeenth century and has recently grown in its application to health care administration. A population is not defined by a fixed, standard number of individuals but by the specific group under study. It is common to associate the concept of a population with the total population, but subpopulations are more often the concern. The students in a school constitute a population, as do the students in a classroom.

Populations are typically defined by geographic boundaries—for example, residents in a country, regions of a country, states, cities, and sections of a city. Within these geographically circumscribed populations are specific subpopulations defined by age, sex, race, and other characteristics. This method of population definition occurs, in part, due to the ease of identifying population membership and the existing infrastructure for health and disease data collection. Geographically defined areas usually correspond to political or governmental units, with their associated public health agencies.

Subpopulations are the basic unit of comparison in epidemiology. The risk of acquiring a disease is studied across subgroups within a population. In a managed care environment, knowledge of health and risk of disease across subpopulations provides essential information for the actuarial estimation of prevention and treatment costs. Managed care focuses on the identification of health and disease characteristics of groups of individuals in a population of covered lives.

An important consideration is that populations differ; traditional methods of measuring health in populations assume that populations are homogeneous (Tsevat, Slozan, and Kuntz, 1996), but this is not the case. Populations can be divided into several categories based on many variables, in addition to demographics. These different categories of patients are correlated with differing health care needs and associated differences in the utilization of health care resources (Kindig, 1997).

An emerging field in epidemiology is social epidemiology. Social epidemiology is defined as the "study of the social distribution and social determinants of states of health" (Berkman and Kawachi, 2001, p. 35). The aim of social epidemiology is to identify socioenvironmental exposures that may be related to physical and mental health outcomes. The principal concern of social epidemiology is the study of how society and social organization influence the health and wellness of individuals and populations. In practice, social epidemiology studies the frequency, distribution, and social determinants of the states of health in a population. Social epidemiology links the traditional epidemiologic concepts with those from economics, sociology, demography, and biology.

Social epidemiology is attempting to explain the pathway between exposure to social characteristics of the environment and its effects on health. Social epidemiology allows for the incorporation of the social experience of populations into the traditional etiologic cause-and-effect relationship. This incorporation allows for a better understanding of how, where, and why social inequalities affect health.

Managing Health Care for Populations and Communities

Encouraged by the rapid growth of managed care, health care managers are in a transition from the traditional role of management to a population health care management model. A population-based orientation is new to many health care executives and will require an additional set of management skills. The "reformed" health care executive will directly interact with the community and its health insurance vehicles in the planning of medical services to be delivered, including allocation of human and material resources to preventive, curative, restorative, and rehabilitative services. The executive's duties include the design of medical interventions and the monitoring and evaluation of medical services and programs. Clinical outcome measurement and comparison will become a major source of information for management decision making. Population health care design and planning will gain importance in the evolving integrated delivery systems of the future.

Due to the community-based nature of health care, the population in a hospital service area can be challenging to describe. By definition, a community is all the people living in a particular area. These people are either loosely or closely associated due to political or economic advantage. Given the combination of the varying characteristics of a community, the different independent providers in an area, and the choice behavior of the consumers of health care, understanding the needs and concerns of the population is a difficult task. Population information is indispensable for planning and targeting the needs of the community. Administrative claims data, disease registries, and clinical information systems are valuable sources of current data for health care executives.

The overall health status of the population is an important concern of the health care executive in the population health care management model. Understanding patterns of health and disease in the population allows for appropriate planning for services and programs to meet legitimate health care needs. Cost containment, with the resulting health promotion and preventive services emphasis of portions of the delivery system, promises at last to align social and economic objectives, such that improving the health of the population has become a measurement of success for integrated providers in the health care system. Contemporary health care executives must be able to acquire data and understand the community by conducting their own investigative studies on the populations served. Such knowledge will be essential to profitability in fully capitated, full-risk-assumption models of care.

Cost containment + health promotion

Objectives of the population health care management model focus on the health of the population and cost containment. Efforts to reduce utilization, which are not emphasized in the facility-based management model, and to shift utilization to low-cost facilities (for example, outpatient settings or home care) are critical executive concerns under conditions of population-based management. Another objective of population health care management is to organize and align providers in network schemes. Clinical improvement focuses on improving the health status of the population and the integration of care across all settings and all providers. Quality of care is documented and studied, and efforts are made to continually improve quality measures.

The change in the role of management is manifested by the modification of management objectives. In the traditional role, management's objectives include the maintenance of high-quality facilities and equipment, achievement of clinical improvement by attracting the "best-quality" health care providers, and increase in market share and volume of delivered services across populations.

In the population health care management model, the management objectives change to include the reduction in volume of services utilized, shift of utilization to lower-cost settings, achievement of clinical improvement by focusing on the health status of the population, integration of health care services, organization of providers into networks, and evaluation and documentation of quality.

The Role of Epidemiology

Epidemiology will play a major role in the twenty-first-century management of health care systems. The evolving nature of health care administration will forever require the principles and application of epidemiology due to the population-based perspective, as is seen in the managed care model. Information about the prevalence of disease and disability in the population will serve as the obvious focal point for planning health care services and organizing health care delivery systems. Likewise, the insurance concept of community rating relative to risk of disease and hospitalization is founded in epidemiology and is dependent on epidemiologic data.

With the continuing threat of emerging infectious diseases, epidemiology will gain renewed prominence in assisting health care managers. New diseases, along with some previously thought to be eradicated, will become common in hospitals and other health care facilities. Severe acute respiratory syndrome (SARS) is a very specific concern. Most cases of SARS have occurred after close contact with SARS patients. The largest number of infected persons was among hospital workers or other types of caregivers. In spite of infection control measures, SARS transmission occurred across many hospital workers. A case-control study of hospital workers in Hong Kong indicated that inconsistent use of goggles, gowns, gloves, and caps was associated with a higher risk for SARS infection. Infection is strongly associated with the amount of personal protection equipment used, the duration of infection control training, and the level of understanding of infection control procedures (Lau and others, 2003). These requirements are known as "universal precautions" and are a mandatory training activity for human resource departments in order to be in compliance with OSHA standards.

Epidemiologic data and information will be crucial for health care managers. Epidemiologic data have become a useful source of information that can guide managerial decisions and outcomes. The relationship of epidemiologic data to the many aspects of managerial epidemiology is illustrated in Figure 1.1.

Summary

Epidemiology—once viewed by health care executives as a fringe element of public health—is in fact an essential discipline for the management of contemporary health systems. Knowledge of health and disease in a population is as important to the health care executive as it is to the public health officer. The ongoing evolution of health care administration requires additional disciplines and tools. Epidemiology provides a wealth of principles and applications that will affect planning, marketing, quality control, and policy formulation, which are fully dependent on epidemiologic data.

The perspective of management in the health care industry is changing from a fee-for-service, individual-patient-encounter, facility-based perspective to managing the health of populations. This population orientation of health care management requires a communitywide understanding of health and disease, with the health care executive participating directly in planning medical services and other interventions.

FIGURE 1.1. EPIDEMIOLOGIC DATA.

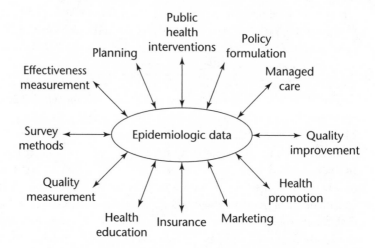

Cost containment (through reduction in utilization of services) and improvement of the overall health of the population are important objectives of the population-based management model. Emerging infectious diseases and the threat of terrorism have resulted in epidemiology becoming thoroughly incorporated into health care administration.

Epidemiologic data are needed to plan and design health care systems, based on communities and groups of communities. Knowledge of epidemiology and an understanding of epidemiologic data are basic requirements for the successful health care executive. The following chapters will introduce terminology, measurements, and techniques of epidemiology. In addition, specific applications to health care management, health care planning, and health care policy will illustrate the benefits of using epidemiology in health care management.

Study Questions

1. Define epidemiology. Give an example of the use of epidemiology, based on this definition, in solving a health care management problem.

2. Discuss epidemiology from a historical perspective. What is the expected next development in epidemiology as a scientific discipline?

3. Identify five other uses of epidemiology, and cite a health care management example of each use.

4. Discuss why health care managers should use population-based data for planning.

CHAPTER TWO

DESCRIPTION OF HEALTH

Chapter Outline

Introduction
Health and Disease
Descriptive Information
Other Descriptive Variables
Sources of Descriptive Information
Reportable Diseases
Reimbursement Approaches
Summary
Study Questions

Learning Objectives

Upon completing this chapter, the reader will be able to do all of the following:

- Discuss what is meant by health and disease
- Explain the uses of descriptive information
- Identify disease classification systems
- Discuss reimbursement approaches
- Describe sources of descriptive information
- Describe person variables
- Describe place variables
- Describe time variables

Introduction

Epidemiology is an observational science that can explain the distribution, determinants, and trends of health and disease in populations. Descriptive information and patterns in descriptive data indicate which factors are associated with the occurrence of disease (causal factors) and provide clues to the origins (etiology) and the causal mechanisms of disease. These data do not establish causal relationships but rather suggest areas for further study and investigation. In the development of epidemiology over time, its use as an observational and descriptive discipline is prominent among the contributions to human health. This chapter will present descriptive epidemiology and its role in designing health care for populations.

Descriptive data offer essential information regarding health, disease, and disease patterns, illuminating disease patterns in terms of person, place, and time. Descriptions of who is affected, where the disease occurs, and when it occurs indicate factors possibly responsible for high or low frequencies of disease in specific groups of individuals. Descriptive data can help identify both high-risk groups of individuals for future interventions and problems to be studied by formal analytic methods.

In addition to aiding in these public health efforts, descriptive data are important to health care administrators because they provide a basis for planning, designing, operating, and evaluating health services. Data describing trends in health and disease provide knowledge about the need and potential demand for health services in populations that is fundamental to effective planning.

Health care planning requires descriptive information about demographics. In fact, age of the population may be the single most important factor in predicting demand for services. Understanding trends in birth rates, death rates, immigration, and emigration is also fundamental to designing and establishing appropriate health care programs.

Descriptive data measurement is insightful because disease is not randomly distributed. Rather, it occurs in specific individuals and groups of individuals in specific geographic areas during specific periods of time. Given this fact, describing health and disease in terms of variables of person, place, and time is the foundation for further evaluation of etiologic and causal mechanisms. If disease were randomly distributed across and among populations, then such description would not help us evaluate and understand its distribution and determining factors.

Health and Disease

Because health personnel focus on disease, health is not typically measured directly; however, descriptive disease measurement is used as an indication of health status. If descriptive data indicate an absence or a relatively low level of disease, the level of health is considered to be high. The measurement of disease is formalized by the use of classification systems for disease, which will be discussed shortly.

Definitions

Health and disease have been defined in a number of ways over the past several decades. Health has been defined as a "state of complete physical, mental, and social well-being and not merely the absence of disease or infirmity" (World Health Organization, 1948, p. 100).

In general, disease has been defined more broadly as the absence of health. This is not always accurate, because an individual with a disease may lead a life that follows the definition of health. For example, an individual with controlled diabetes has a disease but may exhibit optimal well-being and is able to lead a productive life. Disease is best defined as "a pathological condition of a part, organ, or system of an organism resulting from various causes, such as infection, genetic defect, or environmental stress, and characterized by an identifiable group of signs or symptoms" (*American Heritage Dictionary*, 4th ed.).

International Classification of Diseases and Related Problems

In 1910, a World Health Organization (WHO) initiative established a standard classification of diseases that has served as an essential mechanism for national and international comparisons of health and disease. This standard is called the International Statistical Classification of Diseases and Related Health Problems. It is commonly referred to as the International Classification of Diseases (ICD).

The ICD has formed the foundation for disease data collection, presentation, and statistical analysis. The ICD initially classified only data concerning deaths (mortality data) but since 1954 has included data associated with illnesses (morbidity data). Its strength lies, in part, in permitting the study and evaluation of diseases from continent to continent, region to region, country to country, and state to state. Without a standard method to classify diseases, studies and comparisons of long-term trends could not be accomplished.

The ICD is designed to permit international comparability in the collecting, formatting, classifying, presenting, and disseminating of information on mortality. The ICD establishes the format for recording cause of death for vital records systems. Coding rules in the ICD allow for the identification of a single cause of death, which is then recorded on the death certificate.

To keep up with advances in medicine and medical technology, the ICD is revised periodically and has undergone ten revisions since its inception. The revision currently in use in clinical practice is the ninth, known as ICD-9 (Swanson, 2003), with the tenth revision (ICD-10) scheduled soon to replace it.

The ICD was established and is used for epidemiologic reasons (identifying and comparing health and disease trends), but it has recently begun to be used in health care management. The ICD-9, Clinical Modification (ICD-9-CM) is a coding system that is used to classify diagnoses of morbidity in inpatient and outpatient clinical settings. The ICD-9-CM is based on the ICD and is revised every year. The ICD-9-CM is useful in classifying morbidity for medical record storage, medical care review, and health statistics. The ICD-9-CM provides a listing of disease codes, as well as a classification system for surgical, diagnostic, and therapeutic procedures. These codes are used as a basis for reimbursement. Since 1989, physicians have been required by federal law to submit diagnostic codes for Medicare reimbursement. The Centers for Medicare and Medicaid Services (CMS) selected the ICD-9 as the required coding system.

For reasons of statistical tabulation and analysis, the ICD provides three-digit codes for specific disease categories. The classification is based on the anatomical system affected or the agent causing the morbidity or mortality (see Exhibit 2.1). The ICD coding arrangement presents information that may be used to monitor the health of populations and the impacts of causes of mortality and morbidity. The ICD system provides an accurate basis both for the epidemiologist, who needs accurate disease classification for statistical purposes, and the health care administrator, who needs an accurate basis to account for health care services.

Health Status

As was mentioned earlier, health has been traditionally measured as ill health and its severe manifestations. These traditional measures have been morbidity and mortality, which illustrate health at its worst levels. Morbidity and mortality are narrowly focused measures that do not account for disability and dysfunction that affects health.

Health status is a term that describes a measurement of health for a population. Health status has become a multidimensional construct (Patrick and Erickson, 1993). The dimensions of health status include premature mortality, disease symptoms, physiologic states, physical functions, emotional functions, cognitive functions, and health perceptions.

Health status is measured by many different scales and indices that attempt to combine the impact of morbidity and mortality. Health status is typically a measure of the extent to which an individual can function physically, mentally, socially, and emotionally. Health status is actually measuring an individual's health-related quality of life, which has been operationalized as self-administered or interviewer-generated questionnaires. Included in the types of health-related quality-of-life measurements are preference-based measures.

EXHIBIT 2.1. INTERNATIONAL CLASSIFICATION OF DISEASE.

Codes	Disease category
001–139	Infectious diseases
140–239	Neoplastic diseases
240–279	Endocrine, nutritional, and metabolic diseases and immunity disorders
280–289	Diseases of blood and blood-forming organs
290–319	Mental disorders
320–389	Diseases of the central nervous system
390–459	Diseases of the circulatory system
460–519	Diseases of the respiratory system
520–579	Diseases of the digestive system
580–629	Diseases of the genitourinary system
630–679	Complications of pregnancy, childbirth, and the puerperium
680–709	Diseases of the skin and subcutaneous tissue
710–739	Diseases of the musculoskeletal system and connective tissue
740–759	Congenital anomalies
760–779	Certain conditions originating in the perinatal period
780–799	Symptoms, signs, and ill-defined conditions
800–999	Accidents, injury, and poisoning
V codes	Supplementary classification of factors influencing health status and contact with health services—as when a person who is not currently sick encounters the health services for some specific purpose, such as to donate an organ or to receive a vaccination
E codes	Supplementary classification of accidents, injury, and poisoning (external cause)
N codes	Supplementary classification of accidents, injury, and poisoning (nature of injury)

Source: World Health Organization, 1977.

Descriptive Information

Descriptive data occur in two forms—primary and secondary. Primary data are directly collected by a researcher for specific research needs and objectives. The quality of such data is carefully controlled, because data collection is designed to meet the needs of a specific study. Primary data are collected in both large populations and subpopulations. Primary data collection can be time-consuming, expensive, and difficult to accomplish effectively.

Secondary data are collected, usually on a routine basis, by such groups as local, state, national, and international health care agencies. Although they are less expensive and easier to obtain than primary data, secondary data have inherent disadvantages and are often incomplete or inaccurate. Recording and presentation of secondary data can be inconsistent due to the varying methods of data collection used by different collectors. Specific information may be missing, and information may not be recorded in the desired format. Secondary data are typically released several years after being collected.

Descriptive information is typically collected according to person, place, and time. These parameters are described by several measurable variables that indicate health and disease patterns across and within populations and communities. Person variables include age, sex, race, marital status, education, and socioeconomic status. Place variables include country, region of a country, city, and neighborhood. Time variables describe long- and short-term trends.

Person Variables

Individual characteristics are important in describing both health and disease status and trends. Demographic and socioeconomic data provide insights into patterns, etiology, and causation of disease. Major person variables include age, sex, race or ethnicity, marital status, occupation, education, and socioeconomic status.

Age. Age is the most important of the person variables. Disease patterns have been directly correlated with age for many years; typically, disease rates are highest in the very young and the very old. Conversely, disease rates increase or decrease in relationship with age. To describe this trend, rates are often reported as age-specific rates.

For example, age patterns of emergency room visits can be studied for descriptive purposes using 2001 National Hospital Ambulatory Medical Care Survey data (Centers for Disease Control and Prevention, 2001c) to determine the number, proportions, and rate at which women, by age, use the emergency room for injury-related medical care (see Table 2.1). In addition, stratification by age assists in understanding the distribution of patients who experience injuries that require emergency room visits. Descriptive comparisons can be made by age, which can lead to hypotheses that require study for planning purposes.

Table 2.1 shows that most visits to the emergency room for injury-related medical care are made by people in the 25-to-44 age group (32.8%), but the greatest rate of utilization is seen among people aged 15 to 24 (19.1 visits per 100 persons per year). The trend for the rate of injury-related visits across age is not linear. This may be due to many factors, including differing levels of risky activities engaged in by each subpopulation.

Table 2.2 presents information on insurance coverage trends reported in the National Health Interview Survey for the six-month period between January and June 2003. A three-year trend is shown from 2000–2002 with respect to the number of persons who are uninsured. The age categories reflect assumed differences in insurance

TABLE 2.1. NUMBER, PERCENTAGE DISTRIBUTION, AND RATE OF INJURY-RELATED EMERGENCY DEPARTMENT VISITS, BY AGE, 2001.

Age group	Number of visits	Percentage	Rate (visits per 100 persons per year)
All ages	39,389,000	100.00	14.1
Under 15 years	8,137,000	20.7	13.5
15–24 years	7,436,000	18.9	19.1
25–44 years	12,918,000	32.8	15.6
45–64 years	6,629,000	16.8	10.3
65–74 years	1,607,000	4.1	8.9
75 years and older	2,661,000	6.8	17.0

Source: Centers for Disease Control and Prevention, 2001c.

coverage: all people under 65 years of age (those older than 65 are covered by Medicare), people between the ages of 18 and 64 (these people are expected to be employed), and people under 18 years of age. Marked differences can be seen across all years, especially in the under-18 age group.

Table 2.3 presents cancer death rates in the United States, stratified by age, for a three-year period. This three-year trend, 1999–2001, shows that age has an effect on cancer death rates, ranging from 1.8 per 100,000 among people aged less than 1 year to 1,805.8 per 100,000 in the 85-years-and-older category. It is also important to note the linear relationship between age and cancer death rates.

Table 2.4 presents the number of active tuberculosis cases, by age, in the United States during 2002. The data indicate that people in the 25-to-44-year age category have the greatest number of active tuberculosis cases.

Sex. In general, death rates are higher in males in all age groups. By contrast, morbidity rates are higher in females. The number of comorbidities is also significantly higher in females. Disease rates are often reported as sex-specific rates because of the marked differential between mortality and morbidity rates for the sexes. This difference indicates possible etiologic factors, such as genetic and hormonal differences. Occupation may also be a factor, in terms of differences in exposures to risk factors for disease, such as environmental exposures. In recent decades, women have begun to work in all occupations, but in prior periods, certain high-risk job positions (in the military, law enforcement, construction, and industry) were held almost exclusively by men. Over time, sex-specific rates of disease and conditions due to occupational exposure will probably approach insignificance.

TABLE 2.2. NUMBER OF PERSONS LACKING HEALTH INSURANCE, BY AGE, 2000–2002.

Year	Age group	Currently uninsured (millions)	Uninsured for at least part of the past year (millions)	Uninsured for more than a year (millions)
2000	All ages	41.3	51.8	26.6
	Under 65 years	40.8	51.3	26.4
	18–64 years	32.0	39.2	21.3
	Under 18 years	8.9	12.0	5.1
2001	All ages	40.2	50.4	26.1
	Under 65 years	39.8	49.9	25.9
	18–64 years	31.9	38.9	21.4
	Under 18 years	7.9	11.0	4.5
2002	All ages	41.5	51.7	26.2
	Under 65 years	41.1	51.2	25.9
	18–64 years	33.5	40.6	21.9
	Under 18 years	7.6	10.6	4.1

Source: Centers for Disease Control and Prevention, 2003c.

TABLE 2.3. CANCER DEATH RATES PER 100,000 POPULATION, BY AGE, 1999–2001.

Age group	1999	2000	2001
All ages	197.0	196.5	194.4
Under 1 year	1.8	2.4	1.6
1–4 years	2.7	2.7	2.7
5–14 years	2.5	2.5	2.5
15–24 years	4.5	4.4	4.3
25–34 years	10.0	9.8	10.1
35–44 years	37.1	36.6	36.8
45–54 years	127.6	127.5	126.5
55–64 years	374.6	366.7	356.5
65–74 years	827.1	816.3	802.8
75–84 years	1,331.5	1,335.6	1,315.8
85 years and older	1,805.8	1,819.4	1,765.6

Source: Centers for Disease Control and Prevention, 2003d.

TABLE 2.4. TUBERCULOSIS CASES, BY AGE, 2002.

Age group	Number of cases
0–14 years	931
15–24 years	1,595
25–44 years	5,630
56–64 years	4,534
65 years and older	3,295

Source: Centers for Disease Control and Prevention, 2003d.

Table 2.5 presents descriptive information by age and sex detailing discharges from nonfederal, short-stay hospitals in the United States during 1998. This information was collected during the 1998 National Hospital Discharge Survey. It showed that females account for more discharges than males in all age groups, especially in the 15-to-44 and the 65-and-older categories.

Table 2.6 shows data on the number and annual rate of injury-related emergency room visits in the United States during 2001, according to the National Hospital Ambulatory Medical Care Survey. The overall rate is higher for males, 15.8 visits per 100 persons per year, than for females, 12.4 visits per 100 persons per year, with the greatest difference observed in the under-15 age category.

Race or Ethnicity. As with age and sex, disease patterns differ significantly according to race and ethnic group membership. These patterns differ with respect to severity and frequency. Frequency refers to the number of cases of disease, and severity refers to the magnitude of its effect. Table 2.7 presents descriptive information by race. The race categories are black or African American, white, American Indian or Alaska Native, Hispanic or Latino, Asian, and Native Hawaiian or other Pacific Islander.

Research has demonstrated that, in general, African Americans have markedly higher death rates from hypertensive heart disease, cerebrovascular accidents, tuberculosis, syphilis, homicide, and accidental death than other racial and ethnic groups do. Whites have higher death rates from arteriosclerotic heart disease, suicide, and leukemia. In particular, this disparity is seen in cardiovascular disease mortality (Onwuyani, Clarke, and Vanderbush, 2003) and prostate cancer (Crawford, 2003). These findings indicate that disease may occur in a race-specific manner.

Table 2.8 shows information from the 2001 National Hospital Ambulatory Medical Care Survey. The number and rate of injury-related emergency room visits differ significantly according to race and age. The rate for African Americans is 19.3 visits per 100 persons per year, compared to 13.9 for whites. The rate differs according to age across races, with the highest rate among blacks between the ages of 25 and 44.

TABLE 2.5. DISCHARGES FROM SHORT-STAY HOSPITALS, BY SEX AND AGE, 1998.

Sex and age	Number of discharges	Rate per 100,000 population
All persons	31,827,000	116.5
Males (all ages)	12,489,000	93.5
Under 15 years	1,303,000	42.5
15–44 years	2,718,000	44.6
45–64 years	3,286,000	118.8
65 years and older	5,162,000	365.4
Females (all ages)	19,358,000	138.5
Under 15 years	996,000	34.0
15–44 years	7,659,000	125.4
45–64 years	3,410,000	115.9
65 years and older	7,293,000	365.2

Source: Centers for Disease Control and Prevention, 1998.

TABLE 2.6. NUMBER, PERCENTAGE DISTRIBUTION, AND RATE OF INJURY-RELATED EMERGENCY DEPARTMENT VISITS, BY SEX AND AGE, 2001.

Sex and age	Number of visits	Percentage	Rate (visits per 100 persons per year)
All persons	39,389,000	100.00	14.1
Females (all ages)	17,821,000	45.2	12.4
Under 15 years	3,294,000	8.4	11.2
15–24 years	2,977,000	7.6	15.4
25–44 years	5,605,000	14.2	13.3
45–64 years	3,330,000	8.5	10.1
65–74 years	851,000	2.2	8.6
75 years and older	1,764,000	4.5	18.3
Males (all ages)	21,568,000	54.8	15.8
Under 15 years	4,844,000	12.3	15.7
15–24 years	4,459,000	11.3	22.8
25–44 years	7,313,000	18.6	17.9
45–64 years	3,299,000	8.4	10.6
65–74 years	756,000	1.9	9.2
75 years and older	897,000	2.3	15.0

Source: Centers for Disease Control and Prevention, 2001c.

TABLE 2.7. FREQUENCY OF SELECTED RESPIRATORY DISEASES, PERSONS 18 YEARS OF AGE AND OLDER, BY RACE, 2001 (number of cases in thousands).

Race	Emphysema	Asthma	Hay fever	Sinusitis	Chronic bronchitis
White	2,677	18,016	16,614	29,290	9,399
Black/African American	165	2,555	2,026	4,021	1,214
American Indian/ Alaska Native	14	160	174	202	70
Asian	25	466	683	732	157
Native Hawaiian/ other Pacific Islander	10	43	10	28	6
Hispanic/Latino	131	1,874	1,832	2,428	680

Source: Centers for Disease Control and Prevention, 2001b.

TABLE 2.8. NUMBER, PERCENTAGE DISTRIBUTION, AND RATE OF INJURY-RELATED EMERGENCY DEPARTMENT VISITS, BY RACE AND AGE, 2001.

Race and age	Number of visits	Percentage	Rate (visits per 100 persons per year)
All persons	39,389,000	100.00	14.1
Whites	31,552,000	80.1	13.9
Under 15 years	6,314,000	16.0	13.7
15–24 years	6,013,000	15.3	19.7
25–44 years	10,145,000	25.8	15.2
45–64 years	5,347,000	13.6	9.9
65–74 years	1,359,000	3.5	8.7
75 years and older	2,374,000	6.0	16.9
Black/African American	6,752,000	17.1	19.3
Under 15 years	1,587,000	4.0	16.8
15–24 years	1,219,000	3.1	21.9
25–44 years	2,390,000	6.1	21.9
45–64 years	1,121,000	2.8	16.6
65–74 years	206,000	0.5	12.8
75 years and older	228,000	0.6	19.8

Source: Centers for Disease Control and Prevention, 2001c.

Table 2.9 presents information on the frequency of cancer cases by site and race, using the same race categories used in Table 2.7. These data were collected by the Centers for Disease Control and Prevention (CDC) during the National Health Interview Survey in 2001.

Studies have also demonstrated that uncontrolled or poorly controlled hypertension is a major health problem among African Americans. Ischemic heart disease, stroke, and renal failure, major clinical outcomes of hypertension, show significantly higher incidence rates in blacks than in whites. The risk of cardiovascular mortality is greater among black women when compared to white women, which has been shown to be caused by inadequate use of appropriate preventive therapy (Jha and others, 2003). This disparity is also seen among pregnant women, with African Americans demonstrating a higher incidence of hypertensive disorders and a greater risk for severe complications (Zhang, Meikle, and Trumble, 2003).

Death is also directly associated with race or ethnic group. Rates of deaths for homicide are disproportionately higher among minorities. African Americans have higher homicide rates than both whites and Hispanics. Hispanics have significantly higher homicide rates than whites. When these rates are adjusted for age, these same patterns are observed. The death rate for all causes is higher in whites and is significantly higher for diseases of the heart, suicide, malignant neoplasms, and Alzheimer's disease. The death rate for diabetes mellitus, HIV disease, and septicemia is higher in African Americans than in whites (Centers for Disease Control and Prevention, 2003d).

The foregoing observations make it clear, even to the novice, that the planning and delivery of health care services to various populations can be specifically targeted on the basis of race or ethnicity data. Health care organizations seeking to extend programs to underserved populations can focus their efforts in areas of high potential yield. Opening a simple blood pressure screening program at an inner-city church, for example, can detect hypertension inexpensively and permit early referral to appropriate medical care. Current trends of the states toward capitation of Medicaid populations within managed care environments will offer increased motivation for such low-cost screening efforts.

Marital Status. Marital status is associated with varying levels of morbidity and mortality. Death rates are lowest among married individuals and highest among divorced individuals. Marital status is related to differences in women's health status.

Table 2.10 presents data on the number of home health and hospice care discharges in the United States between 1999 and 2000, by marital status. The majority of total discharges are of married persons. Widowed individuals represent the second greatest number of discharges. This trend is seen for both home health and hospice care.

Socioeconomic Status. Socioeconomic status (SES), often referred to as social class, is a term related to occupation, income, education, and overall lifestyle. SES is directly

TABLE 2.9. FREQUENCY OF CANCER IN PERSONS 18 YEARS OF AGE AND OLDER, 2001 (number of cases in thousands).

Race	Total cases of cancer	Breast cancer	Cervical cancer	Prostate cancer
White	12,991	2,047	1,075	1,491
Black/African American	671	149	57	109
American Indian/ Alaska Native	34	3	—	9
Asian	61	17	12	10
Native Hawaiian/ other Pacific Islander	16	—	—	—
Hispanic/Latino	498	168	56	41

Source: Centers for Disease Control and Prevention, 2001b.

TABLE 2.10. NUMBER OF HOME HEALTH AND HOSPICE CARE DISCHARGES, BY MARITAL STATUS, 1999–2000.

Married status at discharge	Total number of discharges	Home health care	Hospice care
Married	3,188,500	2,895,200	293,400
Widowed	2,329,400	2,123,000	206,400
Divorced or separated	411,900	376,700	35,200
Single or never married	1,147,100	1,099,200	47,900
Unknown	723,300	684,900	38,300

Source: Centers for Disease Control and Prevention, 2000d.

related to health and disease; typically, as socioeconomic status declines, morbidity and mortality rates increase. For example, low occupational status is associated with the incidence of hypertension in both African Americans and whites.

The differential prognosis for cancer patients across socioeconomic status has recently been identified as an important factor for cancer survival. The less education and the fewer skills an individual has, the poorer the prognosis. Studies of the relationship of mortality and educational level show several interesting findings. Death rates are higher in groups with lower educational level, as well as in groups with lower income and occupational status. For example, as SES and educational level increase, the rate of mortality from coronary heart disease decreases.

Table 2.11 presents data compiled by the 1997–2003 National Health Interview Survey. Information was collected on uninsured persons under 65 years of age, by age and poverty status—poor, near poor, and not poor. The poor category is defined as persons below the federal poverty threshold. Near poor is defined as individuals with

TABLE 2.11. PERCENTAGE OF UNINSURED PERSONS UNDER 65 YEARS OF AGE, BY AGE AND POVERTY STATUS, 1997–2003.

Age and poverty status	1997	1998	1999	2000	2001	2002	2003 (January–June)
Under 65 years							
All persons	17.4	16.5	16.0	16.8	16.2	16.5	16.7
Poor	32.7	32.7	32.1	32.7	31.0	28.6	29.1
Near poor	30.4	30.8	30.7	31.3	28.6	28.3	30.2
Not poor	8.9	8.0	7.8	8.7	8.4	9.5	8.6
Under 18 years							
All persons	13.9	12.7	11.8	12.3	11.0	10.5	9.4
Poor	22.4	21.6	21.4	20.6	18.8	15.9	13.5
Near poor	22.8	22.5	21.6	21.4	17.0	15.7	14.1
Not poor	6.1	4.9	4.4	5.3	4.4	5.3	4.4
18–64 years							
All persons	18.9	18.2	17.8	18.7	18.3	19.1	19.7
Poor	40.2	40.8	39.9	41.1	39.5	37.0	39.2
Near poor	34.9	36.0	36.3	37.4	35.6	36.2	39.8
Not poor	9.9	9.2	9.0	10.0	9.9	11.0	10.1

Source: Centers for Disease Control and Prevention, 2003c.

incomes of 100% to less than 200% of the federal poverty threshold. Not poor is defined as individuals with incomes of 200% or more of the federal poverty threshold. Since 1997, the percentage of uninsured near poor has increased in the 18-to-64 category and has decreased in the under-18 category. The decrease in the under-18 category is due to health policy changes at the federal and state levels.

Socioeconomic status directly affects health status and disease trends. Growth in children is used as a common indicator of health status, with height measurements used to indicate progress of growth. Differences in height have been related to several factors, including socioeconomic status, parental occupation, employment status, family size, and parental education. Health behavior has been correlated with an individual's socioeconomic status. For example, smoking prevalence rates are high in low-SES groups. This finding could imply that individuals with lower educational levels have less understanding of the relationship between smoking and lung cancer.

Socioeconomic status in general and employment status in particular have been associated with interesting trends in mental disorders. Research found that unemployed women had higher levels of mental depression than employed women. Moreover, when unemployed women were studied across educational levels, women with less education reported more severe depression symptoms.

Table 2.12 presents data on health insurance coverage in the United States in 2003. Among persons aged 18 years and older, as educational level increases, the

TABLE 2.12. PERCENTAGE OF PERSONS LACKING HEALTH INSURANCE COVERAGE, BY EDUCATIONAL STATUS, JANUARY THROUGH JUNE 2003.

Education	Uninsured at time of interview	Uninsured at least part of the past year	Uninsured for more than a year
Did not complete high school	31.1	33.9	25.8
Obtained high school diploma or GED	17.7	21.4	12.1
Continued beyond high school	10.6	13.8	6.4

Source: Centers for Disease Control and Prevention, 2003c.

percentage of individuals without health insurance decreases. Of people with less than a high school education, 31.1% were uninsured at the time of the interview, with 25.8% uninsured for more than a year. This percentage is significantly lower in people with more than a high school education: 10.6% at the time of the interview and 6.4% uninsured for more than a year. As would be expected, as the level of education increases, an inverse relationship is seen with the percentage of individuals who lack health insurance coverage.

The incidence of many diseases is related to socioeconomic status. The risk of end-stage renal disease is significantly higher in African Americans than in whites. The difference is less, but still exists, after adjusting for socioeconomic status (Li and others, 2004). SES is known to create a gradient across many diseases. A thirty-year follow-up study in California found socioeconomic gradients in gender-specific prevalence rates for seven health outcomes. In all seven gradients, an inverse relationship was found between prevalence and SES (Frank and others, 2003).

Population Pyramids. A population pyramid graphically displays the most important demographic features of a population, the distribution of age and sex. Population pyramids are composed of bar graphs that indicate the proportion of the population in each age and sex category. Age is typically divided into five-year increments, with the bar graphs on their sides and the axis in the middle of the graph. Males are illustrated on one side of the pyramid, females on the other. The specific shape of the population pyramid provides insight into the demographic profile of a population. Review of population pyramids over time is a good indicator of future population growth trends. In addition, this information can be used to determine the health needs of the population. Figure 2.1 presents the population pyramid for the United States in 2003.

FIGURE 2.1. POPULATION PYRAMID FOR THE UNITED STATES, 2003.

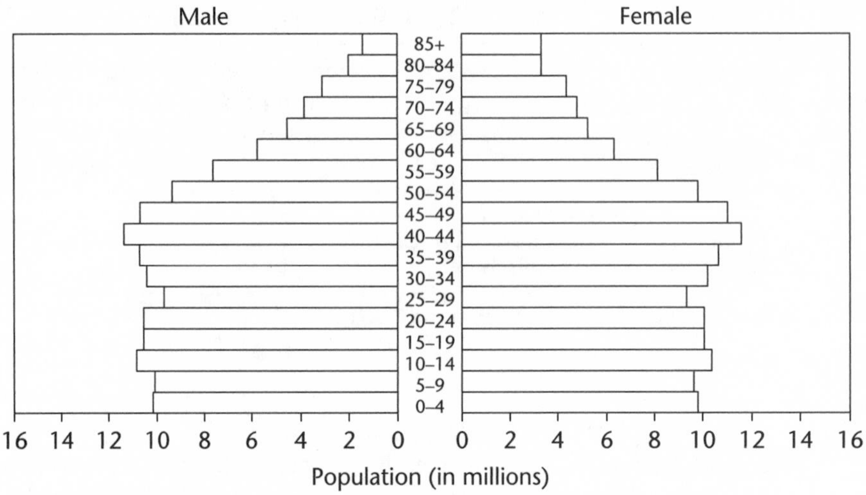

Source: U.S. Census Bureau.

Place Variables

Place data indicate distinct geographic patterns that are useful for understanding possible etiologic factors of disease. Place data are also useful in distinguishing genetic factors of disease causation from environmental factors. Knowing where disease occurs is important for understanding the factors that lead to changes in health. Areas defined by natural boundaries demonstrate varying frequencies of specific diseases. These characteristic patterns occur because of specific environmental factors. In fact, diseases whose occurrence depends on specific environmental conditions are called place diseases. Malaria is a classic example of a place disease because it is found in specific geographic regions of the world.

Table 2.13 presents information from the 1998 National Hospital Discharge Survey. The table shows the number of patients discharged from short-stay hospitals in the United States, by region of the country. It also includes information about the number and type of inpatient procedures performed. The regions are Northeast (Maine, New Hampshire, Vermont, Massachusetts, Rhode Island, Connecticut, New York, New Jersey, and Pennsylvania), Midwest (Michigan, Ohio, Illinois, Indiana, Wisconsin, Minnesota, Iowa, Missouri, North Dakota, South Dakota, Nebraska, and Kansas), South (Delaware, Maryland, District of Columbia, Virginia, West Virginia, North Carolina,

TABLE 2.13. INPATIENT DISCHARGES FROM SHORT-STAY HOSPITALS, BY REGION, 1998 (in thousands).

Region	Total discharges	Discharges without procedures	Discharges after procedures	Discharges after surgical procedures
Northeast	6,818	2,295	4,524	2,998
Midwest	7,366	3,063	4,302	3,211
South	12,022	4,978	7,044	5,385
West	5,621	1,562	4,058	2,876

Source: Centers for Disease Control and Prevention, 1998.

South Carolina, Georgia, Florida, Kentucky, Tennessee, Alabama, Mississippi, Arkansas, Louisiana, Oklahoma, and Texas), and West (Montana, Idaho, Wyoming, Colorado, New Mexico, Arizona, Utah, Nevada, Washington, Oregon, California, Hawaii, and Alaska). The greatest number of discharges and surgical procedures occurred in the South.

The incidence of certain cancers in locations later found to be contaminated by hazardous chemical or radioactive waste is an example of a place variable. There have been instances of successful class-action litigation in which the expected future incidence of disease is estimated. As a result, a hospital could undertake to contract for the future delivery of necessary diagnostic, preventive, curative, and restorative services.

Areas divided by political boundaries are commonly studied and compared for insights into health and disease trends. Political units such as local government agencies routinely collect data and make them available for study and comparison. For example, data on disease cases (collected for administrative purposes) as well as census data are categorized by political units.

An emerging field in epidemiology is the study of the built environment and its relationship to health. Research evidence indicates that physical and mental health problems relate to the built environment. Preliminary results show that there are health benefits from sustainable communities. Studies suggest that coming into regular contact with the natural environment has health benefits (Sriniasan, O'Fallon, and Dearry, 2003; Verderber and Fine, 2001).

Place and socioeconomic status are often related. Lower-SES communities usually have limited access to quality housing. In addition, individuals who are in lower-SES groups have limited access to adequate outdoor facilities and healthy food sources. These lower-SES communities are characterized by inequities in housing, high population densities, and associated higher rates of respiratory disease, developmental disorders, chronic illness, and mental illness (Sriniasan, O'Fallon, and Dearry, 2003).

Place, which has been studied only from a geographic perspective, is now considered important in understanding health impacts that include physical, psychological, social, spiritual, and esthetic outcomes. Place is a public health construct, and this new line of research indicates opportunities for using place to target public health problems. Specific aspects of the built environment—nature contact, buildings, public spaces, and urban form—guide the identification of opportunities (Frumkin, 2003).

It was common, in the recent past, that high densities of low-income individuals were housed in large urban developments, which were typically public housing settings. These situations were the topic of many studies to determine the health impact of living in high-density urban developments. These studies typically centered on the relationship between living in a low-income neighborhood and physical and mental health. Results of these studies indicated that parents who moved from high- to low-density neighborhoods experienced less stress and mental concerns. Boys who moved from low-income to more affluent neighborhoods reported less mental depressive and dependency problems (Leventhal and Brooks-Gunn, 2003).

Time

Time is a descriptive variable that is useful in the explanation of disease trends. The term *endemic* indicates a period of time when the expected incidence of a disease is observed. The term *epidemic* indicates a period of higher-than-expected incidence of disease in terms of place and time. Epidemics are typically defined by a specific time period and are illustrated by a unique graph of the number of cases over time. This characteristic curve is referred to as an epidemic curve. Epidemic curves usually reflect short-term trends—that is, hours, days, weeks, or months. The particular shape of the epidemic curve depends on the type of disease exposure. A point exposure, which occurs in a period of days, will result in a steep, peaked curve. Food poisoning and gastrointestinal problems are examples of point exposure epidemics (see Figure 2.2). The peaked epidemic curve indicates that all cases of the disease, given the same incubation time period, occur in a short amount of time.

Disease trends often parallel seasons of the year. These seasonal epidemics are actually expected fluctuations over a long period of time. This pattern is influenced by the mode of transmission. Chickenpox among school-age children is an example of a seasonal epidemic. Cases of chickenpox typically occur in the winter months because schoolchildren remain indoors for long periods of time each day and this communicable infection is easily transmitted in close quarters. Physicians' offices, clinics, and hospitals will often focus on the almost inevitable influenza epidemic cycle in order to estimate the amount and type of vaccine to have on hand and to predict in-patient staffing requirements resulting from the admission of highly susceptible individuals. A multiyear study indicated that dermatologic disease follows seasonal variations. Specific diseases occur more often in the spring and summer (dyschromia

FIGURE 2.2. GRAPH OF A TYPICAL POINT EXPOSURE EPIDEMIC.

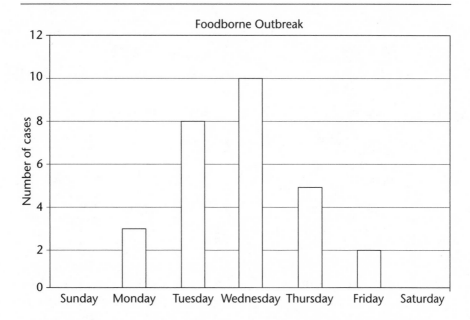

and seborrheic keratosis), while others are seen more frequently in the fall and winter (acne and folliculitis). These variations are related to biological and nonbiological factors (Hancox, Sheridan, Feldman, and Fleischer, 2004).

Disease patterns can also demonstrate long-term trends, usually over a decade or several decades. These are known as secular trends. Secular trends are of utmost importance to both public health and health care policy and planning. These trends indicate information about disease determinants and their influence on morbidity and mortality. Examples of secular trends are hypertensive diseases and coronary heart disease. Since 1940, there has been a continual decline in the incidence of hypertensive diseases. Beginning in 1965, coronary heart disease has also shown a declining trend, which accelerated during the 1970s. The overall decline in coronary heart disease incidence from 1965 to the present has been 50 percent.

It is important for health care managers to understand time patterns in order to plan strategically. Table 2.14 presents data on the number of discharges from U.S. hospitals over a twenty-three-year period, 1975 to 1998, collected by the National Hospital Discharge Survey. The data show that the average length of stay has decreased for all patients and for short-stay patients. In addition, the rates of discharges have

TABLE 2.14. DISCHARGES FROM SHORT-STAY HOSPITALS, 1975–1998.

	1975	1980	1985	1990	1995	1998
Number of discharges (in thousands)	34,043	37,382	35,056	30,788	30,722	31,827
Rate of discharges (per 100,000 population)	159.2	167.7	148.4	122.3	115.7	116.5
Number of days of care (in thousands)	262,389	274,508	226,217	197,422	164,627	160,914
Rate of days of care (per 100,000 population)	1,227.3	1,216.7	957.7	784.0	620.2	589.2
Average length of stay (in days)	7.7	7.3	6.5	6.4	5.4	5.1

Source: Centers for Disease Control and Prevention, 1998.

decreased from 159.2 to 116.5 per 100,000 population, and days of care have decreased from 1,227.3 to 589.2 per 100,000 population. Overall, there have been substantial decreases in both the number of discharges and days of care, which probably indicates that use of hospital care decreased over the period 1975–1998.

Other Descriptive Variables

The risk of health and disease in a population is very important information for scientists and managers. The Behavioral Risk Factor Surveillance Survey (BRFSS) is a large telephone survey, conducted by each state and administered by the CDC, that is used to plan for providing health services to improve the health of people in the United States. The BRFSS started in 1984 as statewide surveys, with several states stratifying information to understand region-specific data trends within those states. The scope of the BRFSS is adults and their personal health behaviors that are thought to have an impact on health and disease. These personal health behaviors believed to be linked with chronic diseases include lack of physical activity, overweight, poor nutrition, tobacco and alcohol use, and low use of preventive health services (Ford and others, 2004).

An extension of the BRFSS is the Youth Risk Behavior Surveillance System (YRBSS). The YRBSS was established in 1990 to survey individuals not included in the BRFSS, namely, youths and young adults. The YRBSS is focused on health behaviors that affect causes of death, disability, and social problems among youths and young adults in the United States. Behaviors of interest include tobacco, alcohol, and drug use; dietary behaviors; lack of physical activity; sexual practices; and behaviors that may result in unintentional injury or violence. The YRBSS is used in estimating the prevalence of health risk behaviors; documenting trends in health risk distribution over time; studying the co-occurrence of health behaviors; and making national and state comparisons and subpopulation comparisons (Grunbaum and others, 2004).

Several additional descriptive variables can be used to understand the populations served by health care systems. One important variable is the payment source. To plan future activities of a health care system, health care managers must know the party responsible for financing health care services, particularly in managed care environments in which a portion of the population are members of a managed care entity. Understanding the payment source distribution across the population can be essential for the health care provider who is responsible for the provision of health care to specific populations within which health plan coverage may have a significant effect.

Table 2.15 presents information about payment sources collected during the 2001 National Ambulatory Medical Care Survey. The largest proportion of people who seek treatment at physicians' offices are those who have private insurance coverage (58.8%), followed by Medicare beneficiaries (21.8%). Other payment source categories, in descending order, are Medicaid/SCHIP (7.2%), self-pay (4.0%), and workers' compensation (1.7%). Medicare and Medicaid figures indicate that the government pays for office visits for 29% of the population.

Sources of Descriptive Information

The process of reporting disease information begins with physicians, hospitals, and other health care providers. Physicians report disease and deaths to local health departments, which in turn report to county and state health departments, which usually tabulate and perform data analysis. Most state health departments maintain disease registries for specific diseases, including tuberculosis, cancer, and HIV/AIDS. State health departments submit periodic reports to the U.S. Department of Health and Human Services, the Public Health Service, and the CDC. The CDC provides reports to the World Health Organization. Clinical diagnoses by physicians, medical chart review, and hospital laboratory results are examples of local data sources.

The CDC processes, analyzes, and publishes periodic reports on death and disease data. The CDC publication *Mortality and Morbidity Weekly Report* (*MMWR*) presents weekly summaries of disease and death data trends. The American Medical Association (AMA) commissions studies of disease patterns for cardiovascular disease in

TABLE 2.15. NUMBER AND PERCENTAGE OF OFFICE VISITS, BY SOURCE OF PAYMENT, 2001.

Payment source	Number of visits (in thousands)	Percentage
All visits	880,487	100.0
Private insurance	517,402	58.8
Medicare	192,139	21.8
Medicaid/SCHIP	63,604	7.2
Self-pay	35,305	4.0
Workers' compensation	14,852	1.7
No charge, charity	3,127	0.4
Other	16,408	1.9
Unknown	37,649	4.3

Source: Centers for Disease Control and Prevention, 2001c.

particular. The CDC, through its National Center for Health Statistics (NCHS), conducts many ongoing surveys, including the National Health Interview Survey (NHIS), the National Hospital Discharge Survey, and the National Health and Nutrition Examination Survey (NHANES). The NHIS collects information about household members' income, education, recent morbidity, and use of health care services. The NHANES conducts physical examinations to determine nutritional status and the presence of chronic diseases.

The CDC has a computerized public health information system to distribute disease data to public health personnel, health care providers, health care managers, and the public. This unified information system, known as CDC WONDER, provides access via telephone and modem to databases containing information on mortality, cancer incidence, reportable diseases, HIV/AIDS, hospital discharges, and the *MMWR*. Data accessed through CDC WONDER are obtained from local and state health agencies and are formatted to simplify management. CDC WONDER is now accessible on the Internet. The data can be used to plan and evaluate health care programs, to request funding from public and private sources, and to conduct research (Friede, O'Carroll, Thralls, and Reid, 1996).

The CDC has a very comprehensive and easily navigated Internet Web site, which can be found at http://www.cdc.gov. This site contains information about CDC publications, software and other products, data, travelers' health, and links to other health-related sites. The Web site is also the source for an electronic version of the *MMWR*. Data that are presented on the Web site include scientific data, surveillance data, health statistics, and laboratory information.

Demographic data are collected every ten years by the U.S. Census Bureau. A census is an official enumeration of the population, with details as to age, sex, occupation, and other demographic characteristics. Census data provide a detailed demographic profile of the U.S. population and subpopulations (subdivided by age, race, occupation, geography, and so on). Denominator data for calculating death and disease rates originate from census data. These periodic population censuses are important sources of data on the size, distribution, and characteristics of the population of the United States. Changes in population can be identified by evaluating demographic trends in census data. Specifically, population density and sex distribution data may suggest potential health problems that should be the focus of health planning.

Vital Statistics

Data on births and deaths have been recorded in the United States since 1930. This recording of vital statistics is required by law and is administered by the NCHS. The data sources are death certificates, birth certificates, and fetal death certificates. All mortality data collected in the United States are culled from the Standard Certificate of Death completed by the attending physician at the time of death. These data are widely accepted because they are universally available and standardized. The certificate records information about the decedent and the cause or causes of death. It contains demographic data, including age, sex, date of death, race, date of birth, location of death, Social Security number, occupation, place of residence, and names of parents. These certificates also contain specific mortality data, including immediate cause of death, contributing conditions, other significant conditions, whether death was accidental, and—if death was due to injury—the circumstances associated with the injury.

A fetal death is defined as death prior to complete expulsion or extraction of the fetus at birth. Fetal death certificates are required by law in all states and are completed by physicians or nonphysician attendants. In addition to demographic data, these certificates include cause of death, maternal conditions, gestational age, and congenital malformations and anomalies. Fetal death certificate data are important for analyzing patterns of fetal deaths by geographic region.

Overall, death certificates have proved to be satisfactory sources of mortality data. However, there are disadvantages to using death certificate data. Because individual physicians are responsible for filling out death certificates, incomplete reporting can occur. The cause of death may be falsified on the death certificate to reduce the chance of embarrassment for the decedent's family (as in cases of suicide or drug overdose). Moreover, analyzing causes of death from death certificate data may be problematic because the ICD changes every ten years. Thus studying long-term trends based on death certificate data may be difficult because the same disease may have different codes over time.

Birth certificates are completed by physicians for every live birth. Typical information collected includes sex, hospital of birth, age of mother, name of mother and father, race of mother and father, birth weight, marital status of parents, educational level of parents, pregnancy history of mother, number of prenatal visits, and pregnancy complications. Birth certificate data reveal patterns of birth weights and severe birth defects and are useful in the analysis of health information on newborns.

Medical Records

The term *medical records* encompasses several different documentation systems. Medical records include hospital inpatient records, emergency room records, physician office and clinic records, school nurse records, and industrial facility employee records. Medical records are used for analyzing disease patterns in specific geographic areas. They are particularly useful because they provide data on diseases that may not be the foci of other descriptive recording systems. However, these data have several disadvantages: clinical diagnoses may vary in quality, authorization is required to access data, searching and abstracting medical records data is costly and time-consuming, defining the population served is difficult because utilization of services may not be geographically bound, and use of medical care is influenced by many factors.

Medical records data are compiled and stored by national health agencies. The NCHS maintains the National Hospital Discharge Survey, which annually summarizes data on two hundred thousand discharges from more than four hundred hospitals. Survey data consist of diagnoses, surgical procedures, and patient characteristics. The Commission on Professional and Hospital Activities (CPHA) compiles data from 40% of U.S. hospitals on discharge diagnoses and patient characteristics. The NCHS also conducts the National Ambulatory Medical Care Survey, which compiles data on diagnosis and characteristics of physician office visits. These data are voluntarily reported by three thousand private medical practitioners.

Reportable Diseases

Some morbidity data are collected as a result of legal mandate. The diseases covered are referred to as notifiable or reportable diseases. Laws regulate which reportable diseases must be disclosed by physicians, hospitals, and other health care providers. Reportable diseases are considered of public health interest and require surveillance. The purpose of this required reporting is to identify the onset of disease outbreaks (epidemics). In addition, the reporting of specific diseases provides information for measuring disease incidence in a population as well as for taking appropriate populationwide actions.

The reporting procedure has several categories. These are mandatory written reporting, mandatory reporting by telephone, reporting of total number of cases, and cancer cases. Each state has a list of reportable diseases, which vary slightly across the country. Exhibit 2.2 presents the reportable diseases included in the listings of all fifty states.

EXHIBIT 2.2. NATIONALLY NOTIFIABLE INFECTIOUS DISEASES IN THE UNITED STATES, 2003.

Acquired immunodeficiency syndrome (AIDS)
Amebiasis
Anthrax
Botulism
Brucellosis
Chancroid
Chlamydia trachomatis
Cholera
Coccidioidomycosis
Cryptosporidiosis
Cyclosporiasis
Diphtheria
Ehrlichiosis
Encephalitis/meningitis, arboviral
Enterohemorrhagic *Escherichia coli*
Giardiasis
Gonorrhea
Hemophilus influenza, invasive disease
Hansen disease (leprosy)
Hantavirus pulmonary syndrome
Hemolytic uremic syndrome, postdiarrheal
Hepatitis, viral, acute (A, B, B virus perinatal infection, C)
Hepatitis, viral, chronic (B, C)
HIV infection
Legionellosis
Listeriosis
Lyme disease

Malaria
Measles
Meningococcal disease
Mumps
Pertussis
Plague
Poliomyelitis, paralytic
Q-fever
Rabies (human and animal)
Rocky Mountain spotted fever
Rubella
Rubella, congenital syndrome
Rubeola
Salmonellosis
Shigellosis
Streptococcal disease, invasive, Group A
Streptococcal toxic-shock syndrome
Streptococcus pneumoniae, drug-resistant, invasive disease
Syphilis
Tetanus
Toxic shock syndrome
Trichinosis
Tuberculosis
Tularemia
Typhoid fever
Varicella (chickenpox—morbidity)
Varicella (chickenpox—deaths only)
Yellow fever

Source: Centers for Disease Control and Prevention, 2004a.

Beginning in 1878, morbidity data have been collected for cholera, smallpox, plague, and yellow fever. Over time, other diseases have been added to this first list of notifiable diseases. In 1912, the first report on notifiable diseases in the United States was distributed. Since 1961, the CDC has maintained responsibility for collection and distribution of information on notifiable diseases. In general, diseases are mandated by law to be reported if they are communicable, they are associated with high rates of mortality, and control measures exist and are available. Reporting of nationally notifiable diseases is voluntary; reporting is mandated in states according to each state's laws governing notifiable diseases. All states comply with the WHO's International Health Regulations and report the internationally quarantinable diseases, which are cholera, plague, and yellow fever. Table 2.16 shows the number of cases of various reportable diseases in the United States in 2001.

TABLE 2.16. INCIDENCE OF NOTIFIABLE DISEASES IN THE UNITED STATES, 2001.

Notifiable disease	Number of cases reported
Acquired immunodeficiency syndrome (AIDS)	41,868
Anthrax	23
Botulism	39
Brucellosis	136
Chancroid	38
Chlamydia trachomatis	783,242
Cholera	3
Coccidioidomycosis	3,922
Cryptosporidiosis	3,785
Cyclosporiasis	147
Diphtheria	2
Ehrlichiosis	403
Encephalitis/meningitis (California)	216
Enterohemorrhagic *Escherichia coli*	3,478
Gonorrhea	361,705
Hemophilus influenza, invasive disease	1,597
Hansen disease (leprosy)	79
Hantavirus pulmonary syndrome	8
Hemolytic uremic syndrome, postdiarrheal	202
Hepatitis A	10,609
Hepatitis B	7,843
Hepatitis C; non-A, non-B	3,976
Legionellosis	1,168
Listeriosis	613
Lyme disease	17,029
Malaria	1,544
Measles	116
Meningococcal disease	2,333
Mumps	266
Pertussis	7,580
Plague	2
Psittacosis	25
Q-fever	26
Rabies (human and animal)	7,150
Rocky Mountain spotted fever	695
Rubella	23
Rubella, congenital syndrome	3
Salmonellosis	40,495
Shigellosis	20,221
Streptococcal disease, invasive, Group A	3,750
Streptococcal toxic shock syndrome	77
Streptococcus pneumoniae, drug-resistant, invasive disease	2,896
Syphilis	32,221
Tetanus	37
Toxic shock syndrome	127
Trichinosis	22
Tuberculosis	15,989
Tularemia	129
Typhoid fever	368
Varicella (chickenpox)	22,536

Source: Centers for Disease Control and Prevention, 2001e, 2004a.

Reimbursement Approaches

Reimbursement methods have been a topic of concern since the beginning of health care reform in 1964. This concern deepened in 1982 with the initiation of the Prospective Payment System for Medicare reimbursement. Many different approaches have been proposed, tested, and used. The common thread is that most of these approaches are based on epidemiologic principles. The following sections will present some of these approaches and the relationship to epidemiology.

Current Procedural Terminology

The Physicians' Current Procedural Terminology (CPT) is not a disease classification system but is very important in designing and managing health care for populations. The American Medical Association, in an attempt to standardize reporting of physician activities, established the CPT in 1963 and three years later published the first listing of terms and codes identifying procedures performed by physicians; these lists are now updated annually. The CPT provides a standardized language to describe medical, surgical, and diagnostic services for reporting needs and for communication among physicians, their patients, and interested third parties.

The nomenclature established by the CPT is the most widely used for reporting physician procedures and services covered by both governmental and private health insurers. The CPT is used for medical care review and administrative medicine; in addition, CPT nomenclature is used in medical education and research because it establishes a basis for local, regional, and national comparisons.

All procedures and services performed by physicians are assigned a five-digit CPT code. Coding is based on consistent contemporary medical practice by physicians in multiple locales. The system was developed and is revised independently of any influence from health insurance coverage or reimbursement policies.

CPT coding permits stand-alone explanation as well as description of medical procedures. Its system is split into six sections, which are further divided into subsections. These subsections are organized according to anatomic, procedural, condition, or descriptor headings. The six sections are evaluation and management; anesthesiology; surgery; radiology, including nuclear medicine and diagnostic ultrasound; pathology and laboratory; and medicine.

Diagnosis-Related Groups

In an effort to reverse the upward trend in Medicare hospital expenditures, Congress in 1982 directed the secretary of health and human services to develop a prospective payment system. The PPS reformed Medicare's cost-based payment scheme, which had seemed to encourage increasing expenditures. Its major changes were a limit on total hospital inpatient costs per discharge, adjusted for hospital patient case mix; a limit on the annual rate of increase of total costs per discharge; and an incentive payment to hospitals whose costs fall below both those limits.

Under the PPS, hospital payment is related to treatment services provided to patients who are categorized into diagnosis-related groups (DRGs). The rate of payment associated with each DRG represents total payment for a Medicare beneficiary's inpatient hospital care. Patient cost sharing, except for mandated coinsurance and deductibles, was prohibited until 1997.

DRGs are based on the ICD-9-CM codes, which are grouped into twenty-three major diagnostic categories (MDCs). DRGs are subsets of MDCs and are intended to describe the patient, the disease condition, and the treatment process. Statistical analysis and clinical judgment are combined to produce case types, which contain patients with similar costs. DRG selection is based on primary diagnosis (ICD-9-CM codes), secondary diagnosis, primary surgical procedures, and complications and comorbidities. Included in the DRG selection is relative resource intensity of medical services.

The effective management of the coding process is a critical determinant of reimbursement for institutional and professional services. Failure to code comorbidities adequately or to identify principal diagnoses properly has the effect of reducing reimbursement. As a result, many consulting firms have developed lucrative product lines focused on the optimization of coding practices. Some firms even furnish this service on a contingency fee basis. At its extreme, this practice has resulted in a phenomenon known as "DRG creep," for which the CMS periodically adjusts its weighting factors. In some cases, upcoding activities have been known to exceed the bounds of ethical management and have resulted in prosecution under civil and criminal statutes.

Reimbursement for each DRG is based on data from the MEDPAR file, the Medicare Cost Report, and the Medicare Discharge file. The MEDPAR file is a sample of Medicare beneficiary bills. The Medicare Cost Report consists of institution-specific cost data as provided to Medicare financial intermediaries. The Medicare Discharge file contains data on the number of Medicare cases treated by hospital and by year. Regional wages and rates for personnel, hospital case mix data, and other factors are used to adjust DRG rates for specific hospitals.

Summary

Descriptive data tell *who, when,* and *where* with respect to a disease or condition. Such data allow the identification of groups of individuals at risk for developing a disease or condition of interest. Given this information, specific health care services or preventive programs can be directed at these targeted groups.

Descriptive data also suggest explanations for why some groups of individuals are at risk for a disease or condition. These data may lead to modifications of existing health services and programs or the provision of new, customized services to those in need of care. Descriptive data thus provide the basis for decisions to implement or modify medical programs and to modify specific aspects of the environment.

Descriptive data are also important in permitting comparison of the effectiveness of new health care services—for example, a new type of immunization, an alternative mode of providing medical care, or a new screening program—to that of existing programs.

Study Questions

1. Discuss the uses, strengths, and weaknesses of the following data sources:
   a. Health insurance data
   b. Special epidemiology surveys
   c. Vital statistics
   d. Disease registries
   e. Absenteeism data from schools or workplace settings
   f. Hospital and clinic data
   g. Reportable disease data

2. Descriptive epidemiology studies the characteristics in a population according to person, place, and time. Discuss the importance of person, place, and time to understanding the distribution of disease.

3. Suppose that the board of directors of a hospital has decided to investigate the feasibility of developing a cancer center. With respect to epidemiologic concepts, answer the following questions:
   a. What information would be important in determining the feasibility of the cancer center? What specific data would you seek?
   b. What are the sources of this information?
   c. What planning significance does each variable represent?

CHAPTER THREE

MEASUREMENT OF HEALTH

Chapter Outline

Introduction
Measures
Measuring Morbidity
Measuring Mortality
Measuring Health
Summary
Study Questions

Learning Objectives

Upon completing this chapter, the reader will be able to do all of the following:

- Explain the use of absolute counts in planning and managing health care services
- Discuss the importance of rates for comparison of health and disease among subpopulations
- Discuss the distinction between and uses of incidence and prevalence data
- Describe the sources and uses of mortality data
- Discuss the distinction between and uses of ratios and proportions
- Describe health-related quality of life
- Describe the sources and uses of morbidity data

Introduction

This chapter will present the constructs used to measure the frequency of health and disease in a population, as well as measures of need for health care services. Epidemiology is a quantitative discipline in which the frequency of disease occurrence is measured to make comparisons among populations with differing characteristics. Disease frequency and death frequency are calculated using specific epidemiologic measures, which will be introduced and discussed in this chapter. Understanding and properly interpreting these measures are important skills for managing, planning, and evaluating health care services.

If a health care manager can accurately predict the future occurrence of health and disease in a population, health care systems and services can be designed to provide adequately for population needs. As a comparison science, epidemiology can be incorporated into forecasting models. Epidemiologic data can thus be used to assist managers in future decision making. Epidemiologic measures, as well as the comparative inference of these measures, are essential for designing and managing health care for populations.

Measures

Basic to measurement of health and disease is quantification of disease in a population. The definition of a case has a clinical aspect, but it also has a dichotomous nature; an individual is a case or is not. In fact, disease manifests itself along a continuous spectrum of severity. Often disease occurs subclinically for an extended period of time before clinical diagnosis can be accomplished.

In epidemiology, the notion of population at risk is related to the occurrence of cases of diseases. Given this notion of risk, several epidemiologic measures are used to quantify the relationship with the occurrence of disease. These measures include counts, rates, ratios, and proportions.

Counts

The simplest method of measuring disease frequency is to count cases of a disease or condition or the number of deaths due to a disease or condition. Absolute counts are commonly performed to study individuals in a population with a specific disease or condition or with a specific set of characteristics.

Table 3.1 presents data on the number of cases of AIDS in the United States in 2002. Based on the data given in the table, can it be concluded that New York and Florida have the greatest need for preventive services for HIV and AIDS? To answer

TABLE 3.1. CASES OF AIDS IN THE UNITED STATES AND SELECTED U.S. TERRITORIES, 2002.

State	Number of cases	State	Number of cases
United States	43,950	Nebraska	70
Alabama	432	Nevada	314
Alaska	33	New Hampshire	41
Arizona	630	New Jersey	1,436
Arkansas	240	New Mexico	88
California	4,264	New York	6,664
Colorado	332	North Carolina	1,061
Connecticut	618	North Dakota	3
Delaware	193	Ohio	780
District of Columbia	927	Oklahoma	204
Florida	5,058	Oregon	301
Georgia	1,471	Pennsylvania	1,811
Hawaii	128	Rhode Island	107
Idaho	31	South Carolina	833
Illinois	2,108	South Dakota	11
Indiana	491	Tennessee	792
Iowa	94	Texas	3,140
Kansas	70	Utah	94
Kentucky	305	Vermont	12
Louisiana	1,167	Virginia	955
Maine	28	Washington	477
Maryland	1,854	West Virginia	83
Massachusetts	810	Wisconsin	187
Michigan	789	Wyoming	12
Minnesota	161	Guam	3
Mississippi	433	Puerto Rico	1,139
Missouri	391	Virgin Islands	58
Montana	17		

Source: Centers for Disease Control and Prevention, National Center for HIV, STD, and TB Prevention, Divisions of HIV/AIDS Prevention, 2004.

this question, it must be stated that counts are useful for describing the actual impact of a disease or condition in a specific population—that is, the number of cases. Counts thus allow for planning for the expected number of individuals who will have AIDS and will subsequently seek treatment. The necessary resources to treat this expected number of individuals can then be allocated for this population. So indeed, more resources, including funding for the provision of treatment services, are required in New York and Florida than other states.

However, a more important question is whether New York and Florida have the greatest need for preventive services to reduce the number of new cases of AIDS. For example, allocation of funding for providing preventive services based on the number of cases may not be appropriate for planning. If you were planning a prevention and health education program to reduce the risk of HIV and AIDS, should you use the information presented in Table 3.1? With respect to this question, counts cannot be used to make comparisons among and across populations. To compare the need for preventive services for states, population numbers of areas or groups to be compared are necessary.

For example, Table 3.2 presents the absolute number of cumulative cases of AIDS in the United States up to 2002, according to age. Without population numbers, inferences cannot be made about which age category has the greatest rate of AIDS. No intercategory comparisons can be made using absolute counts.

Rates

The fundamental measure of disease and death frequency is the rate. Rates differ from absolute counts in that they measure the occurrence of a disease or condition relative to a specific population and during a specified period of time. Rates are used to make comparisons among and across populations and can illustrate differences among and within populations. Rates are the basic units of comparison in terms of morbidity and mortality. A rate is similar to a ratio and is defined as follows:

$$\frac{\text{Number of cases of (or deaths due to)}}{\text{Number of individuals in a population}}$$
$$\frac{\text{a disease or condition}}{\text{during a specified period of time}}$$

The numerator of a rate consists of the cases (or deaths) that are determined from routinely collected data (secondary data) or from specifically designed studies (primary data). Denominators of rates are usually the total number of individuals in a population. A common source of population numbers is the estimated population provided by the U.S. Census Bureau. Other denominator sources, which can be more accurately determined, include military, school, industrial, or health plan enrollment populations.

Rates are expressed in many forms. They may be expressed as a percentage or as numbers per 1,000 or per 100,000 individuals in a population. The form selected depends on convention or the magnitude of population numbers. Fractions are not typically expressed, because it is difficult to understand what is meant by 0.7 cases per 1,000; a more customary form would be to present a rate of 70 cases per 100,000. Several rates have characteristic formats. For example, infant and neonatal mortality rates are expressed as the rate per 1,000 live births. Birth and death rates are presented

TABLE 3.2. CUMULATIVE CASES OF AIDS IN THE UNITED STATES, BY AGE, 2002.

Age group	Number of cumulative AIDS cases
Under 13 years	9,300
13–14 years	839
15–24 years	35,460
25–34 years	301,278
35–44 years	347,860
45–54 years	138,386
55–64 years	40,584
65 years and older	12,868

Source: Centers for Disease Control and Prevention, National Center for HIV, STD, and TB Prevention, Divisions of HIV/AIDS Prevention, 2004.

per 100,000 individuals in a population. Age-specific and cause-specific death rates are expressed as the rate per 100,000 population.

Table 3.3 presents the rate of AIDS cases in the United States in 2002. When a population number is included in the calculation, the order of the magnitude of rates is very different from what is seen with absolute numbers. According to the differences in rates, the District of Columbia has the highest risk of AIDS, by a factor of 5. As was expected, New York and Florida warrant attention. In addition, other localities that do not appear to be a concern using counts may also warrant attention; these include Maryland, the Virgin Islands, Louisiana, Puerto Rico, Delaware, and South Carolina. Thus, when planning, the importance of these areas should be highlighted in a preventive intervention.

Another example of the different information derived from counts and rates involves the number of visits to physician offices. Table 3.4 presents the absolute number of such visits in the United States in 2001, stratified by age, sex, and race. The absolute number of visits to general and family physicians for whites is eleven times greater than for African Americans (777,550,000 compared to 66,141,000). Conversely, this is almost a twelvefold difference in the number of visits. The rate of office visits for whites is only 1.8 times greater than for blacks. Females have a greater number of visits and a higher rate than males (362.3 compared to 264.0 per 100 persons per year). With respect to age, the number of visits among individuals under 15 years of age is slightly higher than among individuals 75 years and older (146,683,000 to 115,452,000). But the rates of office visits show a very different situation, with the rate among individuals 75 years and older three times greater than among individuals under 15 years of age. It may be concluded that the risk of a physician office visit is greater among whites, females, and individuals 75 years of age and older.

TABLE 3.3. AIDS CASE RATE PER 100,000 POPULATION, 2002.

State	Rate	State	Rate
United States	15.0	Nebraska	4.0
Alabama	9.6	Nevada	14.4
Alaska	5.1	New Hampshire	3.2
Arizona	11.5	New Jersey	16.7
Arkansas	8.9	New Mexico	4.7
California	12.4	New York	34.8
Colorado	7.4	North Carolina	12.8
Connecticut	17.9	North Dakota	0.5
Delaware	23.9	Ohio	6.8
District of Columbia	162.4	Oklahoma	5.8
Florida	30.3	Oregon	8.5
Georgia	17.2	Pennsylvania	14.7
Hawaii	10.3	Rhode Island	10.0
Idaho	2.3	South Carolina	20.3
Illinois	16.7	South Dakota	1.4
Indiana	8.0	Tennessee	13.7
Iowa	3.2	Texas	14.4
Kansas	2.6	Utah	4.1
Kentucky	7.5	Vermont	1.9
Louisiana	26.0	Virginia	13.1
Maine	2.2	Washington	7.9
Maryland	34.0	West Virginia	4.6
Massachusetts	12.6	Wisconsin	3.4
Michigan	7.9	Wyoming	2.4
Minnesota	3.2	Guam	1.9
Mississippi	15.1	Puerto Rico	29.5
Missouri	6.9	Virgin Islands	47.0
Montana	1.9		

Source: Centers for Disease Control and Prevention, National Center for HIV, STD, and TB Prevention, Divisions of HIV/AIDS Prevention, 2004

A similar example of the importance of using a rate for comparison would be determining service capacity for emergency department visits. Table 3.5 presents data from the 2001 National Hospital Ambulatory Medical Care Survey. If one reviews the absolute number of emergency department visits in the United States, it appears that the risk of a visit is highest among whites. However, when the population differences between racial groupings are used to calculate the rates of these visits, it becomes apparent that the highest risk of (or future demand for) emergency department services is among African Americans. In the short run, then, a managed care population would be expected to annually incur the normative 63.7 visits per thousand black enrollees. Over the longer term, considerable opportunity exists for managed care

TABLE 3.4. NUMBER OF PHYSICIAN OFFICE VISITS, BY AGE, SEX, AND RACE, 2001.

Characteristics	Number of visits (in thousands)	Number of visits per 100 persons per year
All visits	880,487	314.4
Age		
Under 15 years	146,683	242.7
15–24 years	65,632	168.7
25–44 years	200,636	241.9
45–64 years	112,978	373.3
65–74 years	112,978	624.9
75 years and older	115,452	738.5
Sex		
Female	520,110	362.3
Male	360,377	264.0
Race		
White	777,550	342.6
Black/African American	66,141	189.4
Asian	29,180	263.9
Native Hawaiian or other Pacific Islander	2,929	628.9
American Indian or Alaska Native	1,913	71.9

Source: Centers for Disease Control and Prevention, 2001.

executives to reduce utilization to the mean national rate or less, using copayment or other financial strategies or by assuring ready access to lower-cost service alternatives.

Ratios

Ratios are measures that express a relationship between two quantities. Ratios are useful in making comparisons between groups of individuals or between categories of diseases or conditions. An example is a sex ratio, which compares health and disease experiences among males and females. Another commonly used ratio is a race ratio, which compares whites, African Americans, and other races.

Table 3.6 presents information from the Mississippi State Department of Health, Office of Health Informatics, on male-female death ratios in 2001, stratified by age and race. Overall, the table shows no difference between males and females across race. The table also shows that more males than females die between the ages of 15 and 34. In fact, this trend (more deaths among men than women) is observed in all age categories up through age 74. This is due to the differential in the number of males compared to females who are still alive at ages greater than 75 years. With respect to race, male and female death rates are significantly higher among African Americans at ages 5 to 24 years.

TABLE 3.5. EMERGENCY DEPARTMENT VISITS, UNITED STATES, 2001.

Characteristics	Number of visits (in thousands)	Number of visits per 100 persons per year
Sex		
Female	57,169,000	39.8
Male	50,321,000	36.9
Race		
White	82,012,000	36.1
Black/African American	22,238,000	63.7
Asian	2,099,000	19.0

Source: Centers for Disease Control and Prevention, 2001c.

TABLE 3.6. MALE-FEMALE DEATH RATIOS, BY AGE AND RACE, MISSISSIPPI, 2001.

Age group	Overall male-female ratio	White male-female ratio	African American male-female ratio
All ages	0.98	0.97	0.99
Under 1 year	1.27	1.01	1.44
1–4 years	1.46	1.37	1.55
5–9 years	1.63	1.22	2.00
10–14 years	1.73	1.25	2.30
15–24 years	2.84	3.19	2.56
25–34 years	2.03	2.28	1.82
35–44 years	1.70	2.03	1.42
45–54 years	1.57	1.66	1.46
55–64 years	1.47	1.55	1.34
65–74 years	1.29	1.44	1.02
75–84 years	0.90	0.93	0.80
85 years and older	0.44	0.42	0.51

Source: Mississippi State Department of Health, Office of Health Informatics, 2004.

Table 3.7 presents information from the 2000 National Home and Hospice Care Survey, which annually collects data from home and hospice health agencies in the United States. The survey data are collected on current patients and discharges through personal interview with administrators and staff. The table shows that females use health care 1.7 times more than males, but no such relationship is seen with respect to hospice care (ratio of 0.99 to 1). Whites use home health and hospice care more than eight times more than African Americans and all other nonwhites. Non-Hispanics use these services more than Hispanics by a magnitude of nineteenfold. Married individuals use home and hospice care services more often than widowed, divorced, separated, single, or never-married individuals.

TABLE 3.7. HOME HEALTH AND HOSPICE CARE DISCHARGES, UNITED STATES, 1999–2000.

Discharge characteristics	Total	Home health care	Hospice care
All discharges	7,800,100	7,179,000	621,100
Male-female ratio	0.59	0.56	0.99
Non-Hispanic–Hispanic ratio	19.04	18.89	20.75
White-black ratio	8.48	7.92	10.43
White–all other races ratio	6.50	6.38	8.12
Married-widowed ratio	1.36	1.36	1.42
Married–divorced or separated ratio	7.74	7.68	8.33
Married–single or never married ratio	2.77	2.63	6.12

Source: Centers for Disease Control and Prevention, 2000d.

Proportions

Proportions are ratios that express relationships between two quantified measures. A distinction between ratios and proportions is that in a proportion the numerator is included in the denominator. A second distinction is that proportions are always expressed as a percentage. As in ratios, a unit of time must be expressed in both the numerator and denominator of a proportion.

Table 3.8 presents the distribution of home health agencies and hospices in the United States by type of ownership during 1999 and 2000. This information was collected during the National Home and Hospice Care Survey. The data show that the proportion of proprietary home health and hospice care agencies is 44.7%, making this the major ownership type. The South is the geographic region that has the largest proportion of home and hospice care agencies (42.7%), with the greatest proportion in metropolitan statistical areas.

Measuring Morbidity

Morbidity measurement is a very crucial aspect of planning health care for populations. The rate at which the population becomes ill has an impact on health status, resource utilization, economic development, disease prevention, and medical management. The following sections discuss the epidemiologic measures that are used to evaluate the amount and impact of morbidity within and across populations.

TABLE 3.8. HOME HEALTH AND HOSPICE CARE AGENCIES, BY OWNERSHIP, GEOGRAPHIC REGION, AND LOCATION, 2000.

Agency characteristics	Proportion (%)
Ownership	
Proprietary	44.7
Voluntary nonprofit	42.5
Government and other	12.8
Geographic region	
Northeast	15.9
Midwest	26.1
South	42.7
West	13.3
Location	
Metropolitan Statistical Area	64.8
Other	35.2

Source: Centers for Disease Control and Prevention, 2000d.

Incidence Rate

Incidence rate is a measure that indicates the frequency of morbidity (disease occurrence) among individuals initially without disease over a specified period of time. In other words, the incidence rate illustrates the frequency at which new cases of a disease or condition occur. Incidence is a measure that expresses the continual occurrence of new cases of a disease or condition. The incidence rate may be defined as follows:

$$\frac{\text{Number of new cases of a disease or condition in a specific population over a specified period of time}}{\text{Total number of individuals at risk of developing a disease or condition in a specific population over a specified period of time}}$$

The denominator is typically the average size of the population at the midpoint of the period of time. The specified period of time is the same in both the numerator and the denominator. The period of time is important. For example, an incidence rate for six months should be evaluated differently from an incidence rate for six years.

The incidence rate is a function of the cumulative incidence and the incidence density. The incidence rate as we have just defined it is actually the cumulative incidence rate over the specified time period. The incidence density accounts for the varying time periods during which individuals are followed to determine whether they become new cases. Given this, the incidence density is a more precise measure of the rate of occurrence of a disease or condition in a population. The incidence density can be defined as follows:

$$\frac{\text{Number of new cases of a disease or condition in a specific population over a specified period of time}}{\text{Total person-time of observation}}$$

The denominator is the sum of each individual's time at risk or the sum of the time that each individual in the population remained under observation and disease-free. If the incidence rate is low (as for a chronic disease), the rate is an exact measure of the cumulative incidence.

It is assumed that all individuals in the study population are free of disease at the beginning of the time period. The individuals at risk of developing a disease or condition are typically considered to be the total population of interest. However, this may not always be the case; individuals who currently have a disease or condition are no longer at risk. These individuals should be removed from the denominator if an accurate measurement of those not at risk can be obtained. Often it is impossible to accurately identify individuals who are not at risk, so the total population is, by convention, considered to be at risk.

A rule of thumb that can be used in determining the composition of the denominator is as follows: because a unit of time is included in the incidence rate, it is independent of the length of time under study. If the study is limited to evaluating the first cases of a disease or condition, then the entire population should be considered at risk. If the study period is of short duration, then a small proportion of cases will develop during the study period so it will make little difference to attempt to remove those not truly at risk from the denominator. However, if the study period is of long duration, a significant number of individuals may die or cease to be at risk for other reasons. This should be taken into account when determining the composition of the denominator.

Incidence can be measured as the number of new cases that occur between two points in time, t_0 to t_1. Observation of all new cases of a disease or condition begins at t_0 and continues until t_1. All occurrences of a disease or condition between t_0 and t_1 are known as incident cases. The total number of incident cases is used as the numerator for the incidence rate. The total population at risk between t_0 and t_1 is used as the denominator.

An example of calculating incidence rates will use the data shown in Figure 3.1, which presents data on patients discharged with congestive heart failure from an intensive care unit of a hospital. Assume that five patients are observed from the day of discharge (t_0) for

FIGURE 3.1. INCIDENCE RATE OF READMISSIONS.

	Jan. 1998	July 1998	Jan. 1999	July 1999	Jan. 2000	July 2000	Jan. 2001	July 2001	Jan. 2002	July 2002	Jan. 2003	Total years at risk
A	●- - - - - - - - - - - - - - - -											2.0
B		●- X										3.0
C	●- -											5.0
D			●- -									4.0
E				●- - - - - - - - - - - - - - - - - - - X								2.5
Total years at risk												16.5

●   = Initiation of follow-up
- - - = Time followed
X   = Readmission occurs

a five-year period (the fifth year is t_i) for the occurrence of a readmission. During the observation period, two patients are readmitted, one is lost to follow-up, and the remaining two patients do not experience a readmission. The cumulative incidence rate is 2 cases/5 individuals over a 5-year period of time. This equals 40%, or 40 readmissions per 100 patients. The incidence density is 2 cases/16.5 person-years at risk, or 12.1 readmissions per 100 person-years at risk.

The incidence rate illustrates the risk of developing a disease or condition within a given population. The incidence rate in a population is useful when the etiology of a disease or condition is under study. Incidence offers insight into the factors related to a change in health status, from no disease to disease. An example of this use of incidence rates is shown in Tables 3.9 and 3.10. Table 3.9 presents incidence rates for selected diseases in Los Angeles County. This information allows for the understanding of the most likely infectious disease cases that will occur and require health care services. Table 3.10 shows average annual age-adjusted cancer incidence rates in the United States from 1996 to 1999. The data show that males have a greater overall risk for cancers, especially for the following sites: lung, urinary bladder, oral cavity and pharynx, colon and rectum, and melanoma of the skin. In fact, the risk is twice as high for lung cancer and four times higher for urinary bladder cancer.

Prevalence Rate

Another important measure of disease frequency is the prevalence rate, which measures currently occurring cases of a disease or condition in a specific population. The prevalence rate can be defined as follows:

TABLE 3.9. INCIDENCE RATE OF SELECTED DISEASES BY RACE, LOS ANGELES COUNTY, 2000.

Disease	White	Black/African American	Asian	Hispanic
Amebiasis	1.1	0.5	0.3	1.1
Campylobacteriosis	16.1	7.3	11.3	14.1
Coccidioidomycosis	0.4	0.8	0.1	0.4
Encephalitis	0.4	0.5	0.7	0.4
Giardiasis	5.7	2.0	1.1	5.0
Hepatitis A	7.4	4.6	4.6	9.6
Hepatitis B	0.8	1.8	0.9	0.3
Hepatitis C	0.3	0.3	0.2	0.3
Malaria	0.3	1.8	0.3	0.4
Meningococcal infections	0.4	1.6	0.2	0.4
Pertussis	1.2	1.3	0.6	1.1
Salmonellosis	10.1	9.4	10.4	9.5
Shigellosis	9.8	8.0	1.6	10.7

Source: Los Angeles County Department of Health Services, 2000.

TABLE 3.10. AVERAGE ANNUAL AGE-ADJUSTED CANCER INCIDENCE RATES PER 100,000 POPULATION, BY SEX, 1996–1999.

Site	Overall rate	Males	Females
All sites	470.8	556.1	416.6
Prostate	159.8	159.8	—
Breast	72.3	1.1	131.8
Lung/bronchus	65.2	88.0	48.8
Colon/rectum	56.6	67.3	48.8
Urinary bladder	20.9	37.0	9.5
Melanoma skin	16.2	20.0	13.6
Oral cavity/pharynx	11.7	17.6	6.9
Cervix uteri	9.5	—	9.5

Source: National Cancer Institute, 2000.

$$\frac{\text{Number of existing cases of a disease or condition in a specific population at a designated time}}{\text{Total number of individuals in a specific population at a designated time}}$$

When the designated time is not specified, it is assumed that this construct is measuring the point prevalence rate. The point prevalence rate can be thought of as the probability of having a disease or condition at a given point in time. The point prevalence rate is defined as follows:

$$\frac{\text{Number of existing cases of a disease or condition in a specific population at a specific point in time}}{\text{Total number of individuals in a specific population at a specific point in time}}$$

Often the designated period of time can be extended for a lifetime. This is known as the lifetime prevalence rate and includes individuals known to have had a disease or condition at any time during their lifetime. The lifetime prevalence rate is defined as follows:

$$\frac{\text{Number of individuals in a specific population who have had a disease or condition during their lifetime}}{\text{Total number of individuals in a specific population}}$$

Table 3.11 presents information about the asthma prevalence rate in the United States in 2000.

As an illustration of the use of the point prevalence rate, assume that a local hospital, as part of a marketing campaign, conducts a screening program for hypertension for residents of the community that it serves. During the screening program, which is conducted on the first day of the month, 1,500 individuals have blood pressure readings. Of those screened, 150 individuals are diagnosed with hypertension. The prevalence rate of this screened population is 150/1,500, or 10%. This rate indicates that currently 10% of the screened population has hypertension. No statement about risk can be made on the basis of this screening program. It would be incorrect to assume that 10% of the screening population was at risk of developing hypertension. Prevalence cannot be used to measure risk because it does not provide information about the cases before they were screened. The etiology of hypertension cannot be traced, and risk factors cannot be identified. The incidence rate is what measures the risk in a population.

Table 3.12 presents the results of the 2001 Behavioral Risk Factor Surveillance System (BRFSS) for the prevalence of women, aged 18 years and older, who have had a Papanicolaou test (Pap smear), by age. The survey sample consisted of fifteen states

TABLE 3.11. ASTHMA PREVALENCE RATE, BY RACE AND SEX, 2000.

Characteristics	Lifetime prevalence rate (per 1,000)	Point prevalence rate (per 1,000)
Race		
Non-Hispanic white	115	75
Non-Hispanic black	125	86
Hispanic	95	59
Sex		
Male	108	64
Female	119	83

Source: Centers for Disease Control and Prevention, 2000a.

and territories. The prevalence is highest in the 18–24 age group in Georgia, in the 25–34 age group in Wisconsin, in the 35–44 age group in Wyoming, in the 45–54 age group in Wisconsin and Wyoming, in the 55–64 age group in Wisconsin, in the 65–74 age group in Wisconsin, and in the 75 and older age group in Arizona.

Table 3.13 presents results of the 2001 BRFSS for the prevalence of women, 40 years of age and older, who reported ever having a mammogram during the period 1991–2001. The prevalence increased in all twelve states and territories, with the greatest increase occurring in Mississippi. The smallest increase occurred in Rhode Island.

Prevalence is directly related to the incidence rate. This relationship is manifested by the duration of the disease or condition. Prevalence is affected by both the occurrence of disease (measured by the incidence rate) and the average duration of disease. As both the incidence rate and duration of disease increase, prevalence experiences an associated increase. If incidence and duration decrease, so does the prevalence rate. The relationship can be expressed as follows:

Prevalence rate ≈ incidence rate × average duration of disease.

Using prevalence data for planning and implementation of health care services may not give satisfactory results. Although prevalence helps us assess the impact of a disease, it is not useful in studying the determinants of disease or its etiology. Knowledge of the risk of disease in a population cannot be determined from prevalence data; incidence data are needed to determine risk.

TABLE 3.12. PREVALENCE (PERCENTAGE) OF WOMEN AGED 18 YEARS AND OLDER WHO REPORTED EVER HAVING A PAP TEST, BY AGE, 2001.

State or territory	18–24 years	25–34 years	35–44 years	45–54 years	55–64 years	65–74 years	75 years and older
Arizona	74.0	91.5	98.4	99.1	97.7	96.5	92.6
Arkansas	86.1	97.5	97.9	99.5	96.0	90.9	85.5
Colorado	88.9	93.1	98.6	99.2	—	—	—
Georgia	90.1	98.0	97.4	98.1	97.5	96.5	88.6
Hawaii	81.2	95.3	97.8	97.8	96.2	93.0	89.7
Mississippi	88.7	98.6	—	98.4	—	93.0	92.0
New Jersey	73.1	90.6	96.7	95.0	96.7	94.5	89.4
Oklahoma	85.4	98.1	98.1	94.5	96.0	89.6	89.1
Rhode Island	80.4	96.6	98.1	97.1	97.7	92.6	87.1
South Dakota	87.1	97.7	98.6	99.3	98.6	95.5	84.4
Tennessee	87.9	96.5	97.6	95.3	92.8	88.1	78.7
Wisconsin	81.6	99.6	99.4	99.6	99.2	98.3	83.8
Wyoming	83.8	98.7	99.6	99.6	97.7	97.4	90.7
Guam	68.4	90.9	94.8	90.3	—	—	—
Virgin Islands	75.0	93.6	94.5	94.8	90.6	—	—

Source: Centers for Disease Control and Prevention, 2003a.

TABLE 3.13. PREVALENCE (PERCENTAGE) OF WOMEN AGED 40 YEARS AND OLDER WHO REPORTED EVER HAVING A MAMMOGRAM, 1991 AND 2001.

State	2001	1991	Difference 1991–2001
Arizona	91.4	70.5	29.7
Arkansas	85.3	62.6	36.3
Colorado	87.9	73.9	18.9
Georgia	89.2	72.9	22.4
Hawaii	90.5	74.5	21.4
Mississippi	84.8	61.1	38.7
New Jersey	86.7	70.5	22.9
Oklahoma	84.7	66.0	28.4
Rhode Island	93.0	79.5	17.0
South Dakota	86.5	69.5	24.4
Tennessee	86.7	68.0	27.5
Wisconsin	91.4	76.0	20.2

Source: Centers for Disease Control and Prevention, 2003a.

Period Prevalence

Another extension of the prevalence rate concept is the period prevalence. The period prevalence combines the incidence and prevalence rates and is defined as follows:

$$\frac{\begin{array}{c}\text{Number of existing cases of a}\\\text{disease or condition in a specific}\\\text{population at a specific point in time}\\+\\\text{Number of new cases of a}\\\text{disease or condition in a specific}\\\text{population during a specified period of time}\end{array}}{\begin{array}{c}\text{Total number of individuals in a}\\\text{specific population during a specified}\\\text{period of time}\end{array}}$$

Period prevalence is used if you wish to measure the existing cases of a disease or condition during a designated period of time. If the designated period is a year, the period prevalence rate is the point prevalence rate at the beginning of the year plus the year's incidence rate. The period prevalence can be thought of as the proportion of the population that has a disease or condition during a designated period of time.

An example of period prevalence is as follows. Assume that the number of individuals receiving health care due to an automobile accident-related injury on June 30, 2004, at East Bank Regional Hospital was 75. East Bank Regional Hospital is the only hospital in a community of 100,000 people. The prevalence rate on June 30, 2004, was 75 injuries per 100,000. If the number of individuals receiving health care at East Bank Regional Hospital due to an automobile accident-related injury between July 1, 2004, and December 31, 2004, was 150, the incidence rate of automobile accident-related injury was 150 injuries per 100,000. The period prevalence from June 30, 2004, to December 31, 2004, would be 225 injuries per 100,000.

Measuring Mortality

Attempts to understand who is dying and what the causes are have been central to the study of epidemiology for many years. The following sections present the epidemiologic measures that are used to evaluate mortality in populations.

Death Rates

The overall mortality rate, also called the crude death rate or total death rate, measures the frequency of all deaths in a population. The crude death rate is defined as follows:

$$\frac{\text{Total number of deaths in a specific population during a specified period of time}}{\text{Total number of individuals in a specific population during a specified period of time}}$$

The specified period of time is the same in the numerator and the denominator. The source of numerator data is information abstracted from death certificates. Denominator data originate from estimated population data collected by the U.S. Census Bureau. Table 3.14 presents crude death rates in the United States in 2000 and 2001, by race and sex.

A more specific mortality rate, which measures frequency of death according to cause of death, is known as the cause-specific mortality rate. An example of a cause-specific mortality rate is the heart disease mortality rate. This rate is defined as follows:

TABLE 3.14. CRUDE DEATH RATE, BY RACE AND SEX, UNITED STATES, 2000 AND 2001.

Race	Sex	2000	2001
All races	Both sexes	854.0	848.5
	Male	853.0	846.4
	Female	855.0	850.4
White	Both sexes	900.2	895.1
	Male	887.8	881.9
	Female	912.3	907.9
Black/African American	Both sexes	781.1	773.5
	Male	834.1	823.9
	Female	733.0	727.7
American Indian	Both sexes	380.8	392.1
	Male	415.6	424.2
	Female	346.1	360.2
Asian or Pacific Islander	Both sexes	296.6	303.8
	Male	332.9	335.0
	Female	262.3	274.4
Hispanic	Both sexes	303.8	306.8
	Male	331.3	332.9
	Female	274.6	279.0

Source: Centers for Disease Control and Prevention, 2003d.

$$\frac{\text{Number of deaths due to a specific cause in a}}{\text{Total number of individuals in a specific}}$$
specific population during a specified period of time

Total number of individuals in a specific
population during a specified period of time

The specified period of time is the same in the numerator and the denominator. Again, the sources are death certificates for numerator data and the U.S. Census Bureau for denominator data. Table 3.15 presents mortality rates for the top ten leading causes of death in the United States in 2001. Heart disease is the leading cause of death, with a cause-specific mortality rate equal to 245.8 deaths per 100,000 population. Closely following is death due to malignant neoplasms, with a cause-specific mortality rate of 194.4 deaths per 100,000 population.

Wide variation in cause-specific death rates in a specific population provides motivation for the population-oriented health care executive to explore underlying environmental circumstances, public health practices, or best demonstrated practice in other geographic areas. Illustratively, the use of asbestos as an insulating material was restricted in the United States after it was determined that asbestosis mortality among

TABLE 3.15. CAUSE-SPECIFIC MORTALITY RATES FOR THE TEN LEADING CAUSES OF DEATH, 2001.

Cause	Number	Rate
All causes	2,416,425	848.5
Diseases of the heart	700,142	245.8
Malignant neoplasms	553,768	194.4
Cerebrovascular diseases	163,538	57.4
Chronic lower respiratory diseases	123,013	43.2
Accidents (unintentional injuries)	101,537	35.7
Diabetes mellitus	71,372	25.1
Influenza and pneumonia	62,034	21.8
Alzheimer's disease	53,852	18.9
Nephritis, nephritic syndrome, and nephrosis	39,480	13.9
Septicemia	32,238	11.3

Source: Centers for Disease Control and Prevention, 2003d.

factory workers and installers working unprotected with these products was unacceptably high. Aberrant cause-specific death rates are often sentinel alarms for the quality assurance activities of individual health care providers. Detailed review of institution-specific practices, policies, or procedures will typically reveal procedural changes that can remedy the situation.

Because age is recognized as a major determinant of health and disease, mortality rates are commonly expressed as an age-specific mortality rate, defined as follows:

$$\frac{\text{Number of deaths within a specific age group in a specific population during a specified period of time}}{\text{Total number of individuals in a specific age group in a specific population during a specified period of time}}$$

As with the rates previously discussed, the specified period of time is the same in the numerator and the denominator. Sources of data are death certificates and population data from the U.S. Census Bureau. Table 3.16 presents age-specific death rates for persons with malignant neoplasms in Mississippi in 2002. As age increases, the mortality rate increases, a characteristic of chronic disease, such as malignant neoplasms.

An important measure of mortality used in health care management is the case-fatality rate, which is sometimes used as an indicator of quality of care. The Centers for Medicare and Medicaid Services (CMS) annually ranks hospitals on the basis of case-fatality rates for specific diseases and conditions relative to quality of services provided to Medicare beneficiaries. The local and national press tend to give substantial emphasis to this rate when it is published. The general public tends to use it as a proxy

TABLE 3.16. AGE-SPECIFIC MORTALITY RATE (DEATHS PER 100,000), MALIGNANT NEOPLASM, MISSISSIPPI, 2002.

Age group	Mortality rate
1–4 years	2.4
5–14 years	1.4
15–24 years	3.6
25–44 years	32.2
45–64 years	279.7
65 years and older	1,148.4

Source: Mississippi State Department of Health, Office of Health Informatics, 2004.

for overall quality of hospital care. As with any single measure, case-fatality rates may be misleading because they typically give little emphasis to age or comorbidities. The case-fatality rate is not used as a measure of risk; instead it indicates the frequency of death from a specific disease among individuals with that specific disease. Case-fatality rate is defined as follows:

$$\frac{\text{Number of individuals with disease X who die with disease X}}{\text{Total number of individuals with disease X}}$$

Several specific mortality rates are used to measure the frequency of deaths among maternal and child populations. The most commonly used measure is the infant mortality rate, which is defined as follows:

$$\frac{\text{Total number of deaths among individuals under 1 year of age in a specific population during a specified period of time}}{\text{Total number of live births in a specific population during a specified period of time}}$$

The population and the specified period of time are the same in both the numerator and the denominator. The sources of data in the numerator are death certificates and in the denominator are birth certificates.

Table 3.17 presents data on infant mortality rates in the United States from 1980 to 2001. The trend in rates shows a decrease over the period for all races combined, for whites, and for blacks. Across all races the infant mortality rate decreased from 12.6 to 6.8 deaths per 1,000 live births, approximately a 50% decline. Among whites, the infant mortality rate decreased from 10.9 to 5.7 deaths per 1,000 live births. Again,

TABLE 3.17. INFANT MORTALITY RATE (DEATHS PER 1,000 LIVE BIRTHS), BY RACE OF MOTHER, 1980–2001.

Year	All races	White	Black/African American
1980	12.6	10.9	22.2
1981	11.9	10.3	20.8
1982	11.5	9.9	20.5
1983	11.2	9.6	20.0
1984	10.8	9.3	19.2
1985	10.6	9.2	19.0
1986	10.4	8.8	18.9
1987	10.1	8.5	18.8
1988	10.0	8.3	18.5
1989	9.8	8.1	18.6
1990	9.2	7.6	18.0
1991	8.9	7.3	17.6
1992	8.5	6.9	16.8
1993	8.4	6.8	16.5
1994	8.0	6.6	15.8
1995	7.6	6.3	15.1
1996	7.3	6.1	14.7
1997	7.2	6.0	14.2
1998	7.2	6.0	14.3
1999	7.1	5.8	14.6
2000	6.9	5.7	14.1
2001	6.8	5.7	14.0

Source: Centers for Disease Control and Prevention, 2001e.

this represents a 50% decline. Among African Americans, the infant mortality rate decreased from 22.2 to 14.0 deaths per 1,000 live births.

 Related measures are the neonatal and postneonatal mortality rates. These rates are separated because causes of death during the neonatal and postneonatal periods are quite different. The neonatal mortality rate is defined as follows:

$$\frac{\text{Total number of deaths among individuals under age 28 days in a specific population during a specified period of time}}{\text{Total number of live births in a specific population during a specified period of time}}$$

 The neonatal mortality rate measures the frequency of death shortly after birth. Common causes of death during this period include congenital abnormalities, pregnancy-related problems, slow fetal growth, and trauma at birth. Table 3.18 presents neonatal mortality rates from 1980 to 2001 in the United States, by race.

TABLE 3.18. NEONATAL MORTALITY RATE (DEATHS PER 1,000 LIVE BIRTHS), BY RACE OF MOTHER, 1980–2001.

Year	All races	White	Black/African American
1980	8.5	7.4	13.2
1981	8.0	7.0	12.5
1982	7.7	6.7	12.0
1983	7.3	6.3	11.4
1984	7.0	6.1	10.9
1985	7.0	6.0	11.0
1986	6.7	5.7	10.8
1987	6.5	5.4	10.7
1988	6.3	5.3	10.3
1989	6.2	5.1	10.3
1990	5.8	4.8	9.9
1991	5.6	4.5	9.5
1992	5.4	4.3	9.2
1993	5.3	4.3	9.0
1994	5.1	4.2	8.6
1995	4.9	4.1	8.1
1996	4.8	4.0	7.9
1997	4.8	4.0	7.7
1998	4.8	4.0	7.9
1999	4.7	3.9	7.9
2000	4.6	3.8	7.6
2001	4.5	3.8	7.4

Source: Centers for Disease Control and Prevention, 2001e.

The postneonatal mortality rate is defined as follows:

$$\frac{\text{Total number of deaths among individuals between ages 28 days and 11 months in a specific population during a specified period of time}}{\text{Total number of live births – total number of neonatal deaths in a specific population during a specified period of time}}$$

The postneonatal mortality rate measures the frequency of death of infants who survive past the twenty-eighth day of life. Environmental causes of death are common during this period of time, including sudden infant death syndrome (SIDS) and accidents. Table 3.19 presents postneonatal mortality rates, by year and race.

TABLE 3.19. POSTNEONATAL MORTALITY RATE (DEATHS PER 1,000 LIVE BIRTHS), BY RACE OF MOTHER, 1980–2001.

Year	All races	White	Black/African American
1980	4.1	3.5	7.0
1981	3.9	3.4	6.3
1982	3.8	3.2	6.3
1983	3.9	3.3	6.4
1984	3.8	3.2	6.2
1985	3.7	3.2	5.8
1986	3.6	3.1	5.9
1987	3.6	3.1	5.8
1988	3.6	3.1	5.7
1989	3.6	2.9	6.0
1990	3.4	2.8	5.7
1991	3.4	2.8	5.6
1992	3.1	2.6	5.2
1993	3.1	2.5	5.1
1994	2.9	2.4	4.9
1995	2.7	2.2	4.5
1996	2.5	2.1	4.3
1997	2.5	2.0	4.0
1998	2.4	2.0	4.0
1999	2.3	1.9	4.0
2000	2.3	1.9	3.8
2001	2.3	1.9	4.0

Source: Centers for Disease Control and Prevention, 2001e.

A final measure of frequency of death in child populations is the fetal death rate. The fetal death rate is defined as follows:

$$\frac{\text{Total number of fetal deaths among fetuses of 20 weeks or more gestation in a specific population during a specified period of time}}{\text{Total number of live births + fetal deaths in a specific population during a specified period of time}}$$

An example of a proportion used to understand mortality in a population is the proportionate mortality ratio (PMR). The PMR is used when a population at risk is not available. The PMR indicates whether the proportion of deaths observed from a specific disease is higher or lower than would be expected. The PMR indicates the relative importance of specific causes of death to the total number of deaths in a specific population and is defined as follows:

$$\frac{\begin{array}{c}\text{Number of deaths from a specific}\\\text{cause of death in a specific}\\\text{population during a specified period of time}\end{array}}{\begin{array}{c}\text{Total number of deaths from}\\\text{all causes in a specific population}\\\text{during a specified period of time}\end{array}} \times 100$$

The proportionate mortality ratio is used to evaluate cause-specific death risk when data on deaths are the only available information. Table 3.20 presents PMRs for malignant neoplasms, by age, in Mississippi in 2002.

Table 3.21 shows data from the National Institute of Occupational Safety and Health (NIOSH) mortality summary, the National Occupational Mortality Surveillance (NOMS) system. The data presented are PMRs for selected diseases among white men in general plant systems occupations. These PMRs indicate whether the observed proportion of deaths from specific diseases is higher or lower than would be expected for a specific occupation.

Potential Years of Life Lost

Potential years of life lost (PYLL) is used as an indicator of premature death and represents the number of years that are lost because someone dies prematurely. Premature death is defined in reference to not living to the age of 75 years. Any death between ages 0 and 74 is considered premature. PYLL attempts to quantify the impact of diseases that result in premature death.

The method used to calculate PYLL assigns more importance to deaths that occur at younger ages than at older ages. Using 75 years of age as the reference, deaths of individuals over 75 are not included in the calculation. Infant deaths are included. Table 3.22 illustrates the individual-level calculation method in a population of twelve individuals. In the individual-level calculation method, PYLL is calculated for every individual in the population. The PYLL rate is determined by dividing the total number of potential years of life lost by the total population less than 75 years of age.

Table 3.23 shows the age group calculation method. In this method, the potential years of life lost is determined for each age group by multiplying the number of deaths by the difference between age 75 and the mean age at death in each age group. The PYLL is the sum of these products of each age group. The PYLL rate is determined by dividing the total PYLL by the total population under the age of 75.

TABLE 3.20. PROPORTIONATE MORTALITY RATIOS FOR MALIGNANT NEOPLASMS, BY AGE, MISSISSIPPI, 2002.

Age group	Proportionate mortality ratio
1-4 years	4.2
5–14 years	5.4
15–24 years	3.1
25–44 years	13.3
45–64 years	31.1
65 years and older	20.2

Source: Mississippi State Department of Health, Office of Health Informatics, 2002.

TABLE 3.21. PROPORTIONATE MORTALITY RATIOS FOR WHITE MALE PLANT AND SYSTEM OPERATORS, BY AGE, 1984–1988.

Diseases	Observed	Expected	Proportionate mortality ratio
Malignant neoplasms			
Total cases	199	175	113
Age 20–64 years	70	53	133
Age 65 years and older	129	123	105
Alcohol-associated			
Total cases	3	7	46
Age 20–64 years	2	5	44
Age 65 years and older	1	2	50
Diseases of the circulatory system			
Total cases	343	349	98
Age 20–64 years	72	72	99
Age 65 years and older	271	276	98
Diseases of the heart			
Total cases	289	283	102
Age 20–64 years	67	67	105
Age 65 years and older	222	219	101
Hypertensive disease			
Total cases	6	7	81
Age 20–64 years	6	6	104
Age 65 years and older	0	2	0
Actual myocardial infarction			
Total cases	124	118	105
Age 20–64 years	36	31	115
Age 65 years and older	88	87	102

Source: National Institute of Occupational Safety and Health, National Occupational Mortality Surveillance System., n.d.

TABLE 3.22. CALCULATING POTENTIAL YEARS OF LIFE LOST (PYLL) USING INDIVIDUAL-LEVEL INFORMATION.

Individual	Age at death	Calculation	PYLL
A	9 months	75 – 0.75 =	74.25
B	35 years	75 – 35 =	40
C	58 years	75 – 58 =	17
D	63 years	75 – 63 =	12
E	68 years	75 – 68 =	7
F	79 years	0	0
G	21 years	75 – 21 =	54
H	69 years	75 – 69 =	6
I	82 years	0	0
J	61 years	75 – 61 =	14
K	74 years	75 – 74 =	1
L	70 years	75 – 70 =	5
Total			230.25
Rate		230.25 / 10 =	23.05

TABLE 3.23. CALCULATING POTENTIAL YEARS OF LIFE LOST (PYLL) USING AGE GROUP INFORMATION.

Age group	Number of deaths	Mean age at death	PYLL calculation (75 – mean age)	PYLL (number of deaths × PYLL calculation)
Under 1 year	5	0.75	74.25	371.5
1–4 years	35	2.5	72.5	2,537.5
5–9 years	58	7.0	68	3,944
10–14 years	72	12.0	63	4,536
15–19 years	325	16.5	58.5	19,012.5
20–24 years	425	23	52	22,100
25–29 years	315	27.0	48	15,120
30–34 years	240	32.5	42.5	7,680
35–39 years	182	37.0	38	6,916
40–44 years	128	43	32	4,096
45–49 years	110	48	27	2,970
50–54 years	80	53	22	1,760
55–59 years	87	58	17	1,479
60–64 years	82	63	12	984
65–69 years	65	67.5	7.5	487.5
70–74 years	75	73	2	150
Total				94,143.75

Measuring Health

The health status of a population can be described in various ways, but there is no universally accepted benchmark, and the measure of health status depends on what we value or what is easy and definitive to collect. Common epidemiologic measures that are accepted indicators for population health are natality, mortality, morbidity, communicable disease rates, occupational injury, and illness rates.

Survival Rate

A rate often used to describe chronic disease (cancers in particular) and, conversely, measures of health is the survival rate. Survival rate is an appropriate measure for diseases and conditions characterized by long duration and long-term follow-up. Survival rate defines the probability of survival over a period of time, usually five years, and can be defined as follows:

$$\frac{\text{Total number of cases of a chronic disease or condition who survive over a specified period of time}}{\text{Total number of cases of a chronic disease or condition during the same specified period of time}}$$

Health-Related Quality of Life

Quality of life (QoL) is a concept that represents the overall sense of well-being, including independence and satisfaction with life. QoL is a complex and subjective concept, which makes it difficult to measure and quantify. QoL has different meanings to different people, and a common measurement is not available. Health is only one component of QoL. Other dimensions include culture, employment, neighborhood, housing, and values.

Health-related quality of life (HRQL) is a notion that attempts to merge all aspects of quality of life that affect overall health, both physical and mental (McHorney, 1999). At the individual level these aspects represent physical and mental perceptions, health risks, functional status, and socioeconomic status. At the population level, HRQL measures conditions and resources that affect the perceptions of health and functional status. HRQL expands the concept of health to encompass the physical and mental needs in a population (Stokols, 1992).

HRQL is becoming a popular measurable outcome that evaluates the perceived physical and mental health and function. HRQL is generally considered an appropriate and adequate measure of health care service needs and intervention outcomes (Idler and Benyamini, 1997). HRQL measurements allow for scientific demonstration of the impact of quality of life on health.

HRQL is related to self-reported chronic diseases and risk factors associated with these conditions. The burden of chronic disease can be measured in part by HRQL. The relationship between disease risk factors and the occurrence of preventable diseases can be linked by HRQL. HRQL surveillance can provide insights for the identification of subgroups in a population who have perceived poor health. HRQL can then guide the targeting of subpopulations for interventions.

Due to the complexity of QoL and HRQL, several measures have been used to assess HRQL and related functional status. These include Medical Outcomes Study Short Forms (SF-36, SF-12, SF-10 for Children, and SF-8), the Sick Impact Profile, and Coop Charts. The SF survey series is used by the CMS and the National Committee for Quality Assurance's Health Plan Employer Data Information Set (HEDIS 3.0) to evaluate the quality of care in managed care plans and other health care facilities (Centers for Disease Control and Prevention, 2000b).

Other Rates

Other rates, in addition to morbidity and mortality rates, are of interest to health care administrators. These include the crude birth rate and the fertility rate. The crude birth rate is used as a measure of population growth and can be used to plan age-specific health care services. The rate is defined as follows:

$$\frac{\text{Total number of live births in a specific}}{\text{population during a specified period of time}}$$
$$\frac{}{\text{Total number of individuals in a specific}}{\text{population during a specified period of time}}$$

The source of numerator data is birth certificates and of denominator data is the U.S. Census Bureau. The population and specified period of time are the same in both the numerator and the denominator.

The fertility rate indicates the potential population growth of a specified population and is defined as follows:

$$\frac{\text{Total number of live births in a specific population during a specified period of time}}{\text{Total number of females between the ages of 15 and 44 years in a specific population during a specified period of time}}$$

Summary

Most epidemiologic inference occurs through comparisons of disease frequency among populations who have unique differences of person, place, and time. The representation of disease frequencies as rates allows for these comparisons. Rates are specialized ratios of the number of cases of disease to a specific reference population during a given period of time. The reference population is typically the best estimate of the general population, derived (in the case of the United States) from U.S. census data.

The cases of disease in the numerator of the rate are derived from routinely collected data and specially designed studies. Fundamental to this measurement is the definition of a case based on a set of criteria.

In addition to rates, comparisons are made by using ratios and proportions. Rates, ratios, and proportions all are used to quantify the effect of disease on specific groups of individuals.

Incidence and prevalence rates are the most useful data for management because they measure the impact of disease on the health care system. Incidence identifies the risk of developing specific diseases in the population and thus allows us to forecast expected disease trends. Prevalence indicates the current impact of a disease. This information helps us determine current resource needs for the delivery of health care services.

Study Questions

1. How does the period of follow-up affect the composition of the denominator when determining the incidence rate?

2. In a recent study of acute myocardial infarction, 10,000 males (between the ages of 40 and 60 years) were followed for six months. During this period, 45 males experienced an acute myocardial infarction. What was the incidence rate during this six-month period?

3. You have recently begun the job of executive assistant to the CEO of East Bank Hospital. The county health commissioner has requested that East Bank Hospital consider expanding the number of dedicated beds in the AIDS inpatient unit. What epidemiologic measures are important for evaluating the situation, and how would you use these measures to help make a decision on this recommendation?

4. Define and discuss the contrasts and similarities of crude death rate, cause-specific mortality rate, proportionate mortality ratio, case-fatality rate, infant mortality rate, and neonatal mortality rate.

5. The CMS periodically publishes case-fatality rates for given DRGs in specific hospitals. These rates often appear in the media as a measure of quality of care. As a health

care executive, you may be called on to explain the variation in fatality rates between your hospital and others.

   a. What factors should you be aware of?

   b. If, based on case-fatality rates, your hospital is ranked low in quality of care, how would you respond to the media and CMS concerning this classification?

6. Assume that you are the administrator of a multispecialty medical group composed of thirty physicians. A hazardous waste disposal site in the community has recently been evaluated by the Environmental Protection Agency (EPA). The owner of the site, West Bank Chemicals, has agreed, in an out-of-court settlement, to pay a lump-sum cash payment to all former employees who have already been diagnosed with one of the three classes of cancer or who develop one of these cancers within the next five years. In addition, West Bank Chemicals has agreed to pay for an annual physical examination for each former employee with cancer for the next five years. West Bank Chemicals has approached your medical group about making a single, lump-sum cash payment for provision of the annual physicals. West Bank Chemicals will also pay for treatment of all former employees for a period of ten years after the closure of the disposal site. (The company representative tells you that this lump-sum cash payment can be charged against the company's current year profits on its income statement.) West Bank Chemicals has requested a proposal outlining your group's requested lump-sum cash payment.

   a. How would knowledge of five-year survival rates help you predict the likely future volume of annual physicals for this bid proposal for West Bank Chemicals?

   b. How would incidence information help you predict the likely future volume of patients who will seek treatment?

   c. What other information would be helpful in preparing your medical group's proposal?

7. When would the incidence of a disease equal the prevalence?

8. Discuss the information that is acquired from incidence and prevalence data.

CHAPTER FOUR

DESIGNS FOR STUDYING THE HEALTH AND HEALTH NEEDS OF POPULATIONS

Chapter Outline

Learning Objectives

Upon completing this chapter, the reader will be able to do all of the following:

- Describe experimental study designs
- Discuss the concept of risk
- Discuss the concept of causation
- Describe observational study designs
- Contrast experimental and observational study designs
- Describe descriptive study designs
- Describe analytic study designs
- Explain the method of measuring the association between a suspected causal factor and an outcome
- Define the constructs relative risk, attributable risk, and odds ratio

Introduction

This chapter will discuss the concepts of risk and causation and the study designs and measures used to reveal and clarify their relationship. Epidemiologic studies are used to test the hypothesis that there is a relationship between a suspected causal factor or characteristic and a disease or condition. Such analytic study designs can be used to investigate many suspected relationships, including the associations between smoking and lung cancer, smoking and cardiovascular disease, maternal rubella and congenital malformations, and family history and cancer.

In statistical terms, the disease or condition is known as the dependent or outcome variable. The outcome, hypothetically, is influenced by the causal factor, which is known as the independent variable. The relationship between the dependent and independent variables is shown by using a 2-by-2 contingency table (see Figure 4.1).

The most straightforward example of an analytic study design involves determining whether either the dependent or independent variable, in terms of exposure to the causal factors, is present. With the 2-by-2 contingency table, each study subject can be classified as to whether the disease and exposure are present or absent. The 2-by-2 table relationships will indicate whether there is an association between the disease and the exposure. The table will also show whether the disease and the exposure occur more frequently in the same individual than they would if they were independent of each other. Finally, it can indicate whether the number of individuals who were exposed and have the disease is higher than expected.

There are four possible association situations with respect to the presence and absence of the disease and potential causal factors:

1. Disease is present (dependent variable) and causal factor is present (independent variable).
2. Disease is absent (dependent variable) and causal factor is absent (independent variable).
3. Disease is present (dependent variable) and causal factor is absent (independent variable).
4. Disease is absent (dependent variable) and causal factor is present (independent variable).

Risk and Causation

Risk can be defined as the chance that an event will occur. With respect to health care for populations, risk is the chance that an individual will become sick or die within a specified period of time. The concept of risk cannot be discussed without mentioning

FIGURE 4.1. A 2-BY-2 CONTINGENCY TABLE.

	Dependent Variable	
Independent Variable	**Present**	**Absent**
Present		
Absent		

the notion of causation. Because of the uncertainty of causation, exposure that is associated with a disease or condition is referred to as a risk factor. This uncertainty results from the conclusion that in most cases there are multiple factors that cause a disease or condition. If only one factor causes a disease, as is seen in the bacterial causation of infectious disease, the certainty of its relationship with the disease can be established.

A risk factor is an individual characteristic, lifestyle characteristic, or environmental exposure that is known, based on observed evidence, to be associated with a disease or condition. A risk factor may or may not be a causal factor. A risk factor may be associated with an increased probability of a disease or condition or may actually increase the probability.

In a population of individuals with the same risk factors, there may be a differential, as well as an expected, effect. This differential effect is due to the complex relationship between risk and causation.

Risk is a concept that is based on the association between the presence of disease and a risk factor. Any or all of the following may be observed: individuals with a risk factor will develop a disease, individuals with a risk factor will not develop a disease, individuals without a risk factor will develop a disease, and individuals without a risk factor will not develop a disease.

Rothman (1986) developed a theory of modified determinism that addresses the complex relationship between risk and causation. In this theory, a cause is defined as an act or event that initiates or allows for, singularly or in conjunction with other factors, a sequence of events that result in an effect. The theory further describes a classification of causes; a sufficient cause always produces the effect. This is rarely seen in observations of population health.

A component cause, also called a contributing cause, is one of a group of causes that collectively form the minimum requirement of a sufficient cause. The nature of the relationship is such that the absence of any contributing cause results in the absence of an effect. The importance of this fact is that only one cause need be removed to eliminate the disease. Most causes of disease are component causes.

Two types of causal relationships exist: direct and indirect. Direct causal relationships are characterized by one risk factor that is directly associated with a disease—for example, hemoglobin S and sickle cell disease. Indirect causal relationships are multifactorial, with a nonlinear relationship. An example would be acute myocardial infarction, which is caused by high cholesterol over time, thickening of the coronary arteries over time, hemostatic factors, and lifestyle behaviors.

Following Rothman's theory, there are four types of causal relationships. The first type is a *necessary and sufficient* relationship. In this type, in the absence of the causal factor, the disease will not occur. A classic example is HIV virus and AIDS. The second type of relationship is *necessary but not sufficient*. This type is characterized by multiple factors, one of which is required for the disease to occur. An example is tuberculosis, in which the bacteria must be present, but exposure to the bacteria is not sufficient to cause the disease. Development of tuberculosis is dependent on immunosuppression as well as other factors in addition to exposure to the bacteria.

The third type of causal relationship is *sufficient but not necessary*. This type is characterized by the existence of a factor that can cause the disease, but the disease may occur in the absence of the causal factor. The fourth type of relationship is *neither sufficient nor necessary*. This type is the description of complex models of disease etiology. Examples are high-fat diet and lifestyle behaviors as related to heart disease, hypertension, diabetes, and some cancers.

A notion that is central to causation is exposure. Exposure can be environmental, genetic, or a combination. An important question can be asked about exposure. If an individual is exposed, will that person develop a disease? If this relationship can be established, a second question begs for an answer: if exposure is associated with a disease, does this represent a causal relationship?

Study Designs

To determine whether a causal relationship can be established between an exposure and the occurrence of disease, understanding the disease etiology is an initial task. The second task is to conduct studies in populations. Both of these tasks depend on epidemiologic study designs. Epidemiologic studies can be divided into two broad categories: experimental and observational.

Experimental studies address the first task: what is the disease etiology? Experimental studies include bench and clinical evaluations conducted in human and in animals. For example, in vitro studies and animal studies are used in an attempt to understand disease etiology. These study designs allow for control of exposure, but it is difficult to translate animal study results to human populations.

Experimental and observational studies are used to answer the second task. In experimental studies, the investigator has control over a factor of interest and can manipulate the study population, rather than simply make observations. The experimental study evaluates the impact on the presence of a disease or condition created by experimentally varying some factor. Observational studies involve observing and analyzing contrasts in outcomes among study subjects caused by factors not under the control of the investigator.

Experimental Studies

The framework of a typical experimental study is as follows. First, the investigator selects a number of individuals who are similar in some specific characteristics. Second, the investigator randomly selects a subset of individuals who possess a hypothesized disease-causing factor, known as the experimental group. Then the experimental group and the remaining individuals, known as the control group, are compared for the occurrence of the disease being studied. For many reasons, including costs, experimental studies are not commonly conducted.

Figure 4.2 illustrates the complete array of experimental study designs. These include community and clinical, or medical, trials. Prevention and intervention trials, which are forms of clinical trials, are also examples of experimental studies.

Clinical Trials

Experimental study designs provide strong evidence for the testing of study hypotheses. Experimental studies are difficult and expensive to conduct. The most commonly conducted experimental studies are clinical trials. There are several types of clinical trials: therapeutic trials, prophylactic trials, screening trials, and quality-of-life trials. Therapeutic trials evaluate new treatments, which may include pharmaceutics, surgery, procedures, or combinations. Prophylactic trials test new prevention interventions that may lower the risk of disease occurrence. Screening trials search for optimal methods to identify early stages of a disease. Quality-of-life trials, which are common with chronic diseases, evaluate methods to improve the quality of life of patients.

The need for clinical trials originates from laboratory bench research. After the need has been established, a clinical trial plan, called a protocol, is developed. In practice, clinical trials are organized in phases. Phase I clinical trials investigate the manner of administration of the study methods, the frequency of administration, and

FIGURE 4.2. EXPERIMENTAL STUDY DESIGNS.

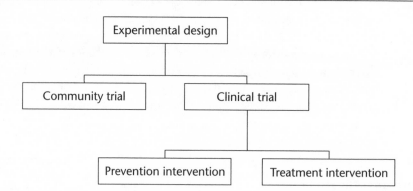

the safety of the clinical trial. Phase I clinical trials typically involve a small number of people. Phase II clinical trials are intended to verify safety and begin to evaluate the effects of intervention. Phase II trials typically target a specific disease or condition. Phase III clinical trials involve large numbers of individuals who are assigned to different study groups (the reason for this will be discussed shortly). Results of Phase III clinical trials are translated into clinical practice.

Clinical trials can be defined as experimental studies that attempt to determine both the efficacy and the efficiency of a therapeutic agent such as a drug or a procedure. The treatment is allocated by the investigator, giving clinical trials their experimental nature. Efficacy measures whether the treatment improves the health of individuals who receive it. Efficiency measures the resources consumed by the treatment. Clinical trials have two overriding objectives: to determine whether receiving the treatment, or prevention intervention, results in a better clinical outcome than not receiving the treatment and to determine whether a treatment is associated with any harmful side effects.

Operationally, clinical trials can be divided into two types: uncontrolled and controlled trials. By definition, uncontrolled trials have no comparison (control) group by which a treatment is evaluated. Treatments are tested on a set of subjects, and results are monitored. Results of these trials cannot be generalized to subpopulations or the overall population. This characteristic limits their usefulness.

In controlled trials, a new treatment is compared with an existing treatment or with no treatment (the control group). Testing a new treatment against no treatment may involve the use of a placebo (an inactive substance masquerading as an active medication).

In controlled clinical trials, selection of control groups is an important concern, both ethically and therapeutically. When the trial seeks to identify whether a new treatment results in an improvement over an existing treatment, control groups are treated by the best existing treatment. If no accepted treatment currently exists, control groups are untreated, and the study question becomes whether the new treatment provides a better result than doing nothing.

Central to the experimental nature of clinical trials is allocation, or assignment of subjects into treatment and control groups. Subjects who receive the new treatment are members of the treatment group. Those who receive no treatment (including placebo) or the existing treatment are members of the control group. There are several methods of allocation in use, including random, nonrandom, and systematic allocation.

Random allocation allows chance to determine assignment to study groups. Randomization has been defined as a process of assigning individuals to study groups in a manner such that all possible assignments and compositions of study groups are equally likely. It eliminates bias because all confounding characteristics of subjects will be equally distributed in both treatment and control groups. The most common method of random allocation is the use of random number generators or random number tables. The problem inherent in random allocation is the associated complexity in operation, as well as relatively high cost. Figure 4.3 presents the framework of a randomized controlled clinical trial.

Nonrandom allocation assigns subjects to study groups by a process other than chance. This method is used when random allocation is not possible or feasible or is unethical. An example is the use of azidothymidine (AZT) in AIDS patients. Another example is the use of an experimental drug therapy for individuals whose medical condition is the most severe.

Systematic allocation is not random but is based on some criterion assumed to be independent of the outcome under study. A common example is the use of subject birth date. For example, all subjects born on an even-numbered date are assigned to the treatment group, and all subjects born on an odd-numbered date are assigned to the control group. The disadvantage with this method is the possibility of bias on the part of the investigator, because he or she may know the birth dates and thus the assigned groups.

Clinical trials must avoid bias. Because clinical trials aim to identify some difference in outcome between the treatment and control groups, any difference in this outcome should be due to the effect of the treatment and not to any other factors. Bias is the difference observed that is due to some factor other than the treatment effect.

One method used to overcome bias is masking. Also known as blinding, masking is used to eliminate bias that may originate from any of the parties involved in the clinical trials: the subject, investigator (observer), or data analyst. Blinding can occur in three ways: in single blinding, the study subjects do not know their study group assignment. In double blinding, neither study subjects nor observers know the study group assignment. In triple blinding, the study subjects, the observer, and the data analyst are all unaware of the study group assignment.

FIGURE 4.3. FRAMEWORK OF A RANDOMIZED CONTROLLED CLINICAL TRIAL.

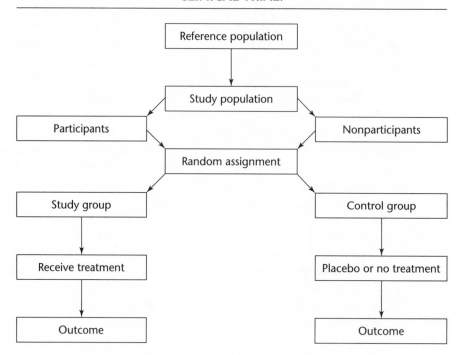

A common type of clinical trial is the randomized controlled clinical trial. In this design, randomization is used to eliminate investigator bias by randomly assigning individuals to treatment and control groups. These trials are either single- or double-blinded and usually result in the most accurate estimate of treatment effect. Randomized controlled clinical trials are the most useful for comparison, because of the use of randomly allocated controls.

The design of a randomized controlled clinical trial is shown in Figure 4.3. The significant characteristic is that both study subjects and controls come from the same subpopulation of individuals who volunteer for the trial. Because of randomization, the volunteer bias should be evenly distributed among both study subjects and controls, so the effect of bias should be less problematic.

Observational Studies

The observational study design is more commonly used in epidemiology. Study subjects are placed into specific groups based on the presence or absence of risk factors. This selection process is not under the control of the investigator; that is, whether a subject has a risk factor is an individual characteristic of the study subjects. The occurrence of a disease or condition is observed in each risk factor–specified study group.

Observational studies investigate the etiology of specific diseases. In this study design, which is known as an analytic study design, the investigator observes but does not manipulate the study population. Observational study designs are presented in Figure 4.4. The different observational study designs can be distinguished with respect to time. Descriptive studies collect data that describe disease according to person, place, and time; they determine rates of health and disease. Ecologic studies collect data according to distinct populations in specifically distinguished areas. Analytic study designs attempt to support hypotheses that exposure to a causal factor is related to the etiology of disease. Analytic studies take the form of cross-sectional, prospective, and retrospective designs. Cross-sectional studies, also called prevalence studies, are concerned with the presence or absence of disease at the present time. Retrospective studies, also known as case-control studies, evaluate the presence or absence of disease in the past. Prospective studies, also called cohort studies, follow study groups into the future to observe the presence or absence of disease.

When investigating the existence of causal relationships between suspected risk factors and the occurrence of a disease, each study design provides important information. Ecologic studies investigate grouped characteristics in populations. Cross-sectional studies evaluate the presence and absence of risk factors and diseases at a specific point or over a specific period of time. Prospective and retrospective studies examine individual characteristics.

Descriptive Studies. Descriptive studies, which can be either prospective or retrospective, evaluate various data, including demographics, morbidity, and mortality. Prospective descriptive study designs include disease registries, mortality data collection, and morbidity data collection, as discussed in Chapter Two. Retrospective descriptive study designs record past measurements of information; included in this category is the decennial census and reviews of other routinely collected data, such as the MEDPAR data file published by the Centers for Medicare and Medicaid Services.

Descriptive studies are not useful for establishing cause-and-effect or exposure-and-result relationships. But descriptive studies, which are inexpensive to conduct, are useful for formulating hypotheses based on the description provided by the study data. For example, assume that census data indicate a higher than expected percentage of individuals over the age of 65 years in a subpopulation. A hypothesis can be formulated from these data that this subpopulation has a higher death rate because of its expected older age distribution.

Cross-Sectional Studies. Cross-sectional studies, also known as prevalence studies, are designed to measure current exposure to risk factors of interest as well as the current health impact of this exposure, disease, or condition in the population. Like

FIGURE 4.4. OBSERVATIONAL STUDY DESIGNS.

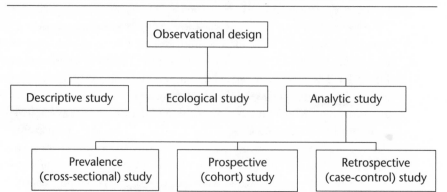

descriptive studies, prevalence studies are usually based on geographically defined populations. This study design results in descriptive data relative to the pattern of disease and the pattern of causal factors in the population at a specific point in time.

The purpose of cross-sectional studies is to obtain a valid estimate of some hypothesized cause-and-effect relationship between a suspected risk factor and a disease or condition. The products of cross-sectional studies are prevalence measures for specific diseases under study.

Cross-sectional studies usually divide the population into exposed and nonexposed groups, based on exposure to a suspected risk factor. At the same time, the presence of disease is evaluated in both exposure groups. It is usually easy to measure the impact of potentially confounding risk factors with this design. The problem associated with this design is that it is very difficult to establish cause-and-effect relationships, for two reasons: the current exposure may not be related to the current disease, and other important prior experiences that may have influenced the disease are usually not known, nor can the timing relationship of exposure and disease be established.

Despite the lack of ability to establish cause-and-effect relationships with this design, cross-sectional studies are useful and provide important information for managers. They can be performed in a relatively short period of time and can study large populations quite easily. Most important, cross-sectional studies provide estimates of the extent of a health problem (that is, the prevalence in a population). These estimates are useful in planning and managing delivery of health care services.

An example of a cross-sectional study involves a large manufacturing company concerned with absenteeism and declining work productivity (Anzalone, Anzalone, and Fos, 1995). The company decided to implement a wellness program at the factory for its employees. A needs assessment and baseline health data were needed before the company could implement the program. A local hospital took histories and conducted physical examinations and cholesterol screening for the company's 2,500 employees. The results of these examinations included prevalence estimates on such employee characteristics as smoking habits, obesity, dietary habits, exercise, and abnormal levels of low-density lipoproteins (LDL cholesterol). This information had two purposes. First, the prevalence of risk factors allowed for proper planning of the components of the wellness program (weight reduction, smoking cessation, and so on). Second, the health effects of the wellness program could be determined by comparing baseline health status data to future wellness program data.

Another example of a cross-sectional study is the Harvard School of Public Health College Alcohol Study (Wechsler and others, 2000, 2002). This study has been conducted at different points in time since 1993. In 1999, the study surveyed more than fourteen thousand college students at 119 four-year colleges in thirty-nine states using mail questionnaires. The results indicated that 44% of college students were binge drinkers of alcohol. These binge drinkers were more likely to experience alcohol-related problems.

Ecologic Studies. Ecologic studies are characterized by use of populations, or groups of individuals, as the unit of analysis. These studies typically use existing data that have been collected for other purposes. The time frame is a point in time across a population, as in cross-sectional studies. Ecologic studies are popular because of the resulting hypothesis generation and the use of easily obtained data. Follow-up or individual contact is not needed.

Ecologic studies can suggest research strategies that may provide insight into the relationship between exposure and the occurrence of disease in populations. As with cross-sectional studies, ecologic study designs do not illustrate the existence of causal relationships. A caveat of ecologic studies is that they may attribute to a population risk characteristics that may be observed in individuals. This is due to the fact that population mean values are used in the analysis.

An example of an ecologic study is an evaluation of the relationship between neurobehavioral diseases and contaminants in the drinking water. This study investigated the association of perchlorate in the drinking water and the prevalence of thyroid diseases and thyroid cancer. The study was conducted in counties in Nevada where known contamination of the drinking water with perchlorate had been previously demonstrated (Chang, Crothers, and Lamm, 2003).

Prospective Studies. Prospective study designs, also known as cohort study designs, have the same purpose as prevalence studies: to obtain a valid estimate of some hypothesized cause-and-effect relationship between a suspected risk factor and a disease or condition. Individuals are identified as being exposed or not exposed to a suspected risk factor and are then followed into the future for a specified period of time. A distinguishing characteristic of this design is that all individuals, in both the exposed and the nonexposed group, are free of the disease or condition when the study begins (t_0).

Cohort studies evaluate individuals in a forward time direction. Individuals in both groups are followed for a specified period of time until the study period ends (t_1).

The number of cases of disease that develop (known as incident cases) in both groups between t_0 and t_1 is determined.

Prospective study design has been used extensively in evaluating the relationship of diet and health. Particular interest has focused on diet and prostate cancer incidence. One study, using a cohort of fourteen thousand men, evaluated the relationship between intake of tomatoes and the risk of prostate cancer (Mills, Beeson, Phillips, and Fraser, 1994). The study findings indicated that high intake of tomatoes is highly correlated with lower prostate cancer risk.

Another study, with a larger sample size of fifty thousand men, centered on lifestyle effects of diet on prostate cancer risk (Giovannucci and others, 1993). In this study, the fat intake of health care professionals was evaluated. The study found that high intake of animal fat from red meat is associated with increased prostate cancer incidence.

Retrospective Studies. The purpose of retrospective study designs is identical to that of other designs: to obtain a valid estimate of some hypothesized cause-and-effect relationship between a suspected risk factor and a disease or condition. Individuals who have been diagnosed with a disease or condition (known as cases) are compared with individuals who have not been diagnosed with the same disease or condition (known as controls). This study design is called the case-control method.

Case-control study designs evaluate individuals in a reverse direction in time, by identifying cases and controls at the present (t_0) and then reviewing and analyzing historical data. The presence or absence of a suspected risk factor in both cases and controls is established in retrospect. Case-control study designs attempt to determine differences in the proportion of cases and controls who have a suspected risk factor or factors.

The presence of a suspected risk factor or factors is determined by reviewing historical data (for example, medical records) and by interviewing study subjects. Because of the dynamics of this study design, case-control studies are usually conducted with relatively small study groups. Advantages of these studies include that they are relatively inexpensive to conduct, are relatively quickly performed, and are useful for studying rare diseases. Disadvantages include that small sample sizes make it difficult to generalize study results and that these studies may incorporate biases (especially recall bias) because the information collected is culled from subject interviews.

Association of Risk Factors and Health and Disease

Association is the presence of a statistical relationship between two or more factors or events. In epidemiology, association is the presence of a statistical relationship between the presence or absence of a risk factor and the presence or absence of a disease or

condition. Risk, in the context of association, is the probability of an i[?]
veloping a disease or condition over some fixed time interval. A concern
association exists between exposure to a suspected risk factor and the o[?]
disease or condition. Worded differently, the question is whether there is excess risk
associated with exposure to a specific risk factor.

Measuring Association in Prospective Studies

Measures of association are used to determine whether an association exists between
a risk factor (that is, exposure to some risk factor) and a disease. The result of the cohort study design is a measure of incidence of a disease or condition in both exposure
groups. Such a measurement allows for the comparison of new cases in both the
exposed and nonexposed study groups. Specifically, a cohort study measures the cumulative incidence of a disease in some exposed group of individuals, as well as the
cumulative incidence. The cumulative incidence measures the risk in a group of individuals over time.

This relative effect of the exposure to a risk factor in groups of individuals is measured by the ratio between the disease occurrence in the exposed group and in the nonexposed group. The construct that measures the relative effect in cohort studies is known
as the relative risk. The relative risk is the ratio of the cumulative incidence in the exposure groups. The relative risk represents the strength of any association and is the
ratio of disease in the exposed to the nonexposed groups. Strength of association refers
to the chance that the occurrence of an outcome is greater for individuals who have
been exposed to a risk factor than for others in the population. The greater the chance,
the greater the strength of association. The relative risk can be defined as follows:

$$\frac{\text{Incidence rate among exposed individuals}}{\text{Incidence rate among nonexposed individuals}}$$

The relative risk is used to express the risk of the exposed group compared to the
nonexposed group. For example, if the risk factor is alcohol consumption, the relative
risk describes how much the risk of an individual who drinks alcohol is increased, compared to an individual who does not drink alcohol. The relative risk also indicates
the amount of benefit, or decrease in risk, that may result if the risk factor is removed.

The value of the relative risk can range from 0 (no individuals in the exposed
group develop the disease) to ∞ (all individuals in the exposed group develop the disease). A relative risk of 1 indicates that the risk of developing the disease is not affected by exposure to the risk factor. A relative risk greater than 1 indicates that
exposure to the risk factor increases the chance of developing the disease; a relative

risk less than 1 indicates that exposure to the risk factor decreases the chance of developing the disease.

The relative risk does not indicate the chance that an individual will develop a disease or condition given exposure to a risk factor. Rather, it measures the magnitude by which the probability is increased in individuals exposed to a risk factor. For example, a relative risk of 5 indicates that the probability is five times greater in individuals exposed to a risk factor than in those who are not exposed. The chance of developing a disease in the exposed individuals may be quite low, but it is five times higher than in those unexposed. The relative risk is best used as a measure of association between a risk factor and a specific outcome, not as a measure of probability of an outcome.

The relative risk can be further explained by reviewing a 2-by-2 contingency table. Table 4.1 demonstrates the calculation of relative risk. The columns of the 2-by-2 table represent the presence or absence of disease. The rows of the table represent the exposure groups (exposed or not exposed to the risk factor). The upper left cell, designated a, gives the number of incident cases in the exposed group, while the upper right cell, designated b, gives the numbers in the exposed group who remained disease free. The lower left cell, designated c, presents the number of incident cases in the nonexposed group. The lower right cell, designated d, presents the number of individuals in the nonexposed group who remained disease free. The relative risk is equal to the ratio of the incidence rate in the exposed group to the incidence rate in the nonexposed group: $(a/a + b)/(c/c + d)$.

The absolute effect of exposure to a risk factor is measured as the absolute difference between the disease occurrence in the exposed and nonexposed groups. This is the absolute difference between the cumulative incidence in the exposed and the cumulative incidence in the nonexposed group. In cohort study designs, a measure of absolute effect is the construct known as attributable risk. The attributable risk measures the amount of absolute risk that can be attributed to a specific risk factor. Absolute risk is the same as the incidence and indicates the rate of occurrence of a disease or condition. The attributable risk is defined as follows:

Incidence among exposed subjects – incidence among nonexposed subjects

Attributable risk measures the excess in the number of incident cases due to exposure to a risk factor and thus illustrates the impact, in number of individuals, of a specific risk factor.

Given data on alcohol use and liver dysfunction, an association can be determined easily. Assume that the incidence of liver dysfunction among alcohol drinkers is equal to 125 cases per 100,000 individuals. Also assume that the incidence rate of liver dysfunction among nondrinkers is 10 cases per 100,000 individuals. The relative risk is equal to the ratio of the incidence rates, or 125/10. This is a relative risk of 12.5, which

TABLE 4.1. CALCULATION OF RELATIVE RISK.

Risk factor	Disease	No disease	Totals
Exposed	a	b	a + b
Nonexposed	c	d	c + d
Totals	a + c	b + d	a + b + c + d

Relative risk = (a/a + b) / (c/c + d)

indicates that alcohol drinkers are 12.5 times more likely to develop liver dysfunction than nondrinkers. The attributable risk is equal to the incidence among drinkers minus the incidence among nondrinkers: $125 - 10 = 115$ per 100,000 individuals. This indicates that 115 cases of liver dysfunction per 100,000 individuals can be attributed to drinking alcohol.

Table 4.2 presents data on the association of smoking and coronary heart disease. The risk factor groups are smokers and nonsmokers. During the study period, of the total population of 765, some 385 developed coronary heart disease. Among these new cases, 210 were smokers. The relative risk calculation (performed using the Centers for Disease Control and Prevention's software, EpiInfo 2000) indicates that the relative risk for this study population is 1.15, with 95% confidence intervals of 1.00 and 1.33. This shows that individuals who smoke have a 1.15 greater chance of developing coronary heart disease than those who do not smoke. In other words, whatever the a priori probability of developing coronary heart disease in this study population, the risk for smokers is 1.15 times greater than for nonsmokers.

Table 4.3 illustrates the framework of retrospective study design. If a higher number of cases (individuals with the disease or condition) are determined to have been exposed to the risk factor than controls (individuals without the disease or condition), an association between the disease and suspected risk factors is established. Tests of statistical significance are done to confirm the association; for example, if $a/a + c$ is statistically significantly greater than $b/b + d$, an association exists. (See the Appendix.)

Table 4.4 presents an example of this process, in which an association between smoking and coronary heart disease (CHD) is under study. Of 321 cases (individuals with CHD), 192 report a history of smoking. Of 337 controls (those without CHD), 156 report a history of smoking. The proportion of cases of CHD who smoke equals 60 percent (192/321), which is greater than the proportion of controls who smoke (156/337, or 46 percent). Using a χ^2 test indicates a significant difference between smokers and nonsmokers ($p < .00051$). This establishes that there is an association between smoking and cases of CHD (see Appendix).

TABLE 4.2. ASSOCIATION OF SMOKING AND CORONARY HEART DISEASE: RELATIVE RISK ANALYSIS.

Smoking status	Disease	No disease	Totals
Smoker	210	180	390
Nonsmoker	175	200	375
Totals	385	380	765

Relative risk $= \dfrac{(210/390)}{(175/375)} = 1.15$ (1.00 < relative risk < 1.33).

TABLE 4.3. RETROSPECTIVE STUDY DESIGN, 2-BY-2 TABLE.

Risk factor	Cases	Controls	Totals
Present	a	b	$a + b$
Absent	c	d	$c + d$
Totals	$a + c$	$b + d$	$a + b + c + d$

TABLE 4.4. ASSOCIATION BETWEEN SMOKING AND CORONARY HEART DISEASE: PROPORTIONS ANALYSIS.

Smoking status	Cases	Controls	Totals
Smoker	192	156	348
Nonsmoker	129	181	310
Totals	321	337	658

Proportion of cases who smoke = 59.8%.

Proportion of controls who smoke = 46.3%.

$\chi^2 = 12.06$, $p = .00051$.

Measuring Association in Retrospective Studies

Retrospective study designs, unlike prospective study designs, do not determine the incidence of a specific disease or condition. Actual incidence rates are the basis for measuring association between exposure to a potential risk factor and a disease or condition; given this fact, the relative risk cannot be determined using a retrospective study design. This is due to the fact that the risk of disease among the exposed and nonexposed individuals is not known because the study evaluates those who are currently cases (in whom the disease has occurred) and controls (in whom the disease has not occurred).

One objective of retrospective study design is to determine whether an association exists between the suspected risk factors and a disease or condition, that is, determination of whether risk factors were present in individuals in the past. This is usually accomplished by interviewing subjects or reviewing records.

The method used in retrospective study design to measure association involves an estimate of the incidence rates among exposed and nonexposed study groups. The retrospective design cannot determine risk, but it can identify how the risk factor is distributed among cases and controls. This distribution can be used to calculate the odds of disease, given exposure to a risk factor. The construct that is usually used to measure the degree of association in retrospective studies is the odds ratio. The odds ratio can also be calculated for cohort studies. In a cohort study, the odds ratio is defined as the odds of developing a disease or condition in exposed individuals compared to the odds of developing the disease or condition in nonexposed individuals.

With respect to the four possible association situations identified earlier in this chapter, the odds ratio is actually the ratio of the product of convergence. The odds ratio is calculated as follows:

Situation when disease is present (dependent variable) and causal factor is present (independent variable) × situation when disease is absent (dependent variable) and causal factor is absent (independent variable)

$\dfrac{a \times d}{c \times b}$

Situation when the disease is present (dependent variable) and causal factor is absent (independent variable) × situation when disease is absent (dependent variable) and causal factor is present (independent variable)

The odds ratio estimates the strength of any association between exposure to a risk factor and the absence and presence of a disease or condition and can be calculated by using a 2-by-2 contingency table. Table 4.5 presents a 2-by-2 contingency table describing a retrospective study. The columns of the 2-by-2 table represent the presence of disease (cases) and the absence of disease (controls). The rows of the table represent the exposure groups (exposed or not exposed to the risk factor). The upper left cell, designated a, presents the number of cases who were exposed to the risk factor. The upper right cell, designated b, presents the number of individuals in the control group who were exposed to the risk factor. The lower left cell, designated c, presents the number of cases who were not exposed to the risk factor. The lower right cell, designated d, presents the number of individuals in the control group who were not exposed to the risk factor. The odds ratio is the ratio of the product of the number of cases who were exposed to the risk factor and the number of controls who were not exposed, compared to the product of the number of cases

TABLE 4.5. CALCULATION OF THE ODDS RATIO.

Risk factor	Cases	Controls	Totals
Exposed	a	b	$a + b$
Nonexposed	c	d	$c + d$
Totals	$a + c$	$b + d$	$a + b + c + d$

Odds ratio = ad / bc

who were not exposed and the number of controls who were exposed to the risk factor.

The odds ratio is a measure of the relationship of the odds of being a case to being a control if exposed to a risk factor, to the odds of being a case to being a control if not exposed to a risk factor. Based on Table 4.5, the odds ratio equals $(a/b)/(c/d)$. However, the odds ratio is usually expressed as the population odds ratio, defined as ad/bc, which is an algebraic equivalent of $(a/b)/(c/d)$. An example of calculating the odds ratio is presented in Table 4.6. The odds ratio is equal to ad/bc, or $(192)(181)/(156)(129)$, or 1.73 to 1, with 95% confidence intervals of 1.25 and 2.38. In other words, whatever the a priori probability of developing coronary heart disease in this study population, the risk for smokers is 1.73 times greater than for nonsmokers.

Application to Population Health Management

A study conducted to investigate racial variation in cesarean section rates among Medicaid beneficiaries (Butcher, Fos, Zúñiga, and Panne, 1997) illustrates the application of a prospective study design to managerial epidemiology. Significant variation occurs in the incidence of cesarean section, due to maternal, physician, and economic factors. Specifically, higher cesarean section rates are seen in mothers with fee-for-service insurance than in Medicaid beneficiaries. This same trend is observed among mothers of high socioeconomic status and those in private hospitals when compared to those in public hospitals.

An objective of this study was to determine whether this trend exists in mothers of different races, controlling for other potential causal factors. Caucasian and African American mothers who are Medicaid beneficiaries were studied, and cesarean section rates were calculated. Theoretically, all Medicaid beneficiaries should be similar with respect to socioeconomic status, provider utilization, and payment sources, differing only by race.

Table 4.7 shows the births and cesarean sections in the study population between July 1991 and July 1993. Table 4.8 presents the total live births among Medicaid

TABLE 4.6. ASSOCIATION BETWEEN SMOKING AND CORONARY HEART DISEASE: ODDS RATIO ANALYSIS.

Smoking status	Cases	Controls	Totals
Smoker	192	156	348
Nonsmoker	129	181	310
Totals	321	337	658

$$\text{Odds ratio} = \frac{(192 \times 181)}{(129 \times 156)} = 1.73 \ (1.25 < \text{odds ratio} < 2.38).$$

TABLE 4.7. BIRTHS AND CESAREAN SECTIONS IN THE STUDY POPULATION.

Time period	Total Medicaid births	Medicaid cesarean sections	Medicaid cesarean section rate (per 1,000 live births)
1991–1992	25,200	6,911	274.2
1992–1993	31,450	8,891	282.7

beneficiaries in the study population. To clarify the relationship between the chance of a cesarean section and the potential causal factors, relative risk calculations were performed. The basis of these calculations was determining the risk of a cesarean section. Table 4.9 presents the cesarean section rates and relative risk of a cesarean section among white and black Americans across age categories. The relative risk is calculated as the ratio of the cesarean rate for blacks compared to the rate for whites. Table 4.10 shows cesarean section rates and relative risk of a cesarean section across geographic locales.

The results of the study indicate that white women had higher cesarean section rates and were at greater risk for a cesarean section than black women when stratified by age and geographic locale. These results imply that within a theoretically similar population, except for race, trends in performing of cesarean sections are quite different. The costs of cesarean sections and reimbursement of providers vary across the study population. This information could be used to argue for the establishment of Medicaid managed care in this population. Managed care would likely reduce the rate of cesarean section among both white and black women and would probably equalize its use across all groups in the population.

TABLE 4.8. TOTAL LIVE BIRTHS AMONG MEDICAID BENEFICIARIES.

Mother's age	Number of births to black mothers	Number of births to white mothers	Total births
Under 15 years	695	89	784
15–24 years	29,480	18,911	43,391
25–34 years	12,487	7,413	19,900
35–44 years	1,003	835	2,738
45 years and older	12	2	14
Totals	43,677	27,677	71,827

TABLE 4.9. CESAREAN SECTION RATE AND RELATIVE RISK, BY AGE OF MOTHER.

Mother's age	Cesarean section rate for blacks (per 1,000 live births)	Cesarean section rate for whites (per 1,000 live births)	Relative risk
Under 15 years	230.2	292.1	0.79
15–24 years	243.5	288.4	0.84
25–34 years	289.2	337.9	0.86
35–44 years	327.9	371.3	0.88
45 years and older	500.0	500.0	1.00
Overall	261.8	302.9	0.86

TABLE 4.10. CESAREAN SECTION RATES AND RELATIVE RISK, BY LOCALE.

Locale	Cesarean section rate for blacks (per 1,000 live births)	Cesarean section rate for whites (per 1,000 live births)	Relative risk
Urban	252.9	301.7	0.84
Rural	290.3	307.9	0.94

Summary

Epidemiologic studies attempt to clarify the relationship between exposure to a suspected causal factor and a disease or condition and are classified as either experimental or observational. In experimental studies the investigator manipulates the study population with respect to exposure to causal factors. In observational studies, the investigator simply observes what occurs and does not manipulate the study population.

Observational studies are the most common and consist of descriptive and analytic designs. The analytic study designs include prevalence, cohort, and case-control studies. Analytic studies attempt to determine whether a suspected etiologic factor and a disease occur in the same individual more often than would be expected if the factor and the disease were randomly distributed in the study population. This relationship is quantified by measures of association: relative risk, odds ratio, and attributable risk.

Study Questions

1. The data in Table 4.11 represent the results of a study on risk factors for falls in an elderly population. The data were collected using a retrospective study design. Select the appropriate measure of association, and calculate it for each risk factor (arthritis, heart disease, diabetes, colon cancer, and unstable gait). Use a 2-by-2 contingency table for each risk factor.

2. The administrator of the only hospital in a community of 150,000 people notices that many patients admitted for salmonella infection indicate that they drink unpasteurized milk from a local dairy. Periodic inspections by the state health department sometimes find milk samples contaminated with salmonella organisms. The dairy has resisted pasteurizing the milk because the state inspections do not always indicate salmonella

TABLE 4.11. RISK FACTORS FOR FALLS IN AN ELDERLY POPULATION.

Risk factor	Cases exposed to the risk factor	Cases not exposed to the risk factor	Controls exposed to the risk factor	Controls not exposed to the risk factor
Arthritis	74	86	30	242
Heart disease	35	107	7	331
Diabetes	38	131	56	282
Colon cancer	9	39	18	91
Unstable gait	25	57	38	255

contamination. The hospital administrator decides to conduct a hospital-based study that may show a strong association between unpasteurized milk consumption and salmonella cases in the community. The following information is abstracted from hospital medical records:

- During the past three years, 10% of the community population was hospitalized at least one day.
- A review of admission forms indicates that of 55,000 admitted patients, 64 were admitted for salmonella infections.
- A total of 3,487 of the 55,000 admitted patients reported that they had consumed unpasteurized milk.
- Thirteen of the patients who reported that they had consumed unpasteurized milk were admitted for salmonella infections.

   a. What study design should the hospital administrator select? Why?
   b. Calculate the appropriate measure of association.
   c. What can be concluded from this hospital-based study with respect to the association of consuming unpasteurized milk and salmonella infection?

3. Discuss the characteristics, strengths, and weaknesses of the following study designs:
   a. Cross-sectional
   b. Retrospective
   c. Descriptive
   d. Prospective

4. Describe an ecologic study, present its strengths and weaknesses, and give an example.

5. When does the odds ratio provide a good estimation of the risk of exposure to a suspected risk factor?

CHAPTER FIVE

STANDARDIZING POPULATION HEALTH INFORMATION

Chapter Outline

Introduction
Stratification
Matching
Standardization of Information
Risk Adjustment
Summary
Study Questions

Learning Objectives

Upon completing this chapter, the reader will be able to do all of the following:

- Discuss the concept of confounding
- Discuss the concept of standardization
- Describe the method of direct standardization
- Describe the method of indirect standardization
- Define the standardized morbidity ratio construct
- Define the standardized mortality ratio construct
- Compare and interpret crude and standardized rates
- Discuss the concept of risk adjustment
- Describe the process of stratification

Introduction

Chapter Three introduced the concept of a rate, which is the basic measure used for comparing disease frequency among and across populations. These crude rates are based on the actual number of events in a specific population during a specific period of time. Crude rates have several inherent limitations. They do not account for the fact that different populations, as well as subpopulations within them, may have significantly different risks for specific diseases and conditions. This situation is particularly problematic in populations with variable age distributions. Behavioral characteristics, such as smoking, coffee drinking, number of sex partners, and drug abuse, also result in varying levels of risk within a population.

Rates are essential in making comparisons across and among populations, because determinants of disease are correlated with the occurrence of health and disease. It is important to identify the determinants, or characteristics, of individuals in the population that are associated with either higher or lower frequencies of health and diseases or conditions. In fact, when making comparisons between two populations (or two or more subpopulations), one seeks to establish whether differences between populations are directly associated with a specific characteristic or set of characteristics and whether the differences are affected by some other characteristic or set of characteristics.

This chapter introduces the concept known as confounding and methods to mitigate its effect. Confounding can be defined as the process of mixing things up or lumping them together indiscriminately. Confounding has the effect of confusing the results of a comparison between two or more populations. The interpretation of differences between two population groups can therefore be misleading and inaccurate as a result of the effect of confounding.

A factor that confounds the comparison of data describing the effect of a population characteristic or characteristics is known as a confounding variable or confounding factor. To satisfy the criteria for classification as a confounding factor, the factor must be a true risk factor for the disease or condition of interest and must be unequally distributed in the two populations. An illustrative example of evaluating the potential effect of confounding on planning and managing health care services follows.

Beginning in 1991, the National Center for Health Statistics has annually collected information about health care services provided in hospital emergency departments in the United States. Ambulatory care services have become the major type of health care services provided. The survey is called the National Hospital Ambulatory Medical Care Survey (NHAMCS) and has two components: emergency department and outpatient department summaries.

Data from the 2001 NHAMCS outpatient summary (Centers for Disease Control and Prevention, 2001d) illustrate that the rate of outpatient department visits among males is 264.0 per 100 persons per year and among females is 362.3 per 100 persons per year. These figures represent a 50% difference between males and females in the United States. Is this comparison correct? Do females use outpatient departments in hospitals twice as often as males? Before we make any inferences, confounding must be considered. Because age is the most common confounding factor, it is important to standardize the rates with respect to age.

Table 5.1 presents a breakdown of outpatient visits according to age categories across sex. Clearly, the utilization of outpatient departments differs between the populations of males and females. First, female visits outnumber male visits by a ratio of 1.52 to 1. Second, females visiting these facilities are slightly older than males, with 16% of females being over 65 years of age, compared with 14% of males. In other age categories, males and females show little variation. In addition, the ratio of crude rates is 1.44 in favor of females. Is this difference sufficient to result in a misleading interpretation of the rates? If the differences in age were accounted for, would this difference in the rates still exist? In other words, what is the true difference between males and females after the potential confounding effect of age is taken into account? Knowing that age is a true risk factor and is unequally distributed across the population suggests that careful study is warranted when making comparisons.

TABLE 5.1. OUTPATIENT DEPARTMENT VISITS, BY AGE AND SEX, 2001.

Age group	Number of visits	U.S. population	Number of visits per 100 persons per year
Males			
Under 15 years	9,613,000	30,854,207	31.1
15–24 years	3,096,000	20,078,818	15.8
25–44 years	6,866,000	42,566,327	16.8
45–64 years	8,561,000	30,144,588	27.6
65–74 years	2,849,000	8,303,274	34.8
75 years and older	3,899,000	6,106,349	36.7
All males	33,183,000	138,053,563	24.3
Females			
Under 15 years	8,706,000	29,399,168	29.5
15–24 years	6,738,000	19,105,073	34.8
25–44 years	13,710,000	42,471,924	32.5
45–64 years	13,029,000	31,810,050	39.5
65–74 years	4,450,000	10,087,712	45.0
75 years and older	70,075,000	10,494,416	40.4
All females	520,110,000	143,368,343	35.2

Source: Centers for Disease Control and Prevention, 2001c; population figures per U.S. Census Bureau, 2000 census.

Stratification

Stratification is a process of dividing data into strata that are defined by the specific confounding factors, resulting in the equalization of the distribution of the potential confounding factors in each stratum. An example of stratification is to divide a population under study for lung cancer risk into two strata: smokers and nonsmokers. The key to minimizing potential confounding is to make certain that the groups being compared are as similar as possible with respect to as many different factors as possible—except, of course, the independent variable being studied.

As an illustrative example, stratification will be used to investigate the association between long-term alcohol use and the incidence of lung cancer. Table 5.2 presents hypothetical data that might result from such an investigation.

The risk of developing lung cancer in this study population relative to exposure to alcohol is determined by calculating the relative risk. The relative risk is 1.5: that is, alcohol drinkers have a 1.5-times greater chance of developing lung cancer when compared to others in the population who do not drink alcohol.

It is known that smoking is also a risk factor for lung cancer. Could smoking be a confounding factor that may be distorting the comparison of individuals who do and do not drink alcohol? Stratification of individuals by smoking status will account for the potential confounding effect of smoking on the risk of lung cancer. Table 5.3 presents the stratification of lung cancer and alcohol use by smoking status.

The risk of lung cancer across categories of alcohol usage can be determined in each stratum. The relative risk of developing lung cancer in the nonsmokers stratum is 1.0. The relative risk of developing lung cancer in the smokers stratum is 1.1.

After controlling for smoking, by stratification, the relative risk for alcohol consumption is very close to 1. The conclusion about the association between alcohol and the risk of lung cancer is that there is no evidence that alcohol use increases the risk of developing lung cancer.

Matching

Matching is a process that accounts for potential confounding factors that can be used in experimental, cohort, and case-control studies. Matching is the application of restraints to a comparison group that make study groups more similar with respect to one or more potential confounding factors. In general, matching consists of selecting controls so that they are similar to cases in characteristics that are potential confounding factors (age, sex, race, socioeconomic status, and so on).

Matching has two major classifications: individual (pair) and group (frequency). Individual matching is characterized by each case being individually matched to a

TABLE 5.2. LUNG CANCER AND ALCOHOL USE.

	Lung cancer	No lung cancer	Totals
Alcohol	60	940	1,000
No alcohol	40	960	1,000
Totals	100	1,900	2,000

TABLE 5.3. STRATIFICATION BY SMOKING STATUS.

	Lung cancer	No lung cancer	Totals
Smokers			
Alcohol	4	396	400
No alcohol	6	594	600
All smokers	10	990	1,000
Nonsmokers			
Alcohol	56	544	600
No alcohol	34	366	400
All nonsmokers	90	910	1,000

subject of similar age, race, sex, and the like. In group matching, there is similar frequency of characteristics among cases and controls. It is important to note that after matching on a potential confounding factor, this factor must be removed from the analysis; it must be controlled for during the analysis. If pair matching is used, a matched-pairs analysis must be conducted on the study.

The purpose of matching is to enhance study efficiency and validity. Study efficiency consists of practical and statistical efficiency. Practical efficiency is governed by practicality. For example, if clinic controls are being used, it is more efficient to select controls who visit the clinic on the same day as cases. Statistical efficiency is governed by sound scientific statistical principles. For example, if you select controls at random for the population in the study of cancer, it will be difficult to stratify by age (or control for age) because cases will be older than controls. In cohort studies, validity is enhanced by matching. In case-control studies, matching enhances efficiency.

Matching is not done without several caveats. First, overmatching is typically done to increase sample size, which will positively affect statistical power. But overmatching may become a problem. Overmatching can make it difficult to identify a sufficient number of controls. In addition, if you match on several factors, the number of variables that can be included in the analysis is reduced. More than two controls per case does not improve the statistical analysis.

Another caveat is that matching may not be efficient. With respect to practical efficiency, matching is expensive and time-intensive. In most situations, matching is not necessary because major potential confounding variables can be adjusted for using other analytic methods. Matching may adversely affect statistical efficiency because matching on a weakly associated potential confounding factor that is strongly correlated with the exposure of interest can reduce efficiency.

Standardization of Information

Because it is known that comparisons using crude rates may lead to incorrect interpretation, a method is needed to ameliorate the confounding of data and overcome the limitations of crude rates. Standardization eliminates the effect of confounding by accounting for differences in populations. Standardization may be defined as the development of a fictitious summary measure of rates of a disease or condition for comparison purposes when evaluating two or more populations. Differences within populations are standardized based on their composition according to age, sex, race, and other characteristics. The most common confounding factor is age. Our discussion will focus on age standardization methods. Later in this chapter, other factors will be discussed and the methods for standardization will be explored.

Two methods of standardization are commonly used. The direct method of standardization develops a summary of rates that can be used to directly compare the populations under study. The indirect method develops a summary of rates that cannot be used to make direct comparisons; indirect inferences can be made to compare populations. Both standardization methods achieve the objective of eliminating the effect of confounding factors.

Direct Method of Standardization

Direct standardization is accomplished by applying crude rates observed in two or more populations to an arbitrarily chosen standard population. The unequal distribution of a potential confounding variable in a study population is *equalized*, or adjusted, by standardization. This equalization is accomplished by applying the distribution of the potential confounding variable in the standard population to each study population. That is, each study population is "forced" to have the same distribution of the potential confounding variable as in the standard population.

The steps of the direct method of standardization are as follows. First, a standard population must be chosen. With respect to age standardization, the most recently estimated U.S. population, obtained from the U.S. Census Bureau, is an example of a standard population. The National Center for Health Statistics used the 1940

U.S. population as its standard for many years (Center for Disease Control and Prevention, 1995). Occasionally, the 1970 U.S. population was used as the standard. Since 2002, the 2000 U.S. population has been used in age adjustment.

Changing the standard population will result in close evaluation of comparisons. This is due to the differences in the 2000 population age distribution. When reviewing long-term trends, it is important to understand the effect of the new standard population. Because the number of people in older age groups is increasing every year, the results of age adjustment will be very different from results in previous years. When one is focusing on cancer, age-adjusted incidence and mortality rates will increase significantly because most cancers occur in older individuals. The risk of cancer has not changed, but because people are living longer, the rate of cancer will increase in the population.

In the event that census data are not available, the aggregate population of the populations under study may be used as the standard population. In this combinational method, each study population is forced to have a distribution of the potential confounding variable similar to that of the aggregate population. In this way, real differences in the distribution of potential confounding variables in each study population will be equalized. If an aggregate standard population is selected, the results cannot be directly compared to other studies using a different standard.

After a reasonable standard population has been chosen and the study population rates are applied to it, the expected number of study events in the standard population is determined. For example, if crude mortality rates are to be standardized, the expected number of deaths in each study population is calculated as if each study population had the same distribution of the potential confounding variable as is found in the standard population. This results in a standardized mortality rate for each study population, which can be defined as follows (where K is the constant used to express the rate):

$$\frac{\text{Expected number of deaths in the study population}}{\text{Total number of individuals in the standard population}} \times K$$

The standardized rates for each study population are then compared to determine if true differences exist between the study populations. Figure 5.1 illustrates the direct method of standardization.

To better understand the direct method of standardization, one of two perspectives can be used. First, the direct method can be thought of as a process of making the study populations exhibit the same distributions of the potential confounding variable. Thus the potential confounding variable is no longer unequally distributed throughout the populations. Second, the direct method can be thought of as a process

FIGURE 5.1. DIRECT METHOD OF STANDARDIZATION.

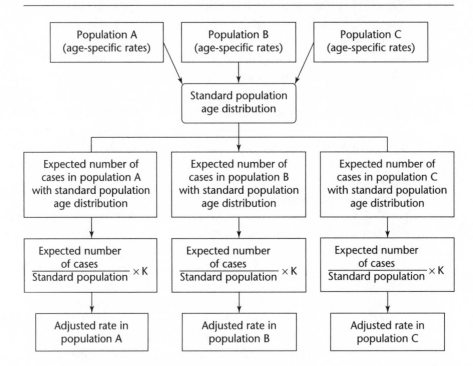

that applies the study population's crude rates to the standard population. Again, each study population will have the same population composition, eliminating the effect of potential confounding variables.

Direct standardization can be used to answer the preceding question concerning the rate of outpatient visits among males and females. Using the 2000 census population as a standard, the rate of outpatient visits among males and females will be adjusted. This standardization process involves applying the standard population numbers in each age category to the crude male and female rates of the study populations. This process will result in standardized rates with respect to the 2000 U.S. population.

Table 5.4 presents the calculation of the standardized rates among males and females. The number of expected visits among males and females in each age category is determined by multiplying the standard population numbers by the study population's rate in each age category. The expected number of visits is 68,808,305 for males and 98,505,906 for females. The standardized, or adjusted, rates are 24.45 per 100 persons per year for males and 35.00 for females. The ratio of adjusted rates, males to females, is 1.43, which is the same as the ratio of crude rates. This indicates that age is not confounding the difference between the rates for males and females.

TABLE 5.4. STANDARDIZATION OF OUTPATIENT DEPARTMENT VISITS, BY SEX, 2001.

Age group	U.S. population	Number of visits per 100 persons per year	Expected number of visits
Males			
Under 15 years	60,253,375	31.1	18,738,800
15–24 years	39,183,891	15.8	6,191,055
25–44 years	85,038,251	16.8	14,286,426
45–64 years	61,954,638	27.6	17,099,480
65–74 years	18,390,986	34.8	6,400,063
75 years and older	16,600,765	36.7	6,092,481
All males	281,421,906		68,808,305
Females			
Under 15 years	60,253,375	29.5	17,774,746
15–24 years	39,183,891	34.8	13,635,994
25–44 years	85,038,251	32.5	27,637,432
45–64 years	61,954,638	39.5	24,472,082
65–74 years	18,390,986	45.0	8,275,944
75 years and older	16,600,765	40.4	6,706,709
All females	281,421,906		98,502,906

Adjusted rate for males = 68,808,305/281,421,906 = 24.45 per 100 persons per year.

Adjusted rate for females = 98,502,906/281,241,906 = 35.00 per 100 persons per year.

Another example of the direct method of standardization focuses on adjusting case-fatality rates among hospitals. The Centers for Medicare and Medicaid Services typically evaluate quality of care by reviewing case-fatality rates within specific diagnosis-related group categories. Table 5.5 presents crude hypothetical case-fatality rates of male patients admitted with myocardial infarction (MI) in two hospitals, East Bank Regional and Westside Memorial. If the crude case-fatality rates are studied, the rate of each hospital is essentially the same. For example, the case-fatality rate for East Bank Regional Hospital is 242.2 deaths per 100,000, compared with a rate of 253.4 deaths per 100,000 for Westside Hospital. Based on these crude rates, the quality of care for inpatient MI patients is identical.

However, if you carefully review the age categories of each hospital's patient population, it becomes clear that there is a significant variation in age distribution. Age is considered a major risk factor for many diseases and conditions, especially heart disease. Given this fact, age is a potentially confounding variable for deaths due to MI, and these crude rates must be standardized before comparisons of the two hospitals can be made. Table 5.6 presents standardized case-fatality rates for each hospital, using the 2000 U.S. population as the standard population. The expected number of deaths due to MI was calculated for each age category using the number of individuals in the

TABLE 5.5. CRUDE CASE-FATALITY RATES, BY AGE.

Age group	East Bank Regional			Westside Memorial		
	Number of cases	Population	Rate	Number of Cases	Population	Rate
19–24 years	12	38,700	0.0003	14	20,900	0.0007
25–44 years	90	32,400	0.003	40	28,900	0.001
45–64 years	68	14,400	0.005	51	20,100	0.003
65 years and older	48	4,500	0.011	119	18,300	0.006
Totals	218	90,000		224	88,200	

Crude case-fatality rate for East Bank Regional Hospital = 242.2 deaths per 100,000 population.
Crude case-fatality rate for Westside Memorial Hospital = 253.9 deaths per 100,000 population.

standard population. The expected number of deaths was then calculated using the death rate for each hospital in each age group. For example, in the 25–44 age group, the expected number of deaths due to MI in East Bank Regional Hospital is calculated by multiplying the age group death rate by the number of individuals in the standard population in this age group (that is, $0.0003 \times 12,500,000 = 150,000$ expected deaths). In essence, the direct method of standardization calculates the number of deaths expected to occur if the age composition of each hospital's cases were the same as the age composition of the standard population.

After the case-fatality rates are standardized for the effect of age, there is a significant difference between the hospitals. The standardized case-fatality rate for East Bank Regional Hospital is almost twice as high as the rate for Westside Memorial Hospital (534.3 deaths per 100,000 versus 284.1 deaths per 100,000). This difference is associated with the age distribution in each hospital's MI cases. Westside Memorial Hospital has a much older group of patients than East Bank Regional Hospital. Thus the effect of age confounds the true difference in case-fatality rates of each hospital, and inferences made from data that are not standardized would very likely result in incorrect managerial action.

There may be times when an appropriate standard population cannot be selected for standardization of rates. In these situations, the combined study populations may be used as a standard population. Table 5.7 presents this aggregate population for the standardization of rates from East Bank Regional and Westside Memorial hospitals. This combined population can be used to standardize the case-fatality rates, following the same calculations used with the 2000 U.S. population.

TABLE 5.6. STANDARDIZED CASE-FATALITY RATES.

Age group	Population (in thousands)	East Bank Regional		Westside Memorial	
		Rate	Expected number of cases	Rate	Expected number of cases
19–24 years	12,500	0.0003	3,750	0.0007	8,750
25–44 years	50,000	0.003	150,000	0.001	50,000
45–64 years	52,000	0.005	260,000	0.003	156,000
65 years and older	35,000	0.011	385,000	0.006	210,000
Totals	149,500		798,750		424,750

Standardized case-fatality rate for East Bank Regional Hospital = 534.4 deaths per 100,000 population.

Standardized case-fatality rate for Westside Memorial Hospital = 284.1 deaths per 100,000 population.

TABLE 5.7. STANDARD (COMBINED) POPULATION.

Age group	Number of cases at East Bank Regional	Number of cases at Westside Memorial	Combined population
19–24 years	38,700	20,900	59,600
25–44 years	32,400	28,900	61,300
45–64 years	14,400	20,100	34,500
65 years and older	4,500	18,300	22,800
Totals	90,000	88,200	178,200

Table 5.8 presents the standardized case-fatality rates using the combined population as a standard. Although a different standard population was used, the trend in differences in the standardized rates is the same. For example, the standardized case-fatality rate for East Bank Regional Hospital is almost twice as high as that for Westside Memorial Hospital, 350.77 deaths per 100,000 versus 192.66 per 100,000. The exact rates using the two different standard populations are not important, but the differences between the rates of each hospital provide a basis for comparison. Either standard population demonstrates the disparity in the clinical outcomes of the two hospitals.

TABLE 5.8. STANDARDIZED CASE-FATALITY RATES USING COMBINED STANDARD POPULATION.

Age group	Combined population	East Bank Regional		Westside Memorial	
		Rate	Expected deaths	Rate	Expected deaths
19–24 years	59,600	0.0003	17.88	0.0007	41.72
25–44 years	61,300	0.003	183.90	0.001	61.30
45–64 years	34,500	0.005	172.50	0.003	103.50
65 and older	22,800	0.011	250.80	0.006	136.80
Totals	178,200		625.08		343.32

Indirect Method of Standardization

The indirect method of standardization can be used for indirect comparisons of crude rates of two or more study populations. The indirect method is indicated when the relative sizes of the study populations are significantly different or when characteristic-specific rates are unknown or are compromised because of the variability of small population numbers.

The steps in the indirect method of standardization are as follows. As in the direct method, the first step is to select a standard population. The standard population is typically the most recently estimated U.S. population. Instead of using the composition of the standard population (the distribution of the potential confounding variable, expressed as the number of individuals in each factor category), the standard population's crude characteristic-specific rates are used to accomplish the standardization (see Figure 5.2). Next, the expected number of study events is calculated for each study population, using the crude characteristic-specific rate of the standard population. The effect of confounding is eliminated indirectly by equalizing the distribution of potential confounding variables by using the same crude characteristic-specific rate for each study population. The distribution of potential confounding variables in the standard population is applied, by way of the standard population's crude rates, to each study population.

Because the study populations' crude rates are not used in the process to determine expected study events, adjustments of the study populations' crude rates are not a product of indirect standardization. Instead, a standardized ratio is calculated. The ratio is called the standardized morbidity or mortality ratio (SMR). If morbidity is the event of interest, then the ratio is called the standardized morbidity ratio and is defined as follows:

$$\frac{\text{Number of observed}}{\text{cases in the study population}}$$

$$\frac{}{\begin{array}{c}\text{Number of expected cases}\\\text{in the study population using crude}\\\text{rates of the standard population}\end{array}}$$

If mortality is the study event, the standardized mortality ratio is the appropriate measure and is defined as follows:

$$\frac{\begin{array}{c}\text{Number of observed}\\\text{deaths in the study population}\end{array}}{\begin{array}{c}\text{Number of expected deaths}\\\text{in the study population using crude}\\\text{rates of the standard population}\end{array}}$$

FIGURE 5.2. INDIRECT METHOD OF STANDARDIZATION.

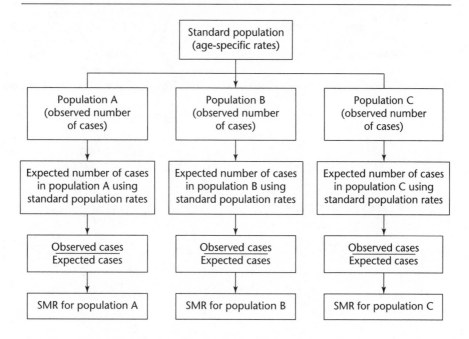

The SMR is calculated for each study population for comparison of the relationship between expected and observed study events.

The following example of the use of the indirect method of standardization concerns outpatient visits among white and black Americans. The NHAMCS Outpatient Department Summary indicates that the rate of outpatient department visits is 48.8 per 100 persons per year among blacks and 27.9 per 100 persons per year among whites (Centers for Disease Control and Prevention, 2001d). This represents an approximate twofold greater rate among blacks when compared with whites. Is this comparison correct? Do African Americans use outpatient departments in U.S. hospitals twice as often as whites?

To determine if this apparent difference is true, confounding must be considered. Age is the most common confounding factor, and these data must be adjusted before making comparisons. Table 5.9 presents data according to age and race. According to the 2000 census, there are 232,529,920 whites and 37,197,000 African Americans in the United States. These populations differ with respect to age. Blacks are younger, with 75% of the population under age 45 and 45% under age 25. In older age categories, whites outnumber blacks, with 14% compared to 8% over age 65. This difference in the number of individuals in each race and in age distribution indicates that the indirect method of standardization should be used to account for potential confounding effects associated with age.

TABLE 5.9. OUTPATIENT VISITS, BY AGE AND RACE, 2001.

Age group	Number of visits	Study population	Number of visits per 100 persons per year
Whites			
Under 15 years	13,163,000	47,047,000	28.5
15–24 years	7,288,000	31,473,000	23.9
25–44 years	15,463,000	68,374,000	23.2
45–64 years	16,421,000	54,392,000	30.5
65–74 years	5,878,000	15,970,000	37.4
75 years and older	5,013,000	15,273,000	35.8
All whites	63,226,000	232,529,000	27.9
Blacks			
Under 15 years	4,328,000	9,953,000	45.7
15–24 years	2,212,000	6,073,000	39.8
25–44 years	4,236,000	11,223,000	41.0
45–64 years	4,351,000	7,007,000	64.3
65–74 years	1,131,000	1,670,000	70.1
75 years and older	774,000	1,271,000	67.3
All blacks	17,032,000	37,197,000	48.8

Source: Centers for Disease Control and Prevention, 2001c.

Table 5.10 presents the calculation of the SMR for whites and blacks. The standard population is the 2000 U.S. population. The U.S. population's rate of outpatient visits in each age category is multiplied by the number of individuals in each age category in the study populations to determine the expected number of outpatient visits if the study populations exhibited the same rates as the standard population. The SMR is calculated by dividing the observed number of outpatient visits by the expected number of visits determined during the standardization of the study populations' rates. For African Americans, the SMR is equal to 17,032,000/10,867,261, or 1.57, whereas for whites it is 63,226,000/69.921,297, or 0.90. This relationship indicates that, using the 2000 U.S. population as a reference population, African Americans make almost

TABLE 5.10. INDIRECT STANDARDIZATION OF OUTPATIENT VISIT RATES.

Age group	Study population	U.S. rate (per 100 persons per year)	Expected number of visits
Whites			
Under 15 years	47,074,000	30.3	14,263,422
15–24 years	31,473,000	25.3	7,962,669
25–44 years	68,374,000	24.8	16,956,752
45–64 years	54,392,000	33.7	18,330,104
65–74 years	15,970,000	40.4	6,451,880
75 years and older	15,273,000	39.0	5,956,470
All whites	232,529,000		69,921,297

$$\text{SMR} = \frac{\text{observed cases}}{\text{expected cases}}$$

$$= \frac{63,226,000}{69,921,297} = 0.90$$

Age group	Study population	U.S. rate (per 100 persons per year)	Expected number of visits
Blacks			
Under 15 years	9,953,000	30.3	
15–24 years	6,073,000	25.3	
25–44 years	11,223,000	24.8	
45–64 years	7,007,000	33.7	
65–74 years	1,670,000	40.4	
75 years and older	1,271,000	39.0	
All blacks	37,197,000		

$$\text{SMR} = \frac{\text{observed cases}}{\text{expected cases}}$$

$$= \frac{17,032,000}{10,867,261} = 1.57$$

Source: Centers for Disease Control and Prevention, 2001c.

twice as many hospital outpatient visits as the U.S. population as a whole. Whites exhibit approximately 10% fewer visits to outpatient departments than the population as a whole. The inference can be indirectly made that African Americans have a rate of outpatient department visits nearly twice that of whites.

Another example of the indirect method of standardization focuses on the incidence rate of invasive carcinoma of the cervix among African American women in the state of New Jersey. The crude incidence rate was determined to be 40.9 per 100,000 in black women in the state, while the rate for African American women nationwide was 34.4 per 100,000 (Holland, Foster, and Louira, 1993). Health officials were concerned by this marked difference. One possible explanation was that black women in New Jersey were at greater risk due to external influences (specifically, chemical plants).

The state health department decided to compare the risk of carcinoma of the cervix among black women in the United States and in New Jersey. A statewide screening program was conducted, and data were collected on the number of cases of this carcinoma. As is seen in all chronic diseases, such as cancers, age is a significant risk factor. Typically, as an individual gets older, the risk for cancer increases. Age is a potential confounding factor, and incidence data must be adjusted with respect to it. Table 5.11 presents the collected screening data, in age categories.

When stratifying the distribution of African American females by age, it is apparent that there were small numbers of females in several age groups, resulting in unstable rates. A change in a few cases of carcinoma could change the rates substantially because of this instability. Given this fact, direct standardization would not be an appropriate method. The instability of rates can be compensated for by indirect standardization. To accomplish this, the standardized morbidity ratio for carcinoma of the cervix for African American women in New Jersey was determined.

To indirectly standardize carcinoma incidence rates, age-specific rates of the U.S. population were used as the standard. These standard age-specific rates were used to calculate the expected number of cases of carcinoma of the cervix if the black women in New Jersey had the same age-specific rates as black women throughout the United States.

Table 5.12 presents the process of indirect standardization. The expected number of cases is determined by multiplying the standard rate by the number of women in each age group. For example, in the 10–19 age group, the expected number of cases equals 0.36 (279×0.0013). The total number of expected cases of carcinoma is 648.4.

After the incidence of carcinoma is standardized for the effect of age, there is a significant difference between the actual observed number of cases (459) and the expected number of cases (648.4). The SMR can be calculated as follows:

TABLE 5.11. SCREENING PROGRAM DATA.

Age group	Number of cases	Number of persons screened
10–19 years	2	279
20–29 years	8	2,792
30–39 years	35	3,017
40–49 years	186	3,350
50–69 years	39	3,071
70 years and older	39	1,396
Totals	459	13,905

Source: Holland, Foster, and Louira, 1993.

TABLE 5.12. INDIRECT STANDARDIZATION.

Age group	Cases	Study subjects	U.S. population rate	Expected cases
10–19 years	2	279	0.0013	0.36
20–29 years	8	2,792	0.0070	19.54
30–39 years	35	3,017	0.0720	217.22
40–49 years	186	3,350	0.1061	355.44
50–69 years	39	3,071	0.0125	38.39
70 years and older	39	1,396	0.0125	17.45
Totals	459	13,905		648.40

SMR = total number of observed cases/total number of expected cases = 459/648.4 = 0.71.

Source: Holland, Foster, and Louira, 1993.

$$\frac{\text{Total number of observed cases of carcinoma of the cervix in the screening population}}{\text{Total number of expected cases of carcinoma of the cervix in the screening population using standard age-specific incidence rates}}$$

The SMR of 0.71, which can be interpreted as the observed number of cases, is much less than should be expected, after standardizing for the effect of age. Based on the results of the statewide screening program, this finding indicates that black women in New Jersey are not exposed to an excess risk of carcinoma of the cervix. Instead, the age distribution of the black women in New Jersey is such that crude incidence rates are higher than the incidence rate among black females in the United States as a whole.

Risk Adjustment

Risk adjustment attempts to account for individual factors that could affect the outcomes of medical interventions. Risk adjustment is intended to account for all factors, excluding the process of delivery of health care services that may be helpful in understanding differences in health outcomes in a population. Risk-adjusted rates are essential when making comparisons of health outcomes across and among hospitals and other health care providers. Risk adjustment is important for studying clinical effectiveness and is used to identify the "algebra of effectiveness," which is based on the notion of health outcomes represented as a function of population demographic characteristics, clinical factors, clinical effectiveness, and quality of care (Iezzoni, 1997).

In practice, risk adjustment is associated with quantifying the risk of short-term outcomes for hospitalized patients and then adjusting rates based on these risks. Severity-of-illness measures are methods that quantify the risks. (More than twelve different methods have been developed to measure severity of illness, all based on unique assumptions and weighting methods. The comparison of these severity-of-illness measurement methods is beyond the scope of this book.)

Risk-adjusted rates can be thought of as clinical outcomes in a population that have been adjusted for demographic and clinical factors. The process of risk adjustment involves several steps. First, the outcomes to be studied and associated risk factors must be identified. The identification of risk factors may include the use of statistical techniques to determine factors that significantly affect the outcomes.

Second, statistical models are developed that control the effect of the risk factors. These models determine the expected outcome, relative to some standard population, for individuals given their specific demographic and clinical characteristics. Finally, the results of individuals are aggregated to represent hospital-specific or health care provider–specific risk-adjusted rates.

The concern for risk adjustment has important implications for Medicare providers since severity of illness has a profound effect on length of stay. Length of stay has served as a basic outcome measurement of resource utilization. But as we mentioned earlier, the impact of severity of illness has been evaluated as a risk factor for unexpected or adverse health outcomes. Case-mix index has been used as a measure of severity.

The rationale for risk adjustment has two foci: clinical and managerial. The clinical focus is on eliminating the confounding effect of severity on health outcomes. This confounding effect is seen in clinical and utilization data. An objective of this adjustment is to understand the impact of the case mix so as to make accurate comparisons across and among providers.

Risk adjustment models can be developed using standardization, stratification, and multivariate statistical techniques. These statistical techniques include multiple linear regression, logistic regression, Markov models, proportional hazards models, cluster analysis, Bayesian models, and artificial neural network models. Stepwise logistic regression modeling is most popular when the relationship of risk factors and the dichotomous outcome of death or not is under study.

An illustration of risk adjustment as provided by the comparison of two hospitals, East Bank Regional Hospital and Riverview Medical Center Hospital, is presented in Tables 5.13, 5.14, and 5.15. Patients are classified in three severity level categories (from best to worst) I, II, and III.

There has been a great deal of discussion in the community that the inpatient care provided at East Bank is of lesser quality than that provided at Riverview. During 2003, some 198 patients were treated for a particular disease at East Bank. Of these, 124 completely recovered (defined as returning to normal activities). The same year, of 502 patients with the same disease treated at Riverview, 222 completely recovered. This information has been used as an indication that Riverview is a superior hospital because 222 patients recovered, whereas only 124 recovered at East Bank.

The administration at East Bank decides to study these differences between the two hospitals. The first thing that is done is the calculation of crude recovery rates. East Bank had a crude recovery rate of 62.8 percent (124/198), and Riverview had a crude rate of 44.2 percent (222/502). Evaluating these crude rates, it appears that East Bank seems to provide better-quality care, which contradicts popular belief.

Risk and severity of illness are directly related. As the severity of illness increases, the risk (or chance) of poor health outcomes

TABLE 5.13. SEVERITY OF ILLNESS DISTRIBUTION.

Severity category	Number	Percentage of patients
East Bank Regional		
I	98	49.5
II	44	22.2
III	56	28.3
Totals	198	100.0
Riverview Medical Center		
I	49	9.8
II	155	30.9
III	298	59.4
Totals	502	100.0

TABLE 5.14. RECOVERY DISTRIBUTION.

Severity category	East Bank Regional	Riverview Medical Center	Totals
I	80	40	120
II	28	88	116
III	18	94	110
Totals	124	222	346

TABLE 5.15. STRATUM-SPECIFIC RATES.

Severity category	Number of patients	Number of recoveries	Recovery rate (percentage per year)
East Bank Regional			
I	98	80	81.6
II	44	28	63.6
III	56	16	28.6
Riverview Medical Center			
I	49	40	81.6
II	155	88	56.8
III	298	94	31.5

also increases. Before comparing the two hospitals, the rates of recovery must be standardized according to severity of illness. It must be determined whether severity of illness is a risk factor for successful recovery, independent of the hospital to which the patient was admitted. If severity of patient illness is shown to be related to recovery rates and at the same time is associated with the type of hospital to which the patient is admitted, then confounding bias is most likely occurring.

Stratum-specific recovery rates can be calculated using severity categories as the stratification criterion. Table 5.15 presents the stratum-specific rates. When stratum-specific recovery rates are reviewed, the hospitals are very comparable. The recovery rates in each severity stratum are the same (that is, there is no statistically significant difference).

Summary

Epidemiologic data are used to compare two or more populations with respect to the occurrence of disease. Mortality and morbidity rates are the quantitative measures used for these comparisons. A concern is whether the comparisons show true differences, because the effect of confounding can cause misleading results. To eliminate this effect, rates must be standardized.

Direct standardization is used to compare rates in populations or subgroups of populations. Crude rates in the study populations are applied to a standard population to obtain expected results in the standard population. Keeping the crude rates in the study populations constant, standard population numbers of individuals are used to determine standardized rates. These rates are calculated based on the distribution of the potential confounding factor in the standard population. The direct standardized rates are compared to determine any differences across the populations.

Indirect standardization calculates a standardized mortality or morbidity ratio (SMR) comparing the standard population to the study populations. To determine the SMR, the rates of the potential confounding factor in the standard population are applied to the number of individuals in the study populations. The SMR measures the excess of the expected cases in the study populations, and indirect inferences are made to determine any differences across the populations.

In other words, in direct standardization, the study population is forced to have the same population distributions as the standard population. In indirect standardization, the study population is forced to have the same age-specific rates as the standard population.

Stratification and statistical techniques are other methods that may be used to account for the effect of confounding. As seen in standardization, these other approaches attempt to account for the effect of different characteristics of individuals in the population. Risk adjustment is a specialization of standardization methods that addresses the effect of the differential distribution of risk and severity of illness across and within populations.

Crude rates should not be used for comparison purposes. Adjusted rates should always be used for the comparison of disease in subpopulations.

Study Questions

1. Tables 5.16 and 5.17 contain information on outpatient department visits in the populations served by two large regional hospital networks, Hancock Regional Hospital Network and Harrison Hospital System.
   a. Compare the crude and age-adjusted rates of visits to the outpatient department in the populations served by Hancock Regional Hospital Network and Harrison Hospital System by completing the tables.
   b. Compare the age-specific rates of visits to the outpatient department in the populations served by Hancock Regional Hospital Network and Harrison Hospital System.
   c. Determine the ratio of the crude rates of the populations served by Hancock Regional Hospital Network and Harrison Hospital System.
   d. The data presented in Tables 5.18 and 5.19 indicate that the population distributions among the populations served by Hancock Regional Hospital Network and Harrison Hospital System are different. Calculate the percentage of the population in each age group in both populations.
   e. Before single summary rates between the populations served by Hancock Regional Hospital Network and Harrison Hospital System can be compared, outpatient department visit rates must be adjusted to account for differences in age distribution. Using the data in Table 5.20, perform a direct adjustment of crude outpatient department visit rates.

TABLE 5.16. CRUDE RATES FOR OUTPATIENT VISITS IN THE HANCOCK REGIONAL HOSPITAL NETWORK

Age group	Population	Number of visits	Crude rates (per 1,000 population)
Under 15 years	44,995	9,224	
15–24 years	27,469	5,329	
25–44 years	67,845	12,280	
45–64 years	41,650	8,330	
65–74 years	16,400	3,772	
75 years and older	11,147	3,099	
Totals	209,506	42,034	

TABLE 5.17. CRUDE RATES FOR OUTPATIENT VISITS IN THE HARRISON HOSPITAL SYSTEM.

Age group	Population	Number of visits	Crude rates (per 1,000 population)
Under 15 years	27,569	6,148	
15–24 years	17,291	5,222	
25–44 years	41,403	10,682	
45–64 years	25,194	7,130	
65–74 years	10,185	3,137	
75 years and older	77,165	2,423	
Totals	198,807	34,742	

TABLE 5.18. POPULATION DISTRIBUTION, HANCOCK REGIONAL HOSPITAL NETWORK.

Age group	Population	Percentage of total population
Under 15 years	44,995	
15–24 years	27,469	
25–44 years	67,845	
45–64 years	41,650	
65–74 years	16,400	
75 years and older	11,147	
Totals	209,506	100.0

TABLE 5.19. POPULATION DISTRIBUTION, HARRISON HOSPITAL SYSTEM.

Age group	Population	Percentage of total population
Under 15 years	27,569	
15–24 years	17,291	
25–44 years	41,403	
45–64 years	25,194	
65–74 years	10,185	
75 years and older	77,165	
Totals	198,807	100.0

TABLE 5.20. STANDARD POPULATION CRUDE OUTPATIENT DEPARTMENT VISIT RATES.

Age group	U.S. population, 2000	Crude outpatient department visit rates
Under 15 years	60,253,375	
15–24 years	39,183,891	
25–44 years	85,038,251	
45–64 years	61,954,638	
65–74 years	18,390,986	
75 years and older	16,600,765	

Source: U.S. Census Bureau, 2000.

The first step is to select a standard population and its outpatient department visit rates. The standard population selected is the 2000 U.S. population (see Table 5.20). The next step is to calculate the expected number of outpatient department visits in each age group. This is accomplished by multiplying the number of persons in each age category in the standard population by the rates of outpatient department visits in each age group in the study populations (the populations served by Hancock Regional Hospital Network and Harrison Hospital System). Using Tables 5.21 and 5.22, calculate the age-adjusted outpatient department visit rates for the populations served by Hancock Regional Hospital Network and Harrison Hospital System by dividing the sum of the expected outpatient department visits by the total standard population.

TABLE 5.21. AGE-SPECIFIC RATE AND EXPECTED CASES FOR HANCOCK REGIONAL HOSPITAL NETWORK.

Age group	U.S. population, 2000	Age-specific rate	Number of expected cases
Under 15 years	60,253,375		
15–24 years	39,183,891		
25–44 years	85,038,251		
45–64 years	61,954,638		
65–74 years	18,390,986		
75 years and older	16,600,765		
Totals	281,421,906		

TABLE 5.22. AGE-SPECIFIC RATE AND EXPECTED CASES FOR HARRISON HOSPITAL SYSTEM

Age group	U.S. population, 2000	Age-specific rate	Number of expected cases
Under 15 years	60,253,375		
15–24 years	39,183,891		
25–44 years	85,038,251		
45–64 years	61,954,638		
65–74 years	18,390,986		
75 years and older	16,600,765		
Totals	281,421,906		

f. What is the ratio of the age-adjusted outpatient department visit rate in the population served by Hancock Regional Hospital Network to the age-adjusted outpatient department visit rate in the population served by Harrison Hospital System?

g. Describe the difference between the ratios of crude and age-adjusted outpatient department visit rates.

2. An alternative method for selecting a standard population for direct adjustment is to use a "combined" population.

a. Complete Tables 5.23 and 5.24 using the population distributions from Study Question 1.

b. What is the ratio of the age-adjusted outpatient department visit rate in the population served by Hancock Regional Hospital Network to the age-adjusted outpatient department visit rate in the population served by Harrison Hospital System?

c. Describe the difference between the ratios of crude and age-adjusted outpatient department visit rates.

d. Do the ratios in part (c) differ from the adjusted rates calculated using the 2000 U.S. population as the standard? What is the significance of any differences?

TABLE 5.23. AGE-SPECIFIC RATE AND EXPECTED CASES FOR HANCOCK REGIONAL HOSPITAL NETWORK USING COMBINED POPULATION.

Age group	Combined population	Age-specific rate	Number of expected cases
Under 15 years			
15–24 years			
25–44 years			
45–64 years			
65–74 years			
75 years and older			
Totals			

TABLE 5.24. AGE-SPECIFIC RATE AND EXPECTED CASES FOR HARRISON HOSPITAL SYSTEM USING COMBINED POPULATION.

Age group	Combined population	Age-specific rate	Number of expected cases
Under 15 years			
15–24 years			
25–44 years			
45–64 years			
65–74 years			
75 years and older			
Totals			

3. Tables 5.25 and 5.26 present data for the number of inpatient complications due to myocardial infarction during 2003 in Jefferson County, the service area for East Bank Regional Hospital, and Washington County, the service area for Westside Memorial Hospital.
   a. Using these data, calculate age-specific inpatient MI complication rates for the two counties per 1,000 population.
   b. Compare age-specific complication rates between Jefferson and Washington Counties. Which county has the higher age-specific complication rates?
   c. Describe the general pattern of the change in complication rate with age.
   d. Calculate the crude complication rate for Jefferson and Washington Counties for 2003.
   e. What is the ratio of the crude complication rate in Jefferson County to that in Washington County?

TABLE 5.25. CRUDE RATE FOR MI COMPLICATIONS IN JEFFERSON COUNTY.

Age group	Number of MI complications	Population	Crude rate (per 1,000 population)
40–49 years	196	80,300	
50–59 years	169	97,400	
60–69 years	623	52,500	
70 years and older	1,920	37,250	
Totals	2,908	267,450	

TABLE 5.26. CRUDE RATE FOR MI COMPLICATIONS IN WASHINGTON COUNTY.

Age group	Number of MI complications	Population	Crude rate (per 1,000 population)
40–49 years	82	34,500	
50–59 years	53	27,600	
60–69 years	436	7,600	
70 years and older	125	5,715	
Totals	696	75,415	

f. Do you draw the same conclusion about the complication rates in Jefferson County versus Washington County when you compare age-specific rates as you do when you compare crude complication rates?

g. What do these age-specific rates indicate with respect to policy and planning for hospital services?

h. The data presented in Tables 5.27 and 5.28 indicate that the population distributions of Jefferson and Washington Counties are quite different. Calculate the percentage of the population in each age group in both populations, and fill in the tables.

i. Based on the preceding calculations, what is the difference between the two counties with respect to their age distributions?

j. Before single summary rates between the two counties can be compared, complication rates must be adjusted for differences in age distribution. Using the data in Table 5.29, perform indirect adjustment of crude complication rates.

The first step is to select a standard population and its MI rates. The standard population selected is the 2000 U.S. population. The second step is to calculate the expected number of complications in each age group. This is accomplished by

TABLE 5.27. POPULATION DISTRIBUTION, JEFFERSON COUNTY.

Age group	Population	Percentage
40–49 years	80,300	
50–59 years	97,400	
60–69 years	52,500	
70 years and older	37,250	
Totals	267,450	

TABLE 5.28. POPULATION DISTRIBUTION, WASHINGTON COUNTY.

Age group	Population	Percentage
40–49 years	34,500	
50–59 years	27,600	
60–69 years	7,600	
70 years and older	5,715	
Totals	75,415	

TABLE 5.29. STANDARD POPULATION CRUDE MI COMPLICATION RATES.

Age group	Standard population rates	Crude MI Complication Rates
40–49 years	0.0035	
50–59 years	0.0025	
60–69 years	0.0075	
70 years and older	0.0095	

multiplying the number of persons in each age category in the study populations (Jefferson and Washington Counties) by the rates of MI in each age category in the standard population. Complete Tables 5.30 and 5.31.

Finally, calculate the standardized morbidity ratio for Jefferson and Washington Counties by dividing the observed cases by the number of expected cases:

$$SMR = \frac{Observed\ cases}{Expected\ cases}$$

k. Discuss the difference in SMR for Jefferson and Washington Counties. What does this difference indicate to you?

TABLE 5.30 EXPECTED MI COMPLICATIONS, JEFFERSON COUNTY.

Age group	Standard population rates	Jefferson County population	Number of expected complications
40–49 years	0.0035	80,300	
50–59 years	0.0025	97,400	
60–69 years	0.0075	52,500	
70 years and older	0.0095	37,250	
Totals		267,450	

TABLE 5.31. EXPECTED MI COMPLICATIONS, WASHINGTON COUNTY.

Age group	Standard population rates	Washington County population	Number of expected complications
40–49 years	0.0035	34,500	
50–59 years	0.0025	27,600	
60–69 years	0.0075	7,600	
70 years and older	0.0095	5,715	
Totals		75,415	

CHAPTER SIX

MEDICAL MANAGEMENT IN POPULATION HEALTH CARE

Chapter Outline

Introduction
Medical Management
Managing Chronic Diseases
Managing Infectious Epidemics
Bioterrorism
Summary
Study Questions

Learning Objectives

Upon completing this chapter, the reader will be able to do all of the following:

- Explain the concept of error in measurement
- Discuss the concepts of validity and reliability
- Make the distinction between validity and reliability
- Define sensitivity, specificity, and predictive values of test results
- Explain the construct of likelihood ratios
- Describe the ROC curve and the area under the curve
- Explain the impact of infectious epidemics
- Discuss the types of epidemics
- Discuss the concept of surveillance

Introduction

The manager's role in today's health care industry consists primarily of planning, organizing, directing, and evaluating clinically related activities. Whether preventive or therapeutic, clinical services must inevitably be allocated and used. Successful managers must therefore understand the importance of clinical aspects of epidemiology and its application to health care for populations. This chapter will discuss clinical epidemiology, clinical effectiveness, and infectious disease epidemiology.

Prevention of disease is an essential component of designing health care for populations. Prevention activities can be categorized as primary, secondary, or tertiary, based on the progression of the disease process from no disease to clinical disease, with its associated disability and possibility of death. Primary prevention is concerned with eliminating risk factors for a disease. Secondary prevention focuses on early detection and treatment of disease (subclinical and clinical). Tertiary prevention attempts to eliminate or moderate disability associated with advanced disease.

Primary prevention intends to prevent the development of disease before it occurs and to reduce the incidence of disease in the population. Primary prevention activities may be considered useful marketing strategies as well as methods to reduce exposure to risk factors. Health promotion is an example of primary prevention. A health care organization may choose to conduct a marketing campaign through the use of media advertising to increase community involvement. For example, hospital-sponsored wellness fairs are commonly undertaken to educate communities about potential risk factors as well as to increase community awareness of available hospital services. Another example of primary prevention is nutrition counseling for children. Because early onset of coronary heart disease has been related to elevated cholesterol levels in children, design and implementation of lower-fat pediatric diets may result in the elimination of a major risk factor for coronary heart disease. Other examples of primary prevention include use of automobile seat belts, condom use, protecting the skin from ultraviolet light, and tobacco use cessation programs.

Secondary prevention is concerned with reducing the burden of existing disease after it has developed, with emphasis on preventing disease complications. Secondary prevention activities are intended to slow progression of disease, eliminate disease, and limit adverse effects of disease, such as disability. An example of secondary prevention is periodic cholesterol testing in children with a familial history of coronary heart disease. The familial history is a nonmodifiable risk factor, so early detection can be accomplished through periodic testing. Other examples of secondary prevention include periodic testing of cholesterol levels in adults, periodic breast and prostate examinations, and Pap smears, because their objectives are early detection of disease.

Tertiary prevention focuses on helping individuals who have suffered irreversible effects of a disease to reach optimal health status. In cases where disease has been associated with adverse effects, tertiary prevention involves rehabilitation and limitation of disability. Physical activity for heart attack patients is an example of tertiary prevention. Physical therapy programs for stroke patients and individuals who have experienced traumatic injuries are another example, as is inpatient respiratory therapy.

Medical Management

Most individuals seek out clinical services after they have begun to experience signs and symptoms. By that time, subclinical disease has been present for a period of time. This self-referral method can result in individuals seeking clinical services late in the progression of a disease. Self-referral also has an effect on cure rates of diseases, especially those that have a proven treatment. The later an individual seeks treatment, the lower the chance for curing the disease. Conversely, the earlier an individual seeks treatment, through early detection, the better the chance for cure.

Clinical Effectiveness

Clinical effectiveness is a concept that investigates the appropriate use of clinical resources: whether tests and treatment are selected appropriately, based on diagnoses. To determine clinical effectiveness, the following questions must be answered: Are the tests accurate? Are the resources used appropriately? What is the impact of testing information? What is the diagnostic ability of the tests?

Accuracy, efficacy, and efficiency are indicators of test performance. Accuracy is defined as the condition of being true, correct, or exact; efficacy is the capacity of producing a desired result or effect (or effectiveness); and efficiency is the ability to accomplish a job with a minimum expenditure of time and effort. Error, which is deviation from the true value, and bias are also important concerns of screening tests. Specifically, evaluation indicators include the constructs of validity, which measures accuracy, and reliability, which measures precision (Mausner and Kramer, 1985).

Diseases or conditions are selected for screening on the basis of several criteria. A disease must have a presymptomatic phase of long duration to be a candidate for screening. Its natural history must be known, and its progression and reversibility must be understood. If a disease is irreversible, screening will not have any beneficial effect on the health status of the individual, although if the disease is communicable, the screened population can still benefit. The disease must cause recognizable changes that can be detected easily. Diseases frequently found in the population and those with an associated severity are typically chosen for screening.

Error, in the context of testing, can be defined as the difference between an observed value and an actual or true value. It can be classified into two categories: random and systematic. Random error, also known as chance error or sampling error, occurs because of variability in the sampling of screening subjects. Systematic error, known as bias, is error caused by anything other than sampling variability and is not random.

Validity

Validity is the construct that measures the accuracy of a test. By accuracy, we mean how often a test correctly identifies individuals with and without a disease. Validity is also thought of as the ability of a test to produce a true measure. Validity is quantified by the parameters known as sensitivity, specificity, and predictive values (of positive and negative test results). Central to the construct of validity is the existence of a well-accepted confirmatory test (to identify the true measure).

Validity parameters are determined by using a 2-by-2 contingency table (see Figure 6.1). The actual disease status is a function of the columns of the table; the test results are represented by the rows. The upper left cell, designated a, represents the number of individuals with the disease who are detected by the screening test; these individuals are called true positives (TP). The number of individuals in the lower right cell, designated d, represents those who do not have the disease for whom the screening test does not detect disease; these individuals are called true negatives (TN). The upper right cell, designated b, represents individuals who do not have the disease but who are incorrectly identified as having the disease by the screening test; these individuals are called false positives (FP). The lower left cell, designated c, represents individuals who have the disease but whom the screening test fails to detect; these individuals are called false negatives (FN). The underlying goal in testing is to minimize the probability of false positive and false negative test results and to maximize the probability of accurate results.

Probabilistic inference is useful in understanding the method of calculating the validity parameters. Each parameter can be thought of as a conditional probability. Sensitivity is defined as the probability of a positive test result (T+) given the presence of disease (D), or p(T+|D). Specificity is defined as probability of a negative test result (T−) if the individual tested does not have the disease (noD), or p(T−|noD). The predictive value of a positive test result is defined as the probability of disease (D) if the test result is positive for the disease (T+), or (D|T+). The predictive value of a negative test result is the probability of no disease (noD) if the test result is negative for the disease (T−), or p(noD|T−). The conditioning event in each conditional probability guides the calculation of each parameter. For example, the source of information from the 2-by-2 table, presented in the margin totals, is dictated for sensitivity and specificity by the disease status (disease or no disease) and for predictive values by the test result (positive or negative). The margin total of the left column, designated $a + c$, represents the total individuals in the study population with the disease (that is, prevalence);

FIGURE 6.1. VALIDITY 2-BY-2 CONTINGENCY TABLE.

	Actual Disease Status		
Test result	**Disease (D)**	**No disease (NoD)**	**Totals**
T+	a TP	b FP	$a + b$
T–	c FN	d TN	$c + d$
Totals	$a + c$	$b + d$	$a + b + c + d$

Sensitivity = $a/(a + c)$.
Specificity = $d/(b + d)$.
PV+ = $a/(a + b)$.
PV– = $d/(c + d)$.

the right column total, designated $b + d$, represents the total individuals in the study population without the disease (that is, $1 -$ prevalence); the top row total, designated $a + b$, represents the total number of test positives; and the bottom row total, designated $c + d$, represents the total number of test negatives.

Sensitivity can be defined as the ability of a test to correctly identify individuals who have a disease. Sensitivity, the true positive ratio (TP ratio), is equal to the ratio of the true positives to the total individuals with the disease. This measures the number of individuals with the disease that the test correctly identifies as positive for the disease and is calculated as $a/(a + c)$. Specificity can be defined as the ability of a test to correctly identify individuals who do not have a disease. Specificity, the true negative ratio (TN ratio), is equal to the ratio of the true negatives to the total individuals without the disease. This measures the number of individuals without the disease that the test correctly identifies as negative for the disease and is calculated as $d/(b + d)$. In probabilistic terms, this is the chance of a negative test result in an individual without the disease, or $p(T-|noD)$. Measures of sensitivity and specificity are functions of the columns of the 2-by-2 table. Given that the sensitivity and specificity are conditional probabilities, their values will be between 0 and 1. The closer the sensitivity is to the value of 1, the more accurate the test is in identifying individuals with a disease. The closer the specificity is to the value of 1, the more accurate the test is in identifying individuals without the disease.

The complements of sensitivity and specificity are the false negative ratio (FN ratio) and the false positive ratio (FP ratio). The FN ratio is equal to the probability of a negative test result (T–) given the presence of disease (D), or p(T–|D). The FN ratio is also equal to 1 – sensitivity. In the 2-by-2 contingency table, the FN ratio is equal to $c/(a + c)$. The FP ratio is equal to the probability of a positive test result (T+) given the absence of disease (noD) or p(T+|noD) and is equal to 1 – specificity. In the 2-by-2 contingency table, the FP ratio is equal to $b/(b + d)$.

The predictive values of test results are functions of the rows of the 2-by-2 table and reflect the predictive ability of a screening test. The predictive value of a positive test result (PV+) is equal to the ratio of the number of true positives to the total number of test positives: $a/(a + b)$. This measures the number of individuals with a positive test result who actually have the disease. The predictive value of a negative test result (PV–) is equal to the ratio of the number of true negatives to the total number of test negatives: $d/(c + d)$. This measures the proportion of test negatives that were correctly identified by the test as not having the disease.

Sensitivity and specificity are unaffected by variations in the prevalence of a disease in the population and remain constant as prevalence increases or decreases. This is not the case with the predictive values of test results. Predictive values of test results are accurate only if the proportion of diseased individuals in the sample used to determine their values is representative of the true proportion of diseased individuals in the population. In fact, as the prevalence of a disease increases, the predictive value of a positive test result increases and the predictive value of a negative test result decreases. When the prevalence of a disease decreases, the predictive value of a positive test result decreases and the predictive value of a negative test result increases. These changes indicate that there is a direct correlation between the prevalence of a disease and the predictive value of a positive test result. In addition, the predictive value of a negative test and the prevalence of a disease exhibit an inverse correlation.

The implications of prevalence for screening can be explained by the following example. Assume that a large internal medicine practice group has decided to screen for arthritis in a screening population of 4,000 individuals. The selected screening test method has an established sensitivity of 66% and specificity of 95%. If the true prevalence of arthritis in the screening population is 3%, 120 individuals with arthritis can be expected among those screened. If the sensitivity is 66%, the number of true positives will be equal to the product of the prevalence and sensitivity (120 × 0.66), or 79. The number of true negatives will be equal to the product of specificity and 1 minus prevalence (0.95 × 3,880), or 3,686. The number of false negatives is equal to 41 (120 – 79), and the number of false positives is equal to 194 (3,880 – 3,686). Continuing these computations, the predictive value of a positive test result (PV+) would be equal to 29% (79/273), and the predictive value of a negative test (PV–) equal to 99% (3,686/3,727). The 2-by-2 table in Figure 6.2 illustrates these calculations.

FIGURE 6.2. VALIDITY PARAMETERS FOR ARTHRITIS SCREENING TESTS WITH A PREVALENCE OF 3%.

Test result	Arthritis	No arthritis	Totals
T+	79	194	273
T-	41	3,686	3,727
Totals	120	3,880	4,000

Sensitivity = 79/120 = 0.66 (66%).

Specificity = 3,686/3,880 = 0.95 (95%).

PV+ = 79/273 = 0.29 (29%).

PV– = 3,686/3,727 = 0.99 (99%).

In addition to validity parameters, an estimated calculation of the prevalence can be determined using test results. The estimated prevalence is equal to the ratio of the total number of test positives (273) to the total in the screening population (4,000), or 6.8% (273/4,000). This estimate is twice as high as the true prevalence, as is expected in the case of low population prevalence. As the true prevalence increases, the accuracy of the estimate also increases.

If the true prevalence were equal to 10%, there would be 400 individuals with arthritis in the screening population. Figure 6.3 presents a 2-by-2 table using the 10% prevalence value. The sensitivity and specificity remain the same, 66% and 95%, respectively. The number of true positives equals 264 (0.66 × 400), and the number of true negatives equals 3,420 (0.95 × 3,600).

The predictive values change as the prevalence changes. In this example, the predictive value of a positive test result is equal to 59% (264/444), and the predictive value of a negative test result is equal to 96% (3,420/3,556). The estimated prevalence is equal to 11% (444/4,000), only slightly higher than the true prevalence. The results of these calculations indicate that as the prevalence increases from 3% to 10%, the predictive value of a positive test result increases and the predictive value of a negative test decreases. In addition, the estimated prevalence and the true prevalence become essentially equivalent.

FIGURE 6.3. VALIDITY PARAMETERS FOR ARTHRITIS SCREENING TESTS WITH A PREVALENCE OF 10%.

Test result	Arthritis	No arthritis	Totals
T+	264	180	440
T−	136	3,420	3,556
Totals	400	3,600	4,000

Sensitivity = 264/400 = 0.66 (66%).

Specificity = 3,420/3,600 = 0.95 (95%).

PV+ = 264/444 = 0.59 (59%).

PV− = 3,420/3,556 = 0.96 (96%).

The predictive value of a positive test result is typically low in screening for disease, but the predictive value of a negative test result is high. Accurate predictive values of test results can be determined if the following are known: (1) the true proportion of diseased individuals in the population, (2) the sensitivity of the test, and (3) the specificity of the test. The use of likelihood ratios (which will be discussed shortly) is an alternative method for evaluating the performance of a test.

Validity can be further explained by using the 2-by-2 contingency table representing the performance of a screening test for colorectal cancer presented in Figure 6.4. Assume that the prevalence of colorectal cancer in the population is 5 cases per 500 individuals (1.0%). If 2,000 individuals are screened and all test positives are given a colonoscopy, what do the sensitivity and specificity of the screening test represent? Sensitivity equals the ratio of true positives to total individuals with colorectal cancer; consulting Figure 6.4 reveals that sensitivity equals 18/20, or 90%. Specificity is the ratio of true negatives to total individuals without colorectal cancer and equals 1,881/1,980, or 95% percent.

The predictive values can also be determined by using Figure 6.4. The predictive value of a positive test result is equal to the ratio of the true positives to total test positives: 18/117, or 15%. The predictive value of a negative test result is equal to the ratio of the true negatives to the total test negatives: 1,881/1,883, or 99.8%. Higher validity levels clearly have the potential to avoid unnecessary procedures with higher cost in terms of money and patient comfort.

FIGURE 6.4. VALIDITY PARAMETERS FOR COLORECTAL CANCER SCREENING.

Test result	Colorectal cancer	No colorectal cancer	Totals
T+	18	99	117
T-	2	1,881	1,883
Totals	20	1,980	2,000

Sensitivity = 18/20 = 0.90 (90%).
Specificity = 1,881/1,980 = 0.95 (95%).
PV+ = 18/117 = 0.15 (15%).
PV– = 1,881/1,883 = 0.998 (99.8%).

Managerial Aspects of Validity

The clinical aspects of epidemiology are applicable to managerial problems, particularly when determining the validity of management tools. An example of a management application of validity is as follows. Preadmission screening has become a fundamental process for Medicaid-supported waiver programs that provide home health and community-based services for the elderly. The purpose of the screening is to identify individuals in the population who are at risk of being institutionalized in a nursing home facility and are subsequently admitted. The Centers for Medicare and Medicaid Services (CMS) are concerned about whether preadmission screening actually identifies those at risk and whether the waiver program functions in a cost-effective manner (Jackson, Eichorn, and Blackman, 1992).

There are well-established techniques for determining the efficacy of screening tests for disease. Similar techniques for determining validity can be used to assess the effectiveness and efficacy of the preadmission screens. The preadmission screen results are analogous to a disease screening test result. Whether an individual is admitted to a nursing home (within six months) is equivalent to the actual disease status. The predictive validity of the preadmission screening tests can be assessed using the parameters of validity: sensitivity, specificity, and predictive values of a positive and negative test result.

Figure 6.5 presents a 2-by-2 contingency table that can be used to calculate measures of predictive validity. The columns represent admission (a and c) or nonadmission (b and d) to a nursing home within six months. The rows indicate eligibility or ineligibility according to the preadmission screening test. The upper left cell, designated a, represents the number of individuals who were admitted to the nursing home within six months and whom the screening test had found eligible. These individuals are the true positives. The lower right cell, designated d, represents the number of individuals who were not admitted to the nursing home within six months and whom the screening test had found ineligible for admission. These individuals are the true negatives. The upper right cell, designated b, represents individuals who were not admitted to the nursing home within six months even though the screening test had indicated that they were eligible for admission. These individuals are the false positives. The lower left cell, designated c, represents individuals who were admitted to the nursing home within six months even though the screening test had indicated that they were ineligible. These individuals are the false negatives.

The margin total of the left column, designated $a + c$, represents the total number of individuals who were admitted within six months. The right column total, designated $b + d$, represents the total number of individuals who were not admitted. The top row total, designated $a + b$, represents the total number of individuals deemed eligible. The bottom row total, designated $c + d$, represents the total number of individuals deemed ineligible.

Sensitivity of the preadmission screening test is calculated as $a/(a + c)$. This represents the ratio of individuals who were determined to be eligible for admission and were subsequently admitted to all those who were admitted within six months. Sensitivity of the preadmission screening can be defined as the ability of the test to correctly identify individuals who will be admitted to a nursing home within six months—in other words, the chance that an eligible individual will have been admitted to a nursing home within six months.

Specificity is the ratio of individuals who were determined to be ineligible by the preadmission screening test and were not admitted to a nursing home within six months to all individuals not admitted. This is calculated as $d/(b + d)$. Specificity of the preadmission screening is the ability to correctly identify individuals who will not be admitted to a nursing home in six months. In probability terms, this is the chance that an ineligible individual will not be admitted to a nursing home within six months, or p(ineligible | not admitted).

Predictive value of a positive test result of the preadmission screening is equal to the ratio of the true positives to the total eligible results, $a/(a + b)$. The predictive value of a positive test result is the probability of an individual's being admitted within six months if the screening test indicates that the person is eligible. The predictive value of a negative test result is equal to the ratio of the true negatives to the total

FIGURE 6.5. PREDICTIVE VALIDITY OF A PREADMISSION SCREENING TEST.

Test result	Admitted	Not admitted	Totals
Eligible for admission	a	b	$a + b$
Ineligible for admission	c	d	$c + d$
Totals	$a + c$	$b + d$	$a + b + c + d$

Sensitivity = $a/(a + c)$.
Specificity = $d/(b + d)$.
PV+ = $a/(a + b)$.
PV– = $d/(b + d)$.

ineligible results, $d/(c + d)$. In probability terms, this is equal to the probability of not being admitted if the screening test indicates ineligibility, or p(not admitted | ineligible).

As the use of standardized treatment protocols in medical practice increases, there will be an increasing need for screening resources of all kinds to guide physicians, physician assistants, and nurse clinicians in the selection of optimal treatment plans. The quantitative tools that have been introduced in this section will be critical to such advances.

Reliability

Reliability is defined as the degree to which repeated observations result in similar results on the same individual, under the same conditions. Reliability is often referred to as precision, reproducibility, and repeatability. Diagnostic and therapeutic testing is dependent on the reliability of measurements used in providing medical care.

Variation in measurements is a common concern and is affected by many independent and interrelated factors. It may result from biological differences among individuals, changes in individuals resulting from therapeutic interventions, and temporal changes within individuals (for example, blood pressure measurements are different in the same individual in the morning and at night). Measurements may vary simply because of random measurement variability.

Variation in measurement may also result from factors unrelated to the testing subjects. Laboratory-based measurement variation may be caused by improper calibration of measuring instruments or inadequately executed testing procedures. Observer-based variation is a common and complex occurrence. Different observers may interpret physical and laboratory examination findings differently or have differing criteria for positive and negative test results. Interobserver variation occurs when measurement results differ between two observers; intraobserver variation reflects varying measurement results by the same observer at different times.

To understand and account for inter- and intraobserver variation, the reliability index (which is known as the overall proportion of agreement) is used to identify levels of acceptable variation. This index quantifies the degree to which two observers' measurements agree with each other or one observer's measurements agree over time. The 2-by-2 contingency table in Figure 6.6 explains the calculation of the reliability index. The upper left cell, designated a, represents the number of times that observers 1 and 2 both identify a positive test result (T+). The upper right cell, designated b, represents the number of times that observer 1 identifies a positive test result (T+) and observer 2 identifies a negative test result (T–).

The lower left cell, designated c, represents the number of times that observer 1 identifies a negative test result (T–) and observer 2 identifies a positive test result (T+). The lower right cell, designated d, represents the number of times that observers 1 and 2 both identify a negative test result (T–). The reliability index is the ratio of the total number of times that both observers agree $(a + d)$ to the total number of observations $(a + b + c + d)$.

An example of the calculation of the reliability index is as follows. Assume that two pathologists review 200 slides microscopically for the presence of abnormal cell morphology in differential white blood cell examination (known as a *diff*). Both pathologists review the same 200 slides prepared from blood specimens collected from 200 different individuals. A management concern is how well these pathologists concur in identification of abnormal white blood cell morphology.

Figure 6.7 illustrates the outcome of this slide review and examination. Of the 200 slides reviewed, both pathologists indicated abnormal white blood cell morphology on 25 slides, and both pathologists indicated normal white blood cell morphology on 137 slides. So out of 200 slides, the pathologists agreed on their interpretation of 162 slides. The reliability index equals the ratio of the times the pathologists agreed (162) to the total number of slides reviewed (200), or 162/200, for an index of 81%.

To determine whether the agreement measured by the reliability index was simply due to chance, the kappa statistic can be used (Cohen, 1960). The kappa

FIGURE 6.6. RELIABILITY INDEX.

Observer 1	Observer 2		
	T+	T-	Totals
T+	a	b	a + b
T-	c	d	c + d
Totals	a + c	b + d	a + b + c + d

Reliability index = $(a + d)/(a + b + c + d)$.

FIGURE 6.7. CALCULATION OF THE RELIABILITY INDEX.

Observer 1	Observer 2		
	T+	T-	Totals
T+	25	20	45
T-	18	137	155
Totals	43	157	200

Reliability index = $(25/137)/200 \times 100 = 81\%$.

statistic, which has been widely used because it is not inflated by chance, is the ratio of the differences between the observed value of the index and the value of the index. The kappa statistic serves as a natural method of accounting for chance-expected agreement in any index. The kappa statistic is a ratio of the observed agreement to the expected agreement on the basis of chance alone. Kappa statistics can range from 1 (complete agreement) to −1, with scores greater than 0.75 indicating excellent agreement beyond chance, 0.40 to 0.75 representing fair to good agreement, and less than 0.40 representing poor agreement.

Impact of Test Information

In addition to the validity parameters we have mentioned, there is another construct that is very useful in describing the performance of a diagnostic test: the likelihood ratio. It is important to understand what impact a test result has on a diagnostic or treatment decision. Likelihood ratios summarize the same performance information as the validity parameters of sensitivity and specificity. The added value of likelihood ratios is that they can be used to calculate the probability of health and disease after a positive or negative test result (Fletcher, Fletcher, and Wagner, 1988).

In a probabilistic sense, likelihood ratios allow for the transformation of prior (pretest) probabilities to posterior (posttest) probabilities. A definition of likelihood ratios can be given in probability terms as follows: a likelihood ratio of a test result is the probability of a test result in the presence of disease divided by the probability of that same test result in the absence of disease. In other words, likelihood ratios express how many more (or less) times a test result will be found in individuals with disease, compared to individuals without disease.

Likelihood ratios can be determined for tests with both dichotomous and polychotomous possible results. Figure 6.8 presents the determination of likelihood ratios in tests with dichotomous results. The 2-by-2 contingency table is used to calculate the likelihood ratio of a positive and negative test result. The likelihood ratios are functions of the sensitivity and specificity and their complements (Fletcher, Fletcher, and Wagner, 1988).

Table 6.1 presents an example of the calculation of likelihood ratios for tests of serum creatine kinase (CK) and its relationship to the diagnosis of acute myocardial infarction (AMI). The test result is dichotomous: abnormal CK (greater than 120) and normal CK (less than 120). If the test result is an abnormal CK, the patient has a 1.38 greater chance of an AMI. If the test result is a normal CK, the patient has a 0.80 greater chance of an AMI.

To understand the impact of test information when there are more than two possible test results, likelihood ratios can be calculated for each result. Again, the

FIGURE 6.8. LIKELIHOOD RATIOS.

Test result	Actual Disease Status		Totals
	Disease	**No disease**	
T+	a TP	b FP	a + b
T-	c FN	d TN	c + d
Totals	a + c	b + d	a + b + c + d

Sensitivity = $a/(a + c)$.

Specificity = $d/(b + d)$.

Likelihood ratio of a positive test result =

$[a/(a + c)]/[b/(b + d)]$ = sensitivity/FP ratio = sensitivity/(1 − specificity).

Likelihood ratio of a negative test result =

$[c/(a + c)]/[d/(b + d)]$ = FN ratio/specificity = (1 − sensitivity)/specificity.

likelihood ratio is determined as a ratio between the probability of the specific test re-sult, given disease, and the probability of that specific test result, given no disease. If a test has K possible results, a likelihood ratio can be calculated for each of the K test results. Computationally, this can be shown as follows (where LR stands for likelihood ratio and TR for test result):

$$LR_K = p(TR_K|D)/p(TR_K|noD)$$

Table 6.2 presents an example of calculating likelihood ratios for tests with mul-tiple results. This example is an extension of the AMI and serum CK relationship pre-sented in Table 6.1. Abnormal CK levels are specified in four ranges: 121–240, 241–380, 381–480, and greater than 480. Likelihood ratios can be calculated for each test result level.

The major benefit of using likelihood ratios to understand the impact of test in-formation is that they allow for summarization of test results at different levels. Likeli-hood ratios can be determined for any number of test results across the set of possible values. The degree of abnormality can be specified and evaluated, relative to normal.

TABLE 6.1. CALCULATION OF LIKELIHOOD RATIOS IN TESTS WITH DICHOTOMOUS RESULTS.

Serum CK result	AMI	No AMI
Abnormal CK	62	315
Normal CK	71	622
Totals	133	937

Sensitivity = 62/133 = 0.46.

Specificity = 622/937 = 0.66.

Likelihood ratio of a positive test result (abnormal CK) = (62/133)/(315/937) = 1.38.

Likelihood ratio of a negative test result (normal CK) = (71/133)/(622/937) = 0.80.

TABLE 6.2. CALCULATION OF LIKELIHOOD RATIOS IN TESTS WITH POLYCHOTOMOUS RESULTS.

Serum CK result	AMI	No AMI	Totals
Greater than 480	12	18	30
361–480	10	15	25
241–360	11	30	41
121–240	15	198	213
1–120	41	621	662
Totals	89	882	971

$LR_{>480}$ = (12/89)/(18/882) = 6.70.

$LR_{361\text{-}480}$ = (10/89)/(15/882) = 6.58.

$LR_{241\text{-}360}$ = (11/89)/(30/882) = 3.62.

$LR_{121\text{-}240}$ = (15/89)/(198/882) = 0.75.

$LR_{1\text{-}120}$ = (41/89)/(621/882) = 0.65.

Given this differential analysis of abnormality, likelihood ratios can be used to support what occurs in clinical practice: more weight is placed on extremely high (and low) test results than others when estimating the chance of disease. The chance of disease is presented in the form of an odds ratio. The pretest probability of disease (that is, prevalence) is converted to an odds ratio as follows:

$$\text{Pretest odds} = \frac{\left(\text{Pretest Probability}\right)}{\left(1 - \text{Pretest Probability}\right)}.$$

The likelihood ratio is used to convert the pretest odds into posttest odds, after the impact of the information represented by the likelihood ratio is applied. This occurs as follows:

$$\text{Posttest odds} = \text{pretest odds} \times \text{LR.}$$

The pretest odds contain the same information as the prevalence, the likelihood ratio contains the same information as the sensitivity and specificity, and the posttest odds contains the same information as the predictive values of a positive test result. The posttest odds can be converted into the posttest probability as follows:

$$\text{Posttest Probability} = \frac{(\text{Posttest Odds})}{(1 + \text{Posttest Odds})}.$$

An additional benefit of likelihood ratios is that they are helpful in describing the overall probability of disease when multiple tests are conducted in either serial or parallel sequences. In serial testing, results from one test determine the need for another test. In parallel testing, all tests are conducted simultaneously. Serial testing is conducted when rapid evaluation of disease is not important or when tests are either risky or expensive. With respect to test performance, serial testing maximizes specificity and the predictive value of a positive test result while decreasing sensitivity and the predictive value of a negative test result. Parallel testing is conducted when rapid assessment of disease is a testing objective. Parallel testing increases sensitivity and the predictive value of a negative test result, with a resulting reduction in the specificity and the predictive value of a positive test result. Parallel testing is a more sensitive diagnostic strategy, with a lower chance of failing to detect disease.

For tests that have a continuous range of possible result values, an important concern in the evaluation of test performance is which test result value indicates the differential between health and disease. In this case, a large set of sensitivity and specificity values can be generated by selecting varying test result values as cutoff points that indicate disease. One method for determining these test result values is the receiver-operating characteristic (ROC) curve. The ROC curve plots the sensitivity and the false positive ratio (1 − specificity) to determine the optimal test result value to use to identify disease. ROC curves illustrate the ability of a diagnostic test to distinguish between diseased and nondiseased individuals, and the trade-off between sensitivity and specificity as the definition of a positive test is modified by varying the cutoff points. Figure 6.9 presents an ROC curve. The diagonal line (called the line of no discrimination) indicates a test that cannot distinguish disease from health; a ROC curve that is well above the diagonal line represents an accurate test.

The quantitative measure of accuracy represented by the ROC curve is a construct known as the area under the curve (AUC). The area under the curve quantifies the

FIGURE 6.9. A RECEIVER-OPERATING CHARACTERISTIC (ROC) CURVE.

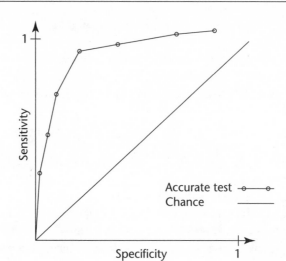

Note: The diagonal line represents chance; a ROC curve that is well above the diagonal line indicates an accurate test.

distance the test performs from the line of no discrimination. A test that has no ability to discriminate between diseased and nondiseased individuals has an AUC equal to 0.5. A test that is perfect has an AUC equal to 1. The better the test performs, the closer its AUC value is to 1. The worse a test performs, the closer its area under the curve value is to 0.5.

Clinical Practice Analysis

Practice analysis is a quantitative method of measuring factors that influence efficiency. Health care providers, including hospitals and physicians, are more efficient when they decrease variation and become partners with their patients. Clinical practice today has many factors that influence success. Practice analysis allows a practice to identify the factors that are the most important drivers specific to that practice.

Practice analysis uses weighted analytic techniques. Factors that are important to clinical practice are defined by the health care providers (and staff). The factors are grouped, ranked, weighted, and analyzed by the practice. In most methods, factors that influence 80% of outcomes are identified for action. The process identifies the areas that need data collection and strategies for change.

Each identified major factor becomes part of the intervention to reorient the practice. The practice typically knows where to place the major emphasis for the change effort. The practice uses this information to develop a strategic plan that will usually include (1) defining the critical measures that validate the change methodology; (2) defining the proper areas for change; (3) creating the desire to effect change; (4) creating the guiding principles of change; (5) developing mission and vision and also strategic action steps; (6) assessing barriers to change; (7) empowering action steps; (8) integrating new processes into the practice; and (9) measuring the effectiveness of the change process (Hiebler, Kelly, and Ketterman, 1998).

Why are formal techniques of practice analysis important? Clinicians are not typically trained in analytic techniques. The health care market changes faster than practice changes. Inefficiency creates increased cost, dissatisfaction, and eventually poorer patient care. It costs more for ongoing inefficiency than to find out what needs fixing and fixing it.

Practice analysis techniques have the capability to evaluate practice performance based on selected criteria. Client-specific evaluation models are used to measure practice performance, and comparison models look at individual practice performance in relation to optimal expectations, as well as local, regional, and national benchmarks. The analysis process includes identification of client-specific measurement parameters, data collection, data analysis and interpretation, comparison analysis interpretation, and recommendations for improvement. A result of a practice analysis is the identification of practice areas that should be targeted to effect improvements in parameters that affect the achievement of optimal performance. Variations in practice performance are identified and evaluated. Causes of the variation are determined, and recommendations to reduce the variation are formulated.

Managing Chronic Diseases

Disease management is a "systematic, population-based approach to identify persons at risk, intervene with specific program of care, [and] measure clinical and other outcomes" (Epstein and Sherwood, 1996, p. 834). An objective of disease management is cost containment, and research indicates that this is occurring. A study of nurse-oriented management of congestive heart failure in an aged population showed significantly lower numbers of readmissions and costs (Rich and others, 1995). Epidemiology plays a major role in disease management because identification of persons at risk is a basic epidemiological activity.

Disease management can be classified as either a contracted carve-out or a primary care model. The carve-out model is characterized by the provision of care to patients by contracting with disease management companies. The term *carve-out* refers to the separation of specialized care from a primary care model.

The primary care model focuses on specialized teamwork within HMOs and other comprehensive health care systems that assist primary care providers in caring for chronically ill patients. The major impact of this model is to help primary care physicians, who are concerned with acute exacerbations of diseases. The less immediate treatment needs of chronic diseases are typically overlooked without an established systematic approach. Disease management teams afford this systematic treatment strategy.

Managing Infectious Epidemics

Transmission of infectious agents, with resulting infection and disease outbreaks, is a serious problem for public health officials. Infectious agents may be transmitted in health care facilities during the delivery of health care services. Transmission may occur between patients, between health care workers, and between patients and health care workers. Such outbreaks are often referred to as having a nosocomial origin. The term *nosocomial* means "beginning or acquired in a hospital or health facility" (Hlady, Hopkins, Ogilby, and Allen, 1993, p. 169).

Nosocomial transmission of hepatitis viruses is common. Typically, transmission results from exposure to infants or young children after the transfusion of blood products. Nosocomial outbreaks of hepatitis B and C viruses have been observed in outpatient settings in New York, Oklahoma, and Nebraska in recent years. These outbreaks occurred from percutaneous or mucosal exposure of blood products from infected patients or health care workers. The cause of all of these outbreaks was unsafe injection procedures, usually from the reuse of needles or syringes (Centers for Disease Control and Prevention, 2003e).

Nursing home facilities are a common location for nosocomial infection outbreaks. An example is the outbreak of *Clostridium difficile* infection that was associated with gatifloxacin usage. Over a two-year period, an increase in the expected number of cases of *Clostridium*-associated diarrhea in a long-term care facility was observed. A case-control study from a sample of 612 admissions to a long-term care facility indicated a statistically significant association between the usage of gatifloxacin and *Clostridium*-associated diarrhea (Gaynes and others, 2004).

Nosocomial infections are a troubling concern when they involved infectious diseases of major public health interest, such as tuberculosis. In 2002, a tuberculosis outbreak in a community hospital affected six persons who were patients or worked in a large community hospital. The outbreak was traced to one patient who was hospitalized for three weeks before being placed in respiratory isolation following diagnosis of tuberculosis (Centers for Disease Control and Prevention, 2004b).

Nosocomial infection outbreaks are associated with high costs to health care facilities. A nosocomial outbreak of adenoviral conjunctivitis infection in a long-term care facility resulted in significant costs because it affected both patients and health care workers. During the outbreak, forty-one people were infected. The direct costs of this outbreak were categorized as medical, investigative, preventive, and lost productivity. The outbreak cost the hospital a total of $29,527: $1,085 in medical costs, $8,210 in investigative costs, $3,048 for prevention, and $17,000 in lost productivity among affected hospital workers (Piednoir and others, 2002).

The impact of nosocomial infections is measured as a major cause of morbidity and mortality at hospitals in the United States and throughout the world. Since 1970, the Centers for Disease Control and Prevention has tracked health care facility–based infections through its National Nosocomial Infections Surveillance (NNIS) system. This system establishes a standard method for collection and comparison of data describing health care facility–based infection rates. In addition, the NNIS system provides benchmark infection rate data for hospitals. As of 2002, more than three hundred hospitals were participating in the NNIS system as sentinel facilities (Jarvis, 2003).

The 2000 Global Burden of Disease study quantified the morbidity, mortality, and disability associated with nosocomial infections involving Hepatitis B virus, Hepatitis C virus, and HIV (Hauri, Armstrong, and Hutin, 2004). This study converted the impact of nosocomial infections into disability-adjusted life years (DALYs). The results indicated that during the time period 2000–2030, contaminated injections are expected to cause 21 million Hepatitis B virus infections, 2 million Hepatitis C virus infections, 260,000 HIV infections, and a burden of disease equaling 9,177,679 DALYs.

Infectious Disease Epidemiology

The traditional concern of epidemiology has been the investigation of the etiology of disease. In fact, the foundation of current applied epidemiology remains the epidemiologic principles from infectious disease. The impact of infectious diseases has gradually declined since the early 1900s, and chronic diseases are now a greater concern to health. However, infectious diseases remain important to health care managers because they are associated with a majority of acute diseases.

Characteristics and actions of infectious agents are indicators of the epidemiology of infections. Intrinsic characteristics distinguish infectious agents and help explain their effects on the infection process. If intrinsic characteristics are known or can be identified, the task of understanding an infectious agent's epidemiology (for example, mode of transmission) becomes quite straightforward.

In addition to studying intrinsic characteristics of infectious agents, we can study agents according to characteristics that result from their interaction with a host. These characteristics include pathogenicity, infectivity, virulence, and immunogenicity. These characteristics are dependent on several factors involving the environment and the individual host.

Pathogenicity is the ability of the infectious agent to cause detectable disease and is quantified by determining the ratio of the number of individuals with clinical disease to the total number of individuals who are infected by the agent. This ratio measures the number of infected individuals who actually become sick due to the presence of the infectious agent. Pathogenicity can be calculated by using the following proportion:

$$\frac{\text{Total number of individuals with clinical disease}}{\text{Total number of infected individuals}} \times 100$$

Pathogenicity is influenced by host characteristics, environmental conditions, dose, portal of entrance, and source of the infectious agent.

Infectivity is the ability of an infectious agent to invade and multiply in a host. The process of multiplication of the infectious agent results in the infection. Infectivity is also defined as the minimum number of infectious agents in half of a group of individual hosts (designated ID_{50}).

Virulence measures the severity of the infection and can be defined as the proportion of cases of clinical disease that result in severe disease or death. The case-fatality rate is typically used to measure the virulence of an infectious agent. The case-fatality rate is defined as follows:

$$\frac{\text{Total number of deaths from an infectious disease}}{\text{Total number of individuals infected}}$$

Virulence is affected by several factors, such as dose of the infectious agent, route of the infection, and individual host factors (such as age and race).

Immunogenicity is defined as the ability of an infection to produce specific immunity. The types of immunity that may result are humoral, cellular, or a combination of both. Immunogenicity is affected by host factors (age, nutrition, and so on) as well as dose and virulence of the infection.

There are two types of transmission mechanisms for infectious agents. The first is called direct transmission, which is the immediate transfer of an infectious agent from one host to another through a portal of entry. Examples of direct transmission activities include kissing, coughing, sneezing, and sexual intercourse. Sexually transmitted diseases (STDs) are infections that result from direct transmission of the infectious agent. Examples of STDs include venereal diseases, chlamydial infections, trichomonal infections, herpes, and AIDS.

The second type of transmission mechanism is called indirect transmission, which occurs by vehicle-borne, vector-borne, and airborne transmission. Vehicle-borne transmission occurs through exposure to contaminated food and water; often the infectious agent does not fully develop into an active agent until it has been introduced into a host. Vector-borne transmission occurs when the infectious agent is transmitted by an organism to a susceptible host. The vector's role in the infection process may be solely for transport or may also be biological. That is, the vector may only carry the infectious agent to the host, or the infectious agent may multiply in the vector prior to transmission (in which case there is an incubation period within the vector).

Infectious agents can be transmitted through the air in the form of dust and drop nuclei. Dust results from the resuspension of particles from household surfaces and soil. Droplet nuclei are tiny particles that have been formed by evaporation of sneezes, evaporation of coughed droplets, and aerosolization of infectious material.

Infectious Epidemics

An epidemic is defined as an unexpected number of cases of a disease or condition in terms of person, place, or time. In epidemics of infectious diseases, the major concern is person-to-person spread of the disease. Central to this is the concept of generation time, which is the period of time between the host's receipt of an infection and its maximum communicability. This concept is analogous to the incubation period. Generation time measures the time interval between cases and is essential in studying the dynamics of the transmission of infection because some infectious agents spread without apparent clinical disease.

The effect of epidemics is described by two epidemiological measures, the attack rate and the secondary attack rate. The attack rate is the incidence rate during the epidemic, which can be further defined by the following ratio:

$$\frac{\text{Number of new cases of a disease or condition}}{\text{Total number of susceptible persons in a group}}$$
$$\text{of individuals during a specified period of time}$$
$$\text{(the epidemic period)}$$

The secondary attack rate is defined as the number of new cases of a disease or condition that develop after the epidemic has ended yet are related to the epidemic. These incident cases result from exposure to infectious agents during the epidemic period. That is, the cases develop during a period of time after the expected number of cases have occurred, but without exposure during the epidemic, the cases would not have developed.

Epidemics, which are referred to as outbreaks, can be categorized on the basis of their duration. Common-source epidemics are those caused by simultaneous exposure of a group of individuals to a common pernicious influence, which is known as a point-source exposure. An example of a common-source epidemic is a foodborne outbreak such as *Salmonella enteritis* infections associated with eggs. Another example of a common-source outbreak is Legionnaires' disease, which is a respiratory infection caused by the *Legionella* bacterium. Figure 6.10 is a graphic representation that describes a common-source outbreak of an epidemic.

Propagated epidemics develop when exposure of susceptible individuals to the infectious agent occurs not simultaneously but over a period of time. These epidemics result from transmission, either directly or indirectly, of an infectious agent from one susceptible host to another. Figure 6.11 presents a graphic illustration of a propagated epidemic.

Severe acute respiratory syndrome (SARS) is a newly recognized global infectious disease that has sparked outbreaks in recent years. A viral respiratory infection caused by a coronavirus, SARS was first reported in Asia in February 2003. It soon spread to North America, South America, Europe, and other parts of Asia. People in the United States had laboratory-confirmed exposure to SARS, but no cases were confirmed in the United States. These individuals had traveled to areas of the world where SARS was actively transmitted.

SARS symptoms include high fever, headache, body aches, and overall discomfort. A small percentage of cases experienced diarrhea. SARS cases develop a deep cough and pneumonia. About 10% of SARS cases end in death. The incubation period can be as long as fourteen days.

FIGURE 6.10. GRAPH OF A COMMON-SOURCE OUTBREAK.

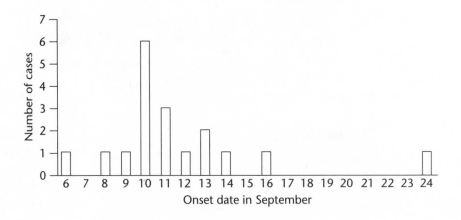

FIGURE 6.11. GRAPH OF A PROPAGATED EPIDEMIC.

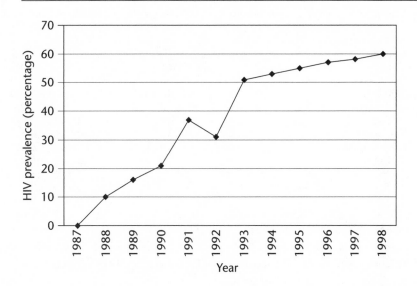

SARS is transmitted by close person-to-person contact and is characterized as a propagated outbreak. The SARS virus can be transmitted directly by respiratory droplets that result from sneezing and coughing at close proximity (up to 3 feet). It is also thought that the SARS virus can be transmitted indirectly by coming into contact with droplets on contaminated surfaces.

As an infectious disease, SARS has an overall deleterious effect on hospital and health care workers. Most SARS cases occur in people who care for or live with SARS patients or have direct contact with infectious materials. There is currently no effective treatment for SARS. The CDC (2003b) has recommended isolation of individuals with SARS but not quarantine. SARS patients are isolated until they are no longer infectious, with seriously affected patients admitted to hospitals. Table 6.3 presents the worldwide impact of SARS in 2003.

West Nile virus was first seen in the West Nile region of Uganda in 1937. The global impact of the virus was first documented in 1957 when it was found to cause severe human meningoencephalitis. West Nile virus was first seen as an equine disease in Egypt and France during the 1960s. Recent human outbreaks have occurred in Algeria (1994), Romania (1996–1997), the Czech Republic (1997), the Democratic Republic of the Congo (1998), Russia (1999), the United States (1999–2003), and Israel (2000).

TABLE 6.3. WORLDWIDE IMPACT OF SARS AS OF JULY 2003.

Country	Number of cases	Number of deaths	Number recovered	Mortality rate (%)
Canada	250	38	194	15.2
China	5,327	348	4,941	6.5
Hong Kong	1,755	298	1,433	16.9
Taiwan	671	84	507	12.5
Germany	10	0	9	0.0
Philippines	14	2	12	14.2
Singapore	206	32	172	15.5
United States	75	0	67	0.0
Vietnam	63	5	58	7.9

Source: World Health Organization, July 11, 2003.

West Nile virus manifests itself as a mild disease in most people, characterized by flu-like symptoms. Fever may be present but lasts for only a few days with no apparent long-term effects. The most severe manifestation of West Nile virus is encephalitis, meningitis, or meningoencephalitis.

Surveillance

Most health care organizations have established disease surveillance programs to continually evaluate the health and disease status of populations. Surveillance is also concerned with continual observation of conditions that increase the risk of disease transmission. These programs are characterized by systematic data collection, aggregation, formatting, analysis, and dissemination. Surveillance programs use structured, systematic methods that outline how and which data are collected. After collection, data are aggregated and formatted into meaningful arrangements for interpretation and detailed analysis in an attempt to describe trends and to test hypotheses about disease occurrence.

Historically, surveillance programs have focused on communicable and infectious diseases. Currently, such programs are being modified to include such areas as the tracking of nosocomial infections in hospitals, marketing efforts for pharmaceutical drugs, and categories of unintentional injuries.

When historical surveillance programs have been applied to control chronic diseases, less than favorable outcomes have resulted. Unlike communicable and infectious diseases, chronic diseases can be linked to no single causal factor. Not only is the etiology of chronic disease associated with multiple factors, but the time between causal exposure and disease occurrence may also be lengthy, measured in years or even decades.

Disease surveillance can be classified as either general population surveillance or sentinel surveillance. In general population surveillance, an entire community or population is the target of study. Such surveillance requires a large amount of resources and manpower and often provides only limited information that varies among subjects and populations. This surveillance is useful in a program of repeated surveys, such as the National Household Interview Survey.

In contrast, sentinel surveillance targets selected sites or subpopulations. Collected data are used to provide impact assessment of intervention strategies and in-depth study of demographics and behavioral aspects of the population. Results of such surveillance are applicable only to the specific study sites and cannot be generalized to the overall population.

Further, two types of disease surveillance can be identified: active and passive. Active surveillance seeks out cases of disease by periodic contact with health care providers. It is expensive and time-intensive but provides complete data. Passive surveillance is initiated by laboratories or health care providers and rarely provides complete information, even over a long period of time. Unfortunately, this is the usual way in which disease surveillance is carried out.

What criteria are used to decide which diseases to place under surveillance? The most important criterion is whether prevention strategies are available for the disease. If they are not, knowledge about the occurrence of disease will not be useful for control. Another criterion is whether the conditions or diseases are work-related. For example, work practice changes that have been established to reduce work-related risk include the use of safety equipment, such as hard hats, steel-toed shoes, and lumbar supports. Work-related diseases may have national public health importance due to their severity and frequency or may be important to individual health care providers. Silicosis and carpal tunnel syndrome are two examples of diseases of local interest.

Bioterrorism

The terrorist attacks of September 11, 2001, have changed the United States in ways that most people would have never anticipated. The increase in military and civil awareness, and its subsequent effect on the lifestyle of Americans, has been accompanied by a change in the view of public health. One result has been a new focus for public health agencies on terrorism preparedness. In addition to providing health services on a routine basis, as well as during outbreaks due to natural causes, federal, state, and local public health agencies are expected to be prepared for terrorism "events."

During fiscal 2001 and 2002, Congress appropriated about $1.8 billion to help the nation's public health system prepare for terrorism. In fact, the Centers for Disease Control and Prevention distributed $940 million in fiscal 2002 and $870 million in fiscal 2003 to state and local public health agencies for public health preparedness. In spite of this funding, a recent evaluation found that states are not significantly more prepared than they were before the events of September 11, 2001 (Trust for America's Health, 2003).

Epidemiology is a core component of terrorism preparedness and response planning. Public health surveillance and epidemiologic response plans for terrorism events are the centerpieces of any local, regional, state, or national system. Public health activities include the integration of disease surveillance and epidemiologic support into terrorism response planning. Surveillance teams are needed to conduct epidemiologic investigations of suspected or confirmed biological or chemical terrorism events.

With respect to changes in disease surveillance that are related to terrorism, new diseases are added to the notifiable disease surveillance systems. Diseases caused by *Variola* and *Francisella tularensis,* as well as *Brucella* species, are examples.

Surveillance data needs of the public health districts, local health departments, and reporting sources, including hospitals and physicians, must be part of the assessment and dissemination plan. Coordination is essential between physicians, hospitals, and public health agencies.

Summary

The traditional use of clinical epidemiology has been in screening the population for disease and in clinical trials. Screening is essential for obtaining descriptive information about the health status of the population. Clinical trials are fundamental for testing therapeutic improvements and advances in treatment methodologies. Bias is an important concern in conducting clinical trials. This problem is mitigated or eliminated by masking subjects, investigators, and data analysts.

Clinical effectiveness is a very important concern for management of medical services. Central to clinical effectiveness is validity, which must be determined in clinical testing to ensure accurate results and interpretations. Validity is quantified by the parameters known as sensitivity, specificity, and the predictive values of test results. The prevalence of a disease is an important consideration in screening tests: as the prevalence increases, the predictive value of a positive test increases and the predictive value of a negative test decreases; conversely, as the prevalence decreases, the predictive value of a positive test decreases and the predictive value of a negative test increases. The likelihood ratios associated with positive test results indicate the impact of testing information on clinical effectiveness and medical management.

Understanding the epidemiology of infectious diseases is necessary for proper management of health care services. Infectious diseases account for a significant demand on such services. Nosocomial infections are prevalent in all health care institutions, and knowledge of their epidemiology, including control measures, can help prevent these infections.

Infectious diseases are the focal point of disease outbreaks. These epidemics may result from a common source or through propagated transmission of infectious agents. Propagated epidemics occur by person-to-person spread of an infectious agent and occur over extended periods of time. Common-source epidemics typically result from exposure to foodborne infectious agents and are of short duration. Emerging infectious diseases are become a major concern and have been associated with recent outbreaks.

Surveillance programs are important components of all health care systems. Surveillance can occur either actively or passively, depending on the infectious disease of interest. Surveillance programs can focus on the general population or subpopulations.

Study Questions

1. East Bank Regional Hospital is considering the purchase of new diagnostic testing equipment, which has a purchase price of $500,000 and an annual maintenance fee of $15,000. In an attempt to evaluate the performance of the equipment, the CEO of East Bank Regional Hospital asks the hospital epidemiologist to gather information from the manufacturer. In tests conducted by the manufacturer, using 100 individuals known to have the disease for which the testing equipment was designed and 200 individuals known to be free of the disease, 90 of the diseased individuals had a positive test result, and 170 individuals without the disease had a negative test result.
   a. Based on these data, determine the sensitivity, specificity, and predictive values of a positive test result.
   b. Should the hospital epidemiologist recommend the purchase of this equipment?
2. Discuss the differences and similarities of a surveillance system and an analytic prospective study design.
3. Describe the different mechanisms of infection transmission. Then contrast the following routes of transmission of infectious agents: vector-borne, vehicle-borne, airborne.
4. Alliance Health System is an integrated delivery system comprising five hospitals, multiple ambulatory care sites, and a closed-panel medical staff of nearly 700 employed physicians. Its South Suburban Hospital has been a subject of much controversy, due to the large number of breast and cervical cancer deaths among patients who are regularly treated by the hospital's medical staff. In fact, the case-fatality rate of breast and cervical cancers is twice that of the rest of the state and three times that of the United States. As CEO, you are particularly concerned about the adverse publicity and notoriety the hospital is receiving. The most recent press release from the regional office of the American Cancer Society has highlighted these facts.

   You have convened the leaders of the hospital's medical staff for an explanation. The chief of staff has hypothesized that the high case-fatality rate is due to either underuse of mammography and Pap smear screening among hospital patients or inaccuracy of screening tests. The chief of staff has informed you that reductions in mortality from breast and cervical cancer depend on early detection and treatment. The idea of underuse particularly upsets you because of a community-based outreach and education program on commonly occurring cancers launched a year ago by Alliance Health System. In conjunction with the community-based program, the hospital began a physician awareness program to inform the medical staff of the availability and benefits of hospital-based cancer screening programs. The chief of staff assures you that any underuse must be patient-created, because the hospital's medical staff is the best-trained and most up-to-date group of health care professionals in the entire state. You are concerned about the possibility that the hospital may be using tests with questionable accuracy.

The chief of staff recommends that the accuracy of screening tests be determined before evaluating the impact of the community-based outreach and physician awareness programs. You hire an epidemiologist to determine the validity of the hospital's screening tests for breast and cervical cancer. The results of the investigation are presented in Table 6.4.

  a. What are the sensitivity, specificity, and predictive values of the mammography screening?
  b. What are the sensitivity, specificity, and predictive values of the Pap smear screening?
  c. What are the clinical and managerial implications of a false positive screening test result?
  d. What are the clinical and managerial implications of a false negative screening test result?
  e. As the prevalence of breast or cervical cancer increases, how are the sensitivity and specificity of the screening tests affected? As the prevalence of breast or cervical cancer increases, how are the predictive values of test results affected?
  f. What can be concluded from your testing analysis?

5. You have been designated the chair of an outbreak investigation and prevention committee by the CEO of South Suburban Hospital. Your committee's charge is to investigate a concern presented by the state health department, which maintains registries for most infectious diseases. Review of these registries revealed that over the past five years, sixteen cases of acute Hepatitis B virus (HBV) infection had a commonality: all sixteen patients had visited the same hospital-based medical practice, housed at South Suburban Hospital, before the onset of the infection.

The state health department conducted an investigation, consisting of the collection of blood samples from health care personnel coupled with a series of comprehensive interviews. Results of the investigation indicated the following: none of the health care personnel had a history of acute hepatitis or HBV immunization, and two physician dermatologists had negative HBV surface antigen tests but positive HBV surface antibody tests, which indicated that the physicians had been exposed to HBV. Further investigation revealed that these two physicians had seen 15,000 patients over the five-year study period (that is, 15,000 patient visits). The majority of these patients were white, female, and over the age of 50 years.

The state health department has issued the following questions to be investigated by your outbreak investigation and prevention committee:
  • What is the source of the Hepatitis B virus outbreak?
  • How did the outbreak begin?

TABLE 6.4. MAMMOGRAPHY AND PAP SMEAR RESULTS FOR FISCAL 2003–2004.

Test results	Cancer	No cancer
Mammograms		
Positive	86	25
Negative	12	352
Totals	98	337 377
Pap smears		
Positive	156	45
Negative	38	1,150
Totals	194	1,195

- Who is the index case?
- Has the outbreak ended?
- What is the hospital's plan to ensure that future outbreaks will not occur?

The state health department has notified local news media about its concern and investigation. A local newspaper suggests that medical practices at South Suburban Hospital will be shut down within thirty days due to substandard treatment practices. The story erroneously reports that the CDC has dispatched an epidemic investigation team and may even close the entire hospital due to patients' acquiring infections while hospitalized.

a. Before investigating the outbreak and searching for answers to the questions posed by the state health department, what preliminary question must be answered by your committee? What methods would you use to answer this preliminary question?

b. What is an appropriate personnel configuration for the outbreak investigation and prevention committee? Why?

c. Which patient records should your committee review?

d. What medical care protocols, if any, should be reviewed?

e. What further testing should be performed, if any? If a comprehensive study is to be designed, discuss and justify potential study designs.

f. Which epidemiologic measures are important in answering the questions posed by the state health department?

g. How would your committee respond to negative news media coverage, and what actions would you recommend that the hospital take?

h. Answer the questions posed by the state health department by drafting a report (three to five pages in length) for submission to the department. Include recommendations for preventive measures.

i. What type of outbreak is occurring?

6. After attending a church dinner, 143 people become ill. About 1,400 had eaten turkey, ham, and oysters at the dinner. One elderly woman dies of salmonella poisoning. Within twenty-four hours, 17 additional people are admitted to the hospital suffering from diarrhea, stomach cramps, nausea, vomiting, and fear.

    a. What is the attack rate of this salmonella poisoning outbreak?

    b. What is the case-fatality rate associated with this outbreak?

    c. What type of outbreak is occurring?

7. What is random error? What factors contribute to random error?

8. What is systematic error? What factors contribute to systematic error?

CHAPTER SEVEN

PLANNING HEALTH CARE FOR POPULATIONS

Chapter Outline

Introduction
The Planning Process
Strategic Planning
Evaluation and Monitoring Population Health
Integrated Health Care Services
Performance Improvement
Planning for Need
Summary
Study Questions

Learning Objectives

Upon completing this chapter, the reader will be able to do all of the following:

- Describe the role of epidemiology in community health assessment
- Discuss the role of epidemiology in strategic planning
- Discuss the new role of epidemiology in performance improvement
- Discuss the impact of epidemiology in planning in the private and public sectors

Introduction

As the saying goes, people don't plan to fail, but they fail to plan. This insight is an important preface to this chapter, which will attempt to present the planning process and the role of epidemiologic methods and data. It will not discuss planning theory in any detail but will instead develop the notion that planning for health services consists of efficient and effective alignment of resources (or capacity), based on expected health needs. Expected health needs are identified on the basis of epidemiologic-based demand and contact with an environment. This contact is measured by the burden of disease (Murray and Lopez, 1996).

The Planning Process

Planning health care for populations is a straightforward and often simple task. Rushed and inconsistent planning can result when information is imperfect, assumptions are educated guesses at best, and limited financial resources prohibit acquisition of the necessary capacity to meet the entire current and future burden of disease. The planning process, properly approached, consists of two primary activities: (1) aligning available resources (new resources as well as the existing capacity of the environment) in the most efficient path between the decision and the outcome and (2) implementing an intervention when resources and capacity are adequate to accomplish the task or support the decision. In health planning, the environmental component is included as the environmental burden of disease, years of life lost due to premature mortality, and years lived with disability (Murray and Evans, 2003).

The core elements of planning are related to resources and objectives: which resources are available and what objectives are of interest in the plan. An underlying question is whether the environment is such that the planning intervention can achieve its objectives. The available resources must be inventoried to assess existing capacity and compare it to necessary capacity. This process includes identification of all stakeholders and their perspectives.

Strategic Planning

Strategic planning is defined as the development of the most efficient and effective plan that optimizes the available new resources and existing capacities into a decision model. The strategic planning process should include evaluation of the planning organization's strategic position, analysis of the internal and external environment, generation of alternative strategies, optimization of choices through decision science, a logical implementation plan, and identification of the milestones that need to be measured to gauge the effective implementation of the plan.

SWOT (strengths, weaknesses, opportunities, and threats) analysis is an example; it provides a good framework for understanding strategy and assessing the direction of the planned project or intervention. It can help planners focus on the strengths and opportunities of the environment in which the plan will be implemented. As with all decision support tools, the greatest strength is the underlying recognition, inclusion, and addressing of components of the decision rather than the final answer. Planners must be certain that they have identified all of the necessary resources, existing capacity, and demands of the project.

For successful strategic positioning of a health care delivery entity or system and to improve its functioning in a population-based paradigm, health care services must be packaged to correspond to population needs (Zelman and McLaughlin, 1990). These customized packages of services have been referred to as clinical lines or population segments (Gray, 1988).

Strategic planning is most beneficial when it includes both human and financial resources. Budgeting and planning for delivery of health care services is best served by reviewing and evaluating decisions strategically. This is true in both private and public health care systems. In fact, it may be more important in public health care systems. For example, state public health agencies are charged with providing and overseeing the management of basic public health services on a populationwide basis.

A significant tension is felt in budgeting and planning in statewide public health care systems, which may not be very different in large private and not-for-profit systems, given the diverse population constituencies that are served in each state. State health agencies must be prepared to allocate finite resources in a more formal manner to be able to provide basic public health services on a routine basis as well as during outbreaks. The issue of funding is a constant concern for state health agencies.

The demands from the population served have been exaggerated by the events of September 11, 2001. The terror attacks changed the functions of statewide health agencies to include preparedness planning for possible terrorism. Federal, state, and local health agencies are required to inventory resources and to understand their capacity to provide health services on a routine basis as well as during outbreaks caused by natural and bioterrorism events (Marmagas, King, and Chuk, 2003).

It is important to understand the role of epidemiology, because if a heterogeneous population is to be served adequately and appropriately, demographic information must be considered. Large populations will be very different with respect to important demographic characteristics, including age, sex, race, and socioeconomic factors such as unemployment rate.

Budgeting and planning are complex activities that are affected by economics, health considerations, and politics. Managers and planners must be able to manage the tensions between these factors in order to budget for facilities configuration and support, staffing, and other needs (Reinke, 1998). Development of a budget is planning, and budgets are often the major planning and control tool used in organizations (Koontz, O'Donnell, and Weihrich, 1986). One advantage of developing a budget is that people are forced to plan, using data, and to evaluate the use and impact of allocation of funding.

Evaluation and Monitoring Population Health

A basic activity in planning is the evaluation and monitoring of future and existing interventions and programs. The core of evaluation and monitoring is information in the form of data, which is then converted to knowledge for future planning.

Data Types

An important question is whether to use variables data or attributes data. Variables data quantify measurable units, such as time, weight, and money. Variables data also reflect counts or ratios of total output of a specific process. Examples of variables data are length-of-stay days, surgery time, number of readmissions, and total number of patients treated in the emergency room daily. Variables data are typically continuous and may be transformed into attributes data.

Attributes data are counts of a characteristic or an event that may or may not occur. Examples of attributes data are mortality rates, percentage of population infected, percentage of inpatients with pneumonia, and number of false positives in a screening test. Attributes data may be dichotomous, categorical, and discrete. Inferences from attributes data are not as insightful because they provide less information than variables data do.

Another important question is whether to use retrospective or prospective data. Retrospective data are easier to collect but are often inaccurate or incomplete. Prospective data are difficult to collect but are usually accurate and complete. Deciding whether retrospective or prospective data will be used has study design implications; data needs dictate the choice of study design.

Community Health Status Evaluation

Analysis of health status, effects of lifestyles, and disease trends in the population will determine the array and distribution of health care services that are required to meet a population's needs. The success of a health care delivery system will be measured, in part, by improvement of the health status of its population. If the health care delivery system can help its population remain healthy, there will be an associated decrease in the use of resources.

To effect health status improvement, the health care delivery system will be required to work with its population, community agencies, and providers to encourage lifestyle behaviors that promote improved health. Strategic planning will originate in basic population health needs. Development of the health care system's strategic and marketing plans will be directed primarily at addressing the needs of the population.

Central to improving the health of the population is promoting wellness and lifestyle behavior modification. If members of a health care delivery system's population change their risky behavior and remain healthy, there will be a resultant savings in systemwide health care costs. Across the entire system, this change in risky behavior and improved health will be seen as a reduction in the use and need for human resources.

Data should be selected to answer evaluation study questions. Evaluation study questions should not be developed to fit existing data, but existing data should be reviewed for accuracy, ease of collection, and match to the evaluation concerns. If existing data do not match well, primary data must be collected.

Integrated Health Care Services

Hospital-specific product lines have existed for years to emphasize the business perspective of segmented services. Success has been measured on the basis of the performance of specific product lines provided by hospitals and other health care facilities. In the recent past, product line management has been replaced with the concept of service lines. The intent of service line management is to attempt to match the strengths of a hospital or health care facility to market demands.

When the health care for a population is the focus, a change in service line planning must take place. Specific services or physicians are no longer highlighted in planning efforts because the entire hospital or health care system becomes the focus. Physicians, hospitals, payers, and insurance programs must work together in population-based health care management. The objective is to provide the highest-quality health care for a population at the lowest possible cost. Planning efforts are concentrated on an integrated health system approach; that is, the entire integrated health system is the focus of planning, not individual hospitals or service lines.

Performance Improvement

It is important to monitor the performance of programs and interventions to understand whether they are meeting established objectives. After determining the performance of programs and interventions, the next managerial objective is to improve them by increasing their efficiency and effectiveness.. The following sections will discuss performance improvement methods and examples.

Rapid Cycle Improvement

The rapid cycle improvement process is a continuous quality improvement method that can accomplish targeted improvement goals more effectively and efficiently than approaches that are informal in nature. Its intentionally rapid timeline has proved to be one of its best assets. Given the short-term process, pilot interventions can be tested, new interventions can be compared to the status quo, multiple pilot interventions can be tested simultaneously, and success can be seen early in the process.

The rapid cycle improvement process is, of course, cyclical, consisting of the following main steps: setting time-specific performance goals, establishing quantitative performance measures, making changes after real-world testing, and evaluating results based on scientific methods. This is an iterative process: after results are evaluated, new performance goals are set, and the improvement intervention continues through another cycle (Fos and others, 2005).

The rapid cycle improvement process is becoming very popular in health care administration and medical management. A clinical process improvement intervention was performed on the prevention of pneumothorax in a neonatal intensive care unit (NICU). The goal was to decrease the incidence of pneumothorax and decrease the NICU days. This intervention consisted of a multidisciplinary quality improvement effort based on evidence-based clinical care. The result was a significant decrease in pneumothorax, NICU days, and mortality (Walker and others, 2002).

Another use of the rapid cycle improvement process involved increasing immunization for influenza and pneumonia among high-risk patients in critical care hospitals. Patients who were admitted for reasons other than influenza and pneumonia were targeted for immunization before discharge. The purpose of the intervention was to improve documentation of immunization status at discharge. The result was significant improvement of documentation and development of standardized charting for immunization status for inpatients. This indicates that quality improvement interventions can be successful in critical care hospitals (Ellerbeck and others, 2003).

Statistical Process Control

Statistics and epidemiology are essential to planning because they focus on description, analysis, and interpretation of data. Statistical methods are used to provide the basis of inference for decisions characterized by uncertainty and incomplete information, such as missing data. Probability theory allows for the estimation and description of the uncertainty inherent in most marketing and quality assurance decision problems. Knowledge of the probability of an event provides the rational basis for analyzing and making decisions. The laws of probability are the foundation of sampling, confidence intervals, and hypothesis testing.

Statistical process control is a technology whose goal is to detect "out of control" conditions and to determine whether the processes involved are stable and statistically "in control." If a process is found to be "out of control," then it is a target area for improvement. Statistical process control technology establishes the "bounds of control," typically within ±3 standard deviations around the mean value. This can be visualized using quality control charts. Quality control charts can be developed by analyzing process data retrospectively for a given period of time or by implementing an online statistical process control system in which charts are continuously updated in real time as new data become available (Farnum, 1994). Statistical process control as a tool for measurement of health outcomes will be discussed in Chapter Eight.

With respect to quality control problems, two issues exist: deviation from target expectations (described by using the mean, μ), and excessive variability around the target expectations (described by using the standard deviation, σ). Standard quality control charts analyze these two problem issues. These charts consist of X-bar and R charts. The X-bar chart, which describes deviation from the target expectations, plots the data items along the x-axis and the sample mean values along the y-axis. The center line represents targeted mean value. The R chart, which describes excessive variability, plots the data items along the x-axis and the range of values along the y-axis. The center line represents the acceptable range of values. The greater the variability in the data, the more variable the range of values on the quality control chart.

Figures 7.1 and 7.2 present the results of a rapid cycle improvement process. Figure 7.1 shows a quality control chart for completion of the recommended medication regimen for latent tuberculosis infection. Figure 7.2 presents a more traditional graph of the changes in the mean and standard deviation over the improvement intervention time period.

In Figure 7.1 the y-axis of the quality control chart is the percentage of people who completed their medication regimen, and the x-axis is time. Data points are the percentage of patients completing the medication regimen in different health facilities over time. For the study period, the mean medication completion percentage was 90.03%, with a standard deviation of 4.23, compared to a mean of 84.1% (standard deviation of 4.5) in the month before the quality improvement intervention began. During the study period, the mean rose to a high of 96.5% and the standard deviation decreased to 2.59. The quality control chart analysis indicates that a significant improvement was observed as a result of the quality improvement intervention (Fos and others, 2005).

FIGURE 7.1. QUALITY CONTROL CHART.

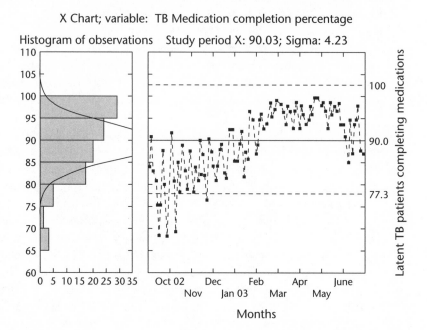

Figure 7.2 reveals the changes in the means and standard deviations of the latent TB medication completion rate. The mean medication completion rate of 79.8% was its lowest before the improvement intervention began, and the variation, 7.7%, was the greatest. During the improvement intervention, the means increased and standard deviations decreased in a constant manner.

Planning for Need

Planning for need is a critical aspect of managing the health care of populations. An important consideration is the perspective from which need will be determined and planned to be met. It may be a public, private, public-private, philanthropic, or advocacy perspective. The public perspective is what public health agencies use for planning and managing health care services. The private perspective is employed in for-profit health care delivery systems. The private-public perspective is typically seen in not-for-profit health care delivery systems that compete with private systems (such as acute care hospitals). The philanthropic perspective is seen with wealthy individuals or foundations that are attempting to improve the common good. And the advocacy perspective is commonly observed in groups that are passionate in the treatment

FIGURE 7.2. CHANGING PATTERN OF MEAN AND STANDARD DEVIATION OF LATENT TB MEDICATION COMPLETION RATE.

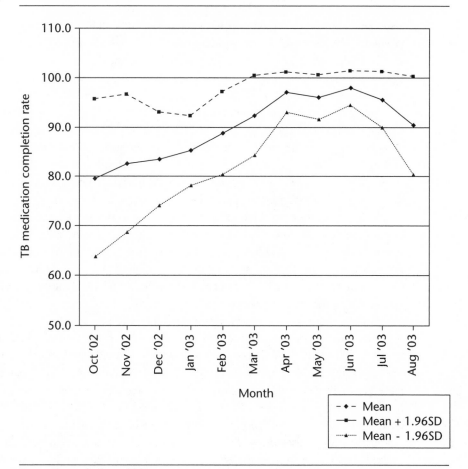

Source: Fos and others, 2005.

or prevention of diseases and conditions, based on personal experience or hardships (Mothers Against Drunk Driving is a good example).

The intent of health planning and health regulatory activities is to improve the health of the population. To achieve improved health, health planning and regulation have the following objectives:

- To increase access to care
- To increase continuity of care
- To increase acceptability of care
- To increase quality of care

- To prevent unnecessary duplication of services
- To encourage cost containment

 An example of health regulation characterized by these objectives is the certificate of need (CON) process, which is used in many states in the United States.

One application to planning taking the public perspective in a large state health agency involved the use of epidemiology and decision sciences for budgeting and planning (Fos and others, 2005). Decision science theory was used to develop a county planning model that highlighted, quantitatively, areas of need for services in each county across several planning and budgeting variables in Mississippi. In Mississippi, as in all state governments, the state legislature has authority over the spending of all state agencies. Regardless of the funding source (federal funds, self-generated fees, and so on), state agencies cannot expend funds without having first received authorization to do so through the legislative appropriation process.

Mississippi has a centralized public health care delivery system, serving more than 2.8 million people through 107 county health clinics. Centralized public health systems have been defined by local health departments functioning directly under the state's authority and are operated by a state health agency or board of health (Association of State and Territorial Health Officers, 2002). Only fifteen states have a centralized public health delivery system.

A multicriterion decision model was developed to assist in budgeting and planning for health services across the state. The planning model constructs a numeric score that is used to rank counties in their ability to provide public health services. Model parameters consist of routinely collected information, including demographic, mortality, morbidity, and resource data. The planning model was weighted using expert input, and the scores were determined using objective data. The planning model's benefit is that it indicates a county's ability, relative to other counties using the same funding sources, to provide public health services. The model information can then be used to allocate resources, to distribute funds for health care services, and to guide policy formulation and implementation.

Table 7.1 presents the weighted variables used in the model. Major variable categories were populations at higher risk of disease or death, access to health care, quality of care, and health outcomes. Each major category had explanatory variables, usually collected, updated, and made available by state and federal agencies. Populations at high risk were described by childhood poverty (the proportion of children under 15 years of age living in families at or below the poverty level), births to adolescents (10 to 17 years of age) as a percentage of total live births, prevalence of low birth weight (percentage of live born infants weighing under 2,500 grams at birth), unemployed population, and high school graduation rate. Note that several of these variables cannot be affected by a health care system, but nevertheless, they have a profound effect on health and the use of health services.

TABLE 7.1. WEIGHTED VARIABLES USED IN THE PLANNING MODEL.

Category and indicator	Weight
High-health-risk populations	0.26
Child poverty	0.09
Adolescent births	0.05
Low birth weight rate	0.05
Unemployed	0.04
High school graduation rate	0.03
Health care access and resources	0.29
Prenatal care	0.09
Health professional shortage area coverage	0.07
Physician-to-population ratio	0.06
CHIP enrollment	0.06
Medicare enrollment	0.02
Health care quality	0.27
Child immunization	0.15
Adult immunization	0.05
Cesarean section rate	0.03
Skilled nursing facility infection rate	0.02
Skilled nursing facility staff ratio	0.02
Health outcomes	0.18
Heart disease mortality rate	0.08
Infant mortality rate	0.03
Breast cancer mortality rate	0.03
Potential years of life lost	0.03
Motor vehicle deaths	0.01

Health access and resources were explained by percentage of pregnant women receiving prenatal care in first trimester, physician to population ratio, percentage of the county population covered by a health professions shortage area, physician-to-population ratio, percentage of Children's Health Insurance Program (CHIP) enrollment, and percentage of Medicare + Choice enrollment. Quality of care is illustrated in the model by child immunization coverage, adult immunization coverage, cesarean section rates per 1,000 live births, percentage of nursing home residents with infections, and mean nursing home nursing staff hours per resident per day. Health outcomes are reflected in cardiovascular disease deaths per 100,000 population, race-specific infant mortality, breast cancer incidence per 100,000 women, potential years of life lost (to age 75), and motor vehicle crash deaths per 100,000 population.

The planning model has been found to be very effective in many ways. The major benefit of the planning model is establishment of a relative comparison of counties. The planning model has the ability to distinguish counties that are achieving established clinical, public health, and managerial objectives from those that are experiencing less success. A second benefit is that the planning model can be used to prospectively evaluate whether funding will result in an expected or desired improvement in an area.

The planning model can identify potential areas for intervention and improvement. Coupled with financial analysis, funding requirements in each county to achieve desired outcomes can be determined.

Alternatively, the planning model has the ability to identify situations in which improvements will not result, independent of funding. Many variables are not under the control of a health agency. These factors confound and interfere with public health agency efforts to provide services and improve the health of the population. These situations occur often, and the planning model can not only identify these but also suggest better uses of funds to achieve planning goals and objectives.

Certificate of need programs attempt to ensure access to essential health services for all citizens in a state. They are usually administered by state health agencies or state health commissions. One purpose of CON programs is to balance the growth of health care delivery systems and facilities and services with the need for these services. The decision to apply for a CON by the health care delivery system must be established on the need for the services planned. The decision to grant a CON must be founded on the anticipated need for the services. A dilemma occurs when the perspectives are different and the definition of need is not congruent.

Summary

This chapter presented an overview of the planning process and the role of epidemiologic methods. The core elements of a successful plan are related to new and existing capacity of resources, environment as represented by burden of disease, epidemiologic data, utilization of health services, demographics of general and populations at risk, and identification of and input from all stakeholders. The strategic planning process incorporates the planner's perspective as a strategy. This is accomplished by weighing each choice from the planner's perspective and then optimizing the outcomes by prioritizing the choices.

Epidemiology serves as crucial information if we are to match present and future health needs to health services. The incidence, prevalence, and burden of disease contribute to the health risk of both general and target populations. The health status of communities, demographics, and socioeconomics factors provide additional information useful in the planning process. Continuing reassessment can provide prospective data for ongoing improvement of the performance of health care services.

The rapid cycle improvement process and statistical process control have helped large organizations visualize quality assurance, quality improvement, and quality maintenance. The most useful tool in the planning process is multiple attribute decision analysis or decision science. Making the best decisions as components of any plan will ensure optimization of the match between health capacity and health demand. The need for optimization is critical in a world where the latter is always greater than the former.

Study Questions

1. You live in a state with a certificate of need program. The CON program attempts to balance the growth of health care facilities and services with need. Need is determined from many perspectives, based on multiple and conflicting objectives. Assume that there are three stakeholders in the CON planning process: the state regulatory agency that issues the CON, a group of oncologists who wish to invest in a freestanding cancer treatment center, and the CEO and board of directors of a very competitive acute care hospital that wishes to deliver cancer treatment using a new machine that has not yet been purchased. The regulatory agency can issue only one CON for cancer treatment this fiscal year: to either the oncology group or the acute care hospital.

   a. Identify the types of data you would require to determine need from each stakeholder perspective.

   b. Discuss the information and insight each stakeholder would receive from each type of data.

   c. Rank the importance of each type of data from each stakeholder perspective.

   d. Select the perspective of either the oncology group or the acute care hospital. Write a two- to three-page report that will be submitted to the regulatory agency in support of the application of the stakeholder.

2. A philanthropist wishes to bequest $500,000 for a cancer program. After some investigation, the philanthropist decides that the following interventions are possible: donate to building a new cancer treatment facility, initiate a comprehensive cancer screening program, purchase an MRI scanner to diagnose cancer, or purchase the latest cancer therapy equipment. You have been selected to recommend one of these options to the philanthropist.

   a. What types of information would you require to make a recommendation?

   b. What additional information would you require, if any, from the philanthropist to make your recommendation?

   c. Write a two- to three-page report to the philanthropist supporting your recommendation.

CHAPTER EIGHT

POPULATION HEALTH OUTCOMES AND QUALITY OF CARE

Chapter Outline

Introduction
Assessing Health Outcomes
Monitoring Health Outcomes
Managing with Health Outcomes
Quality of Health Care
Quality of Life and Global Burden of Disease
Summary
Study Questions

Learning Objectives

Upon completing this chapter, the reader will be able to do all of the following:

- Explain the concept of health outcomes
- Discuss the methods of population health status assessment
- Explain the concept of best practices
- Discuss the benchmarking process
- Discuss the concept of quality
- Explain the role of epidemiology in health outcomes assessment
- Explain the role of epidemiology in quality-of-care assessment

Introduction

Epidemiologic data have been used for years to plan, implement, and evaluate health care services. With respect to payment mechanisms, epidemiologic indicators of morbidity and mortality are of particular interest. For example, in fee-for-service and indemnity insurance methods of payment, these indicators provide the information necessary for third-party payers to assume organizational viability.

The prospective payment system introduced in 1982 and the expansion of capitated methods of reimbursement for health care services created further opportunities to use epidemiologic information resulting from a population management orientation. Reimbursement constraints and ethical concerns associated with advancing medical technology require that health care managers analyze and synthesize information with enhanced epidemiologic models in order to plan services and evaluate payment models.

Epidemiology can help identify the health care services that are fulfilling expectations and demonstrate the benefits that result from the monies invested. Health care administrators must consider how to control costs while preserving and enhancing quality and must make strategic decisions about which services to expand, modify, or eliminate.

This chapter will present the concepts of health outcomes, benchmarking for best practices, and quality of care. The relationship of epidemiology to measuring and analyzing outcomes, identifying best practices, and defining and measuring quality will be discussed.

Assessing Health Outcomes

The approach that addresses the concerns of this chapter is known as outcomes assessment. Outcomes assessment usually focuses on establishing effectiveness and assessing the quality of the results of health care services. Outcomes are "bottom line" measures of how well the health care delivery system works; some optimal measures include health improvement, decreased morbidity or mortality, and recovery and control of disease states (such as high blood sugar).

Outcomes assessment has two broad objectives: to establish effectiveness of care and to assess quality of care. The first objective involves evaluating and identifying the most effective care for individuals with specific characteristics. This evaluation uses epidemiologic data collected in the routine, uncontrolled conditions of health care delivery.

The second objective involves using information to compare quality of care delivered across providers. The Centers for Medicare and Medicaid Services (CMS) report hospital data (case-fatality rates) that are used to compare quality of care among providers, including hospital- and physician-associated mortality rates for cardiac patients. The principal objectives of the CMS in this regard are to evaluate the quality of providers over time, identify high-quality providers, identify low-quality providers for improvement, and identify the most cost-effective providers.

Currently, the CMS is sponsoring the National Voluntary Hospital Reporting Initiative, providing Internet-based information on the quality of care in hospitals that have volunteered to report their data for selected clinical conditions. CMS goals for the publicly available Internet hospital information source are to "increase public awareness and understanding of health care quality; inform quality improvement activities in hospitals; give health care providers information they can use to educate patients; and promote public accountability" (Centers for Medicare and Medicaid Services, 2004).

Other determining factors of health and disease are important to accomplishing health outcomes assessment initiatives. These include demographics, socioeconomic factors, environmental influences, individual susceptibility, and use of health care services (for example, hospitalizations, prescriptions, and per capita health care expenditures). The Institute of Medicine clearly emphasizes the ecologic approach as a guide to thinking about population health. According to the Federal/Provincial/Territorial Advisory Committee on Population Health, population health refers to "the health of a population as measured by health status indicators and as influenced by social, economic and physical environments, personal health practices, individual capacity and coping skills, human biology, early childhood development and health services" (Institute of Medicine, 2002, p. 1).

The assessment of quality of care is based on three distinct functions of outcomes assessment: measurement, monitoring, and management. These functions are interdependent. A core set of outcome domains has been defined, along with measures of evaluation, including clinical states, functional status, quality of life, adverse events, patient satisfaction, and costs of care—all parts of effectiveness research and all connected with patients, residents, or users of care services. These measures include routinely collected epidemiologic data, as well as medical care information.

Outcomes measurement is the assessment of one or more variables that describe results of some health care intervention. For example, outcome measures of physical and mental symptoms indicate an individual's clinical state. These measures allow for the assessment of severity of illness, course of illness, and effect of interventions on possible clinical states.

Avedis Donabedian's incorporation of quality measures into the structure-process-outcomes triad has provided useful methods for assessing health care quality. According to Donabedian (1988), structural measures of health care settings are characterized by the availability of human and material resources. Some characteristics of the health care setting are the presence or absence of nurse practitioners, board-certified specialists, on-site laboratories, accredited facilities, and parking facilities.

Process measures relate to the providers' and staff's personal behavioral and technical characteristics, including the courtesy shown to patients and patients' perceptions of time spent with the provider. Some technical process measures are the provision of preventive counseling, patterns of use of drugs, surgical rates, and referral patterns. Outcome measures involve current and future health status and are represented by functional status, competence to perform the activities of daily living (ADL), and satisfaction with care. These measures are used to evaluate the impact of health programs on the health status of different groups; assess the ADL of elderly and chronically ill persons; measure physical health in terms of function, mental health, social health, and general health perceptions; and distinguish the concepts of physical and mental health and identify the five indicator categories of clinical status, functioning, physical symptoms, emotional status, and evaluations and perceptions.

Studying clinical outcomes has focused on evaluation of administrative claims data. Claims data are commonly used because they are readily available and easily accessible, but it is not certain that data collected for reimbursement purposes is valid for studying clinical care. This question has been studied in detail, and specific findings are that administrative claims data lack important diagnostic and prognostic information. Also, coding schemes used in administrative claims data (ICD-9, DRG, and CPT) often do not accurately describe the clinical aspects of care. One conclusion is that administrative claims data are inappropriate for identifying clinically relevant patient groupings and for adjusting for risk in outcome assessment studies (Jollis and others, 1993).

Given the concern with administrative claims data, an alternative source of data is medical records. Medical records contain information about patient histories, clinical signs and symptoms, clinical assessments, diagnostic laboratory findings, diagnoses, and discharge plans. Medical records are very useful in the study of quality of care for many projects. Quality improvement organizations use medical record reviews to assess performance on a set of quality-of-care indicators.

Another example is the Pneumonia National Project, a quality improvement initiative that recognizes that pneumonia causes substantial morbidity and mortality for Medicare patients. The focus of this initiative is to modify processes of care to improve health outcomes for Medicare beneficiaries admitted to the hospital with pneumonia. Furthermore, an increase in inpatient vaccination rates against influenza and pneumococcal disease is encouraged. The medical review process identifies quality indicators using the following medical record documentation: initial antibiotic therapy consistent with current guidelines; collection of blood cultures within twenty-four hours of hospital arrival; collection of blood cultures prior to the initial antibiotic dose; screening for influenza and pneumococcal immunization status and vaccination prior to discharge, if indicated; smoking cessation counseling during hospitalization; and arterial oxygenation assessment within twenty-four hours of hospital arrival.

By collecting relevant clinical data, risk adjustment can be performed before comparing providers. Providers, both physicians and hospitals, can be ranked on the basis of unadjusted risk, risk-adjusted clinical information, and risk-adjusted patient comorbidities. After risk adjustment, rankings of providers often undergo significant modification.

Health Status Assessment

Historically, mortality rates have been used as health status indicators for populations. Mortality rates actually measure death (which is often a result of disease or injury), not health. At best, mortality rates are a proxy measure for health. Health is a concept that is broader than simply the absence of disease; it encompasses physical, social, mental, and emotional well-being. This limitation has resulted in the development of more comprehensive health status indicators (McDowell and Newell, 1996).

Health status is determined by several factors, including physical health and functional status, and its measurement involves these dimensions and associated objective and subjective measures. Health status measurement is accomplished as either a health status index or a profile. An index is characterized by a single score representing health status. Conversely, a health status profile provides a multidimensional evaluation of all the aspects of health. Health profiles are popular in situations where the interaction of the physical, social, mental, and emotional determinants of health are of interest. Health indices are useful in health policy and economic evaluation because a single score is helpful in making choices and decisions.

The Medical Outcomes Study (MOS) "Short-Form 36" health survey is one of the many health indices that have been developed since 1950. The SF-36, as it is commonly known, is designed for population health surveys and as an evaluation tool for health policy. The SF-36 was initially developed in 1970 during the Health Insurance Experiment conducted by the RAND Corporation. The SF-36 was further refined in 1990 (Ware and Sherbourne, 1992). In its current form, the SF-36 addresses both physical and mental aspects of health.

The SF-36 consists of thirty-six items, divided into eight dimensions: physical functioning, role limitations due to physical health, bodily pain, social functioning, general mental health, role limitations due to emotional problems, vitality, and general health perceptions. The SF-36, available in two versions (with wording and scoring differences but comparable in output), is self-administered or administered during personal or telephone interviews; self-administration is the most common and feasible approach for most patients. The need to capture data from large population groups led the developers of the SF-36 health survey to evaluate the feasibility of decreasing the number of questionnaire items to minimize the survey administration respondent burden. These efforts led to the development of the SF-12 and SF-8 surveys. The

SF-12 survey produces two summary scales (of physical components and mental components). The SF-8 survey produces eight scales and two summary scales comparable to the SF-36 health scales.

Other health status assessment surveys in use today include the Quality of Life Index (Spitzer, 1988), developed to measure the general health and well-being of terminally ill individuals; the COOP Charts for Primary Care Practice (Greenfield and Nelson, 1992), used to assess health and function in primary care patients; the Functional Status Questionnaire (Jette and Cleary, 1987), a self-administered general health and social well-being survey for ambulatory patients; the Duke Health Profile (Parkerson, Broadhead, and Tse, 1990), which evaluates health status in primary care patients; the Sickness Impact Profile (Bergner, 1993), which was developed to measure changes in an individual's behavior as a result of illness; and the Nottingham Health Profile (Hunt, McEwen, and McKenna, 1985), developed as a measure of perceived general health status for primary care patients and general population health surveys.

For example, consider this application of the SF-36 in population health surveying. The SF-36 was used in the city of Merida, in the state of Yucatán, Mexico, to evaluate the health status of municipal workers (Zúniga and others, 1999). The SF-36 was translated into Spanish following approved guidelines. This health status information was intended to serve as a baseline measure from which the impact of future interventions could be determined. Overall, 488 municipal workers from all city departments completed the survey. These city departments included administration, finance, public services, social services, urban planning, and public works.

The resulting health profiles established baselines for municipal workers in general, individual workers, and workers across city departments. These baselines were intended to be used by Merida's department of human resources to plan health interventions for municipal workers. In addition to identifying areas of need for intervention, the baselines will be used to evaluate the impact of these future interventions. The SF-8 health survey was also used to measure health status in residents of Hidalgo County, Texas (Zúniga, Blakely, and Tromp, 2003), as part of an intervention to improve access of community residents to available health care services.

Patient Satisfaction and Expectations Assessment

Patient satisfaction with health care has been operationalized to assess quality of care from the patient's perspective. The shift of care from hospital to outpatient settings, including home care, has made the patient's opinions increasingly important. Most satisfaction surveys measure several aspects of health care delivery, such as costs of care, ease of access to care, and interpersonal skills of health care providers and others. Cost measures include not only costs of care but also costs related to lost work productivity in both patients and family members, as well as cost-effectiveness of specific types of treatment.

Quality measures may vary with the specific quality assessment program because they are both objective and subjective. Rates of occurrence of disease or conditions (incidence and prevalence) are used to measure the quality of prevention programs. Rates of detection of disease or conditions (prevalence and yield) are measures of the quality of diagnostic and screening methods. Patient satisfaction is a very important measurement of quality of care. Patients' perceived access to care, time spent with the health care personnel, and conveniences of the provider's location are measured by patient surveys. The patient's general well-being is measured by surveying the patient's perceived health status.

At the point-of-service level, patient satisfaction evaluation remains a fundamental source of quality improvement information. It also provides valid data to affect provider behavior by highlighting individual performance compared to peer provider performance. For example, the Visit Specific Satisfaction (VSS) and Outpatient Satisfaction (OPS) surveys, available from the Group Health Association of America Consumer Satisfaction Survey, were used to compare performance of ambulatory care settings (Zúniga, Babo, and Fos, 1996). Four ambulatory care clinics in an urban academic medical center served as the study site, with 688 patients participating in the survey. Participants indicated their level of satisfaction by responding to eight VSS or twenty-two OPS statements about ambulatory care services, on a five-point scale ranging from excellent to poor.

Results of the study indicated that patient satisfaction was multidimensional. Respondents assigned statistically significant positive ratings to appointment scheduling wait, telephone access, wait time at the clinic, explanation of what was done, and overall visit satisfaction. This study showed that health care organizations should consider using available tools for measuring patient satisfaction. The information from this measurement tool is essential for planning and quality assurance efforts. Organizations respond to patient satisfaction information by addressing areas for improvement—for example, enhancing telephone system technology and telephone etiquette or automating the scheduling of appointments and other provider encounters.

A continued initiative to assess ambulatory care visit-specific patient satisfaction during a five-year period showed that the satisfaction of 19,276 respondents from twenty-one ambulatory care clinics varied but remained within statistical confidence limits (Zúniga and Frentz, 2001). Patient satisfaction reports are useful at the point of service to assess physician performance. In this visit-specific assessment of patient satisfaction, physician-specific scores were used to allocate physician reimbursement bonuses for those with managed care payment contracts. The graph presented in Figure 8.1 is a control chart that illustrates the proportion of excellent responses to the assessment of visits overall. The confidence limits vary from quarter to quarter to adjust for different response rates. (Control charts are described in more detail later in this chapter.)

Variability in measuring user satisfaction is widespread; health care organizations collect patient satisfaction data at different levels, for different purposes, and with

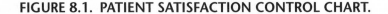

FIGURE 8.1. PATIENT SATISFACTION CONTROL CHART.

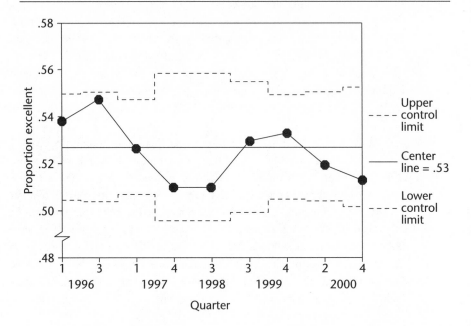

different methods. Standardization for the assessment of patient satisfaction is beginning to show results. Initiatives that are demonstrating the value of standardization of survey process, analysis, and reporting are exemplified by the Department of Health and Human Services–sponsored hospital and health plan report card initiatives. This survey methodology uses standardized data collection instruments, data analysis, and reporting. Two surveys are used to create publicly available consumer-based report cards, the Consumer Assessment of Health Plan Survey (CAHPS) and its spin-off, the hospital-specific HCAHPS (Agency for Healthcare Research and Quality, 2003).

The CAHPS is a comprehensive survey that includes the following domains: getting needed care, getting care without long waits, how well doctors communicate, courtesy and helpfulness of office staff, and customer service of the health plan. The HCAHPS is being tested in a three-state pilot program. Its domains include nurse communication, nursing services, doctor communication, physical environment, pain control, communication about medicines, and discharge information.

CAHPS data collection and reporting was adopted nationally in 1988, and an additional initiative called the National CAHPS Benchmarking Database (NCBD) was implemented to provide a resource for benchmarking and research related to consumer assessments of care. All CAHPS survey users pool their data in the national database and receive a customized report that compares their individual results to NCBD benchmarks. A recent analysis of the NCBD 2003 data yielded several important findings. First, the majority of survey respondents rate their medical care providers and overall health care highly. More than half of all respondents in all sectors gave their personal doctors and specialists either 9 or 10 on a ten-point scale where 0 is the worst possible and 10 is the best possible (National CAHPS Benchmarking Database, 2004, p. 7).

In general, other findings indicated that respondents rate their health plans lower than they rate their personal doctors and specialists. The exception to this is among SCHIP enrollees, who give their health plans higher ratings. Respondents in all sectors report the most positive experiences for questions related to getting needed care. In contrast, questions related to getting care quickly receive the least positive responses. Parents responding about their children generally report more positive experiences than adults responding about their own care, except for Medicare enrollees (CAHPS Consortium, 2003).

The pilot HCAHPS survey tested a sixty-six-item data collection instrument in 109 hospitals in three states from June through August 2003. This initiative to standardize the perceptions of hospital care will add a valuable and useful tool to benchmark perceptions of quality in U.S. acute care hospitals. The CAHPS family of surveys offers the opportunity to standardize data collection, analysis, and reporting efforts. Benchmarking national and regional organizations and groups of individuals will aid the quality improvement team's understanding of areas of strength and areas needing improvement while meeting external review and accreditation requirements by the National Committee for Quality Assurance (NCQA) and the Joint Commission on Accreditation of Healthcare Organizations (CAHPS Consortium, 2003).

Monitoring Health Outcomes

Outcomes monitoring is the repeated assessment of variables defined as outcomes, or results of interactions between a patient and the health care delivery system, that allow for causal inferences about what produced the observed results.

Using the 1999 study by Patrick and others, introduced in Chapter Seven, Table 8.1 presents the results of twenty-four- and forty-eight-month follow-ups of the study participants with respect to mortality in the treatment and control groups. An interesting finding was that the mortality rate was higher in the treatment group than in the control group. This difference was seen at both the twenty-four- and the forty-eight-month follow-up. Age stratification showed no significant difference in patients 65 to 74 years of age. This was not the case for those 75 years and older, where a significant difference was found between the twenty-four- and forty-eight-month follow-ups.

TABLE 8.1. MORTALITY AT TWENTY-FOUR-MONTH AND FORTY-EIGHT-MONTH FOLLOW-UPS IN THE COSTS AND OUTCOMES OF MEDICARE REIMBURSEMENT FOR HMO PREVENTIVE SERVICES.

	24-month follow-up		48-month follow-up	
Study group	Alive (%)	Dead (%)	Alive (%)	Dead (%)
All participants				
Total	95.6	4.4	90.7	9.3
Treatment	94.5	5.5	89.6	9.8
Control	96.7	3.3	91.2	8.2
Age 64–74 years				
Total	97.2	2.8	94.1	5.9
Treatment	96.7	3.3	93.7	6.3
Control	97.6	2.4	94.5	5.6
Age 75 years and over				
Total	92.5	7.5	84.0	16.0
Treatment	90.0	10.0	81.4	18.6
Control	95.0	5.0	86.5	13.5

Source: Data from Patrick and others, 1999.

Another outcomes monitoring effort sponsored by the CMS is the Medicare Health Outcomes Survey (HOS). This is the first outcomes measure used in Medicare managed care. The HOS is a longitudinal self-administered survey that uses the SF-36 health survey and additional case mix and risk adjustment variables (Cooper and others, 2001).

The Medicare program states that for each health plan with Medicare + Choice contracts, "One thousand Medicare beneficiaries, who were continuously enrolled for a six-month period, are randomly sampled from each plan and surveyed every spring (i.e., a survey is administered to a different baseline cohort, or group, each year). Two years later, these same respondents are surveyed again (i.e., follow-up measurement). Cohort I was surveyed in 1998 and was resurveyed in 2000. Cohort II was surveyed in 1999 and was resurveyed in 2001. Cohort III was surveyed in 2000 and was resurveyed in 2002." (Centers for Medicare and Medicaid Services, 2004). A timeline of HOS adminstration is available on the Centers for Medicare and Medicaid Service Web site (www.cms.hhs.gov). Managed care organizations are using these results to track and manage variability of health outcomes from the member's point of view.

Managing with Health Outcomes

The approach of managing what you can measure affords health care organizations the opportunity to quantify outcomes and assess their variability in the epidemiologic triad of person, time, and space so as to better manage processes and outcomes.

Uses of Outcomes Assessment

Outcomes can be used for many management objectives. Managing with outcomes can be defined as the use of information obtained from outcomes monitoring in clinical decision making, patient care management, and organization of health care services, with the goal of achieving optimal patient outcomes.

Public and private payers, hospitals and other health organizations, individual providers, patients, and the general public all have an interest in and are affected by outcomes assessment and research. The uses of outcomes information vary according to the needs of specific interest groups. Epidemiology provides the summary measures and evaluation methods needed for interpreting outcomes assessment and research. This information can be used in managing fee-for-service and managed care environments.

An emerging use of outcomes measurement is in making reimbursement decisions based on quality assessment. Payers can relate clinical care outcomes with reimbursement for care and with incentive mechanisms for rewarding or penalizing hospitals and other providers.

Outcomes data can be used in decisions about rationing of care, based on results of cost-effectiveness studies. In addition, patients may use effectiveness results to rank different types of care and may pay only for those above a particular cutoff. The state of Oregon has used cost-effectiveness analysis to develop a priority list of reimbursable health care services delivered to Medicaid patients. This list is based on a ranking methodology that uses both the input of the community and the relative cost-effectiveness of all services. A cutoff of ranked services is used to select which services on the priority listing will be reimbursable.

Outcomes can be used to guide the selection of providers by payers of health care services. For example, an HMO may use outcomes to evaluate potential providers for contracting purposes. Benchmarking and "report card" approaches are useful in deciding which providers satisfy objectives of the health care payer. Outcomes can also be used to monitor the performance of HMO-contracted providers.

How can outcomes assessment aid the managers of hospitals and health care organizations? First, effectiveness results can be used to establish local guidelines. Clinical guidelines developed locally are often easier to implement because they address acceptance-dominated decisions. However, conducting outcomes research on a local scale is difficult because obtaining and maintaining an adequate database locally can be a formidable task.

Second, data on quality outcomes can be used for marketing purposes. Such strategies are evaluated and implemented after thorough analysis of quality-of-care data. Health service quality can be assessed using both quantitative and qualitative methods, with interviews of physicians and staff and surveys of patients as the sources of qualitative data.

Once hospital managers and other health care providers understand current health status, outcomes assessment data can be used to identify areas to target for improvement. After targeting, continuous quality improvement strategies can be monitored for effect. The improvement process involves both modifying procedures and identifying best practices for clinical treatments.

Another benefit of outcomes assessment is that it can provide information to patients in the selection of health plans and providers. For example, a patient may use outcomes information to select a hospital with a high rate of favorable outcomes. Alternatively, patients may exclude from consideration a hospital with high rates of unfavorable outcomes. The same is true in the selection of individual physicians who will provide health care services.

Benchmarking

A benchmark is a measurement that is used to evaluate the performance of a specific health care provider relative to other providers. By comparing and studying benchmarks, a health care provider can set goals for performance improvement. This evaluative process is known as benchmarking.

Benchmarking is defined by the American Society for Quality as "an improvement process in which a company measures its performance against that of the best in class companies, determines how those companies achieved their performance levels and uses the information to improve its own performance. The subjects that can be benchmarked include strategies, operations, processes and procedures" (American Society for Quality, 2004). Benchmarking is a continuous process that occurs over an extended period of time and can illustrate the dynamic nature of organizational performance over time.

The benchmarking process results in learning to adapt best practices, leading to process improvements and a healthier population. *Best* is a relative term and indicates what is best for a given population according to a set of accepted objectives. Benchmarking for best practices is a clinical and administrative improvement process, not a rigorous scientific method. Benchmarking also has a place in evidence-based management. Using epidemiologic data to effect cost reductions is a practical approach to benchmarking. Some cost reduction opportunities can be realized by creating benchmarks to adjust staffing levels, optimize procurement efficiency, minimize materials consumption, decrease telecommunications costs, adjust employee benefits to the market, reduce costs through outsourcing, and optimize technology investments, among other managerial issues identified through the use of epidemiologic tools.

Benchmarking has its greatest impact in evaluating current health care services for populations and in planning for the future. Benchmarking is a core component in strategic planning, forecasting future needs of the population, the generation of new concepts for servicing population needs, comparative and competitive analyses of the delivery of health care services, and goal setting.

Benchmarking is a challenging process to adopt because it is not a onetime activity but an ongoing process. The concept of continuous improvement is essential to successful benchmarking. The process of identifying and understanding "best practices" is, by its very nature, dynamic because of the changing state of the health care delivery industry.

Benchmarking is not intended to provide simple answers to short-term questions, but it does provide valuable information that can be used to plan and design the health care services system. Benchmarking identifies the best practice providers who should be used as models for improvement. Once the best practice providers have been identified, it is not appropriate to simply adopt their practice patterns. Instead, information obtained from the best practice providers must be adapted to the style and culture of each organization to ensure improvement.

There are five stages in the benchmarking process: (1) determine what to benchmark, (2) form a benchmarking team, (3) identify benchmark partners, (4) collect and analyze benchmarking information, and (5) take action (Spendolini, 1992). The process is iterative; this is essential in practice to ensure success. Benchmarking is thus not a linear but a continuous, cyclic process.

The first stage of the benchmarking process is concerned with identifying who will be interested in the information and what their objectives are. The specific measures and the intended use of the information must be defined before beginning data collection and specification of the benchmarking process. Benchmarking must be a broad-based search for information, but it should encompass specific objectives and discrete activities to achieve those objectives.

Benchmarking is a team effort. The second step of the benchmarking process is to assemble the benchmarking team. Team membership is not limited to individuals inside the health care organization; external experts should be enlisted to assist in the process. In addition to internal benchmarking experts, others in the organization should be members of the team. The rationale is twofold: those affected by any changes should be part of the process of measurement selection and data collection, and team members should have input in the local benchmarking process. Because benchmarking is a continuous process, a stable team membership is essential. Involving as many individuals as possible who are associated with the health care organization ensures the continuous process dynamic.

This next stage of the benchmarking process is the identification of sources of information and best practice providers. Sources of information are both internal and external to the organization. During this stage, available information sources are determined, and best practice providers are identified on either a relative or a comparative basis. One method for identifying best practices is to use industry norms, such as the Malcolm Baldrige Award criteria (discussed later in this chapter).

Data make up a fundamental component of the benchmarking process. Primary and secondary data are collected following the selected method, and the information is analyzed and interpreted according to the users' benchmarking objectives. The results of the analysis are formatted in such a manner that the users can understand them and apply them to decision making.

The final stage of the benchmarking process is to take action based on the conclusions of data analysis. The action taken is guided by the initial objectives of the users of the benchmarking process. The array of possible actions includes simply writing a report of the activities, identifying a new set of objectives, and establishing a revised protocol of practice (that is, making some change in the way the organization or provider conducts its business). Some health care organizations sponsor physician profiling activities to enhance their ability to communicate with providers about their practice behaviors. The measurement of physician performance is an important quality improvement activity. The performance profiling tools used are generic to epidemiologic analysis and reporting.

Benchmarking by external organizations producing report cards is another widely used mechanism to describe top performers or best practices. *Consumer Reports* ("How Safe Is Your Hospital?" 2003) noted that report cards are becoming increasingly popular among health plans and other health organizations. However, no standardized data collection and reporting methods yet exist. This fact leads to criticism of results presented in report cards because ratings may vary widely, depending on the data analysis methodologies used.

Another quality improvement report card effort leading to improved outcomes and improved consumer awareness is the New York State Cardiac Advisory Committee report, titled "Coronary Artery Bypass Surgery in New York State" (New York State Department of Health, 2004). This report card, prepared every two years since the early 1990s, presents adjusted mortality outcomes from all facilities and surgeons certified to perform coronary artery bypass grafts (CABGs). The results assess performance of hospitals and surgeons over time, independent of the severity of individual patients' preoperative conditions. This report has been used to evaluate the "higher volume, better outcomes" theory. This theory implies that facilities and surgeons with more numerous CABG procedures will have better mortality outcomes compared to low-volume facilities and surgeons. Managerial epidemiology plays a major role in interpreting risk-adjusted results. The report states that "extreme outcome rates may occur due to chance alone. This is particularly true for low-volume providers, for whom very high or very low mortality rates are more likely to occur than for high-volume providers. To prevent misinterpretation of differences caused by chance variation, confidence intervals are used" (p. 11).

Best Practices and Practice Guidelines

A best practice can be defined as a service or process that has been improved and implemented to produce superior outcomes (Hiebler, Kelly, and Ketteman, 1998). Best practices result in benchmarks that meet or exceed an existing performance standard. A guideline reflects the state of current knowledge regarding clinical effectiveness and appropriateness of practices.

The notion of "best" indicates optimal performance as a relative comparison across providers. The purpose of the identification process is to enable implementation of modifications that allow practicing hospitals and health care professionals to begin to perform similarly to optimal providers. The goals of best practices are to improve clinical outcomes, improve administrative efficiency, and reduce health care costs.

Best practices may not be evidence-based. Evidence-based practices use available evidence in an attempt to provide clinically effective and cost-effective care to a population. This evidence is derived from rigorous scientific research and evaluations of health care interventions.

When health care practice patterns are related to provider performance, it is important to review several perspectives. First, cause and effect should be assessed; for example, infant mortality and neonatal mortality must be separated because of differing sources of causation. Second, classifying health issues by disease results in information with respect to morbidity, mortality, and cause.

Health resource utilization is also important to evaluating performance. Resources refer to areas of human, physical, and financial resources. An inventory must be established of all three types of health resources, including a survey of the geographic distribution of resources.

Practice guidelines are gaining in popularity, in the managed care arena in particular. Most guidelines are based on clinical and process evidence that has been observed in the population. The intent of these practice guidelines is to explicitly assist physicians in diagnosis and treatment. The result of the application of practice guidelines is the efficient use of time and resources and the optimal management of medical processes.

The use of practice guidelines can be illustrated with antiviral treatment to prevent cytomegalovirus disease in adults after renal transplantation (Jassal and others, 1998). The practice guidelines were based on evidence collected from physicians, patients, epidemiologic information, experts in the field, and meta-analyses. The specific guidelines were as follows: recommended prophylaxis for seropositive recipient and seropositive or seronegative donor, recommended prophylaxis for seronegative recipient and seropositive donor, no recommendation for seronegative recipient and seronegative donor, and prophylaxis left to the discretion of the physician for recipients and donor with conventional immunosuppression.

Several concepts and notions are typically mentioned in the context of best practices. These are practice standards, critical pathways, and clinical protocols. A practice standard is a statement that outlines performance expectations or processes that must be implemented to enhance the quality of care. A critical pathway is a patient management tool related to clinical practice guidelines. Critical pathways outline the process, timeline, and benchmarks for fulfilling the patient's clinical needs. Hospitals often use them as a cost control method to meet fixed and capitated payment systems. Critical pathways involve the entire patient's care team, from preadmission through discharge. A protocol, or algorithm, is an organized method of analyzing and treating a disease or condition. These concepts may be considered a best practice if they produce superior outcomes and are clinically efficient and cost-effective.

Application of Best Practice Assessment

Best practice assessment has been applied to the development of an analytic scoring model that can be used to identify best practices in delivery of neonatal intensive care services. Performance of neonatal intensive care systems is of great concern to providers, payers, and recipients of care. This model allows for the ranking and rating of associated parameters according to their relative impact on performance (Fos, Bowen, and Zúniga, 1999).

The establishment of priorities is a focal point of health care decision making and evaluation. After establishing priorities, every subsequent activity constitutes progress toward desired goals. A necessary skill for establishing priorities is the ability to balance the importance of very different and multidimensional variables. Establishment of priorities is intuitive and subjective, requiring insight, experience, and wisdom. Therefore, this task is optimally accomplished during a very structured and well-defined exercise. The method used to assess performance focuses on the development of a scoring system that assigns a numeric score to each hospital's performance. This score represents a hospital's current performance according to the measurement parameters, by which a hospital may be ranked relative to all hospitals in the health care system to reflect relative performance.

Not all variables have an equal influence on outcomes (Edwards, 1970). Given this variation, there must be some mechanism to account for the variance of influence among variables. One method is to assign weights to each variable to reflect the relative influence of each variable on the outcome of interest (Keeney and Raiffa, 1976). In other words, weights assigned to variables reflect their percentage of the overall performance score. The best practice scoring model was tested on a subsample of hospitals of a large national neonatal intensive care health care system. Thirty hospitals were selected from the sample based on geographic, hospital size, and hospital type characteristics.

Performance scores ranged from 72.317 to 14.540 (with 100 the highest possible score and 0 the lowest), indicating a rather wide distribution. The optimally performing hospital had a performance score that was seven times higher than that of the lowest-scoring hospital.

If the scoring of hospitals is distributed in thirds (top, middle, and bottom), the occurrence of outliers, costs associated with outliers, and the chance of an outlier can be studied. There were 265 outliers in the study period, with each outlier having a cost equal to $70,000. The optimally performing hospital experienced no outliers during the one-year study period, and the lowest-scoring hospital had 3.5% of the outliers in the thirty-hospital system. When the top ten hospitals in terms of performance were compared with the bottom twenty hospitals, the top ten had a significantly lower proportion of outliers ($p = 0.02$). When the middle ten hospitals were compared with the bottom ten hospitals, the same relationship was seen, with the middle ten having a significantly lower proportion of outliers ($p = 0.04$).

Relative risks were calculated for the different scoring categories of these thirty hospitals. Similar differences between scoring categories were seen. Hospitals in the middle and lower thirds had a 1.5 times greater chance of an outlier when compared to hospitals in the upper third. This represents an increased probability of 50%. Hospitals in the lower third had a 1.55 times greater chance of an outlier when compared to hospitals in the middle third. Again, this represents an increased probability of 50%. Hospitals can be encouraged to improve their performance to reduce the probability of the occurrence of an outlier.

Quality of Health Care

Monitoring and evaluating the quality of medical services requires that the investigator collect and analyze information. Quality assurance, or quality control, and associated clinical improvement activities focus on using information to achieve quality medical care and clinical improvement. Central to this process is interpreting useful information from final outcomes and process data. Epidemiologic methods are used to identify, collect, analyze, and interpret these data.

Performance of medical services is measured with respect to several parameters. One parameter is actual quality of care. Quality variables, including satisfaction and final health outcomes, are important components of the evaluations of clinical performance. The intermediate process outcomes also affect performance.

Quality measurement is based on establishing and using a method for information generation. Information is generated from data that are collected using epidemiologic study designs. Following the population-based management approach, outcomes measures should include population data. Necessary information includes population health data, functional status at the time of discharge, patient satisfaction, and process data (length of stay, number of readmissions, postoperative complication rate, number of diagnostic tests, and so on).

Quality assessment involves defining quality measurements, selecting performance criteria, identifying expected performance levels, and establishing a data collection and analysis plan. Epidemiologic data are indispensable in assessing quality of care. Process and final health outcome variables include epidemiologic data. Process variables measure intermediate outcomes throughout the health care delivery process, including compliance data. Final health outcomes variables measure the health status of patients resulting from health care services, including patient satisfaction data.

Quality indicators are used in an attempt to measure and quantify quality of care. A valid indicator must have the ability to measure what it is intended to measure. In addition, an indicator must be evaluated as to how well it measures the intended concept. Validity and reliability of an indicator are important aspects whenever quality-of-care concerns arise.

Quality measures include mortality rates, case-fatality rates, readmission rates, average length-of-stay days, patient satisfaction, and discharge status. The CMS's use of hospital mortality rates to describe quality of care is one example. Mortality and case-fatality rates are commonly used as quality indicators, but questions arise as to the validity of using mortality rates as an indicator of hospital performance. Many factors in addition to quality of care affect mortality rates.

Quality of care is a concept that is not easily defined. One widely accepted definition is that of the Institute of Medicine (2001, p. 79), which defines quality as "the degree to which health services for individuals and populations increase the likelihood of desired health outcomes and are consistent with current professional knowledge." This definition was instrumental in providing the framework for the adoption of the three-way classification of quality problems. These classification categories are (1) underuse, which is the "failure to provide an effective health care service when it would have produced favorable outcomes" (for example, missed prenatal care or proportion of patients with diabetes type II not detected early); (2) overuse, which is the "provision of a health service when its risk of harm exceeds its potential benefit" (for example, indiscriminate antibiotic prescribing or a high rate of laboratory tests); and (3) misuse, which is defined as "avoidable complications of appropriate health care" (Institute of Medicine, 2001, p. 194).

Historically, quality of medical care has been measured by reviewing medical records and administrative claims data for unexpected complications and outcomes. Medical record review is a less than optimal method to measure quality because of problems with record interpretation (Jollis and others, 1993). Recently, several alternative methods have been established to review and analyze quality of medical care by focusing on the correlation of outcomes to quality.

Since 2003, the CMS has sponsored the Hospital Quality Incentive Demonstration Project. The goal of this three-year program is to determine whether economic incentives have an effect on improving the quality of hospital inpatient care. The CMS is measuring and paying incentives for high-quality inpatient care among a group of 278 hospitals. Five conditions are targeted for optimal quality-of-care services: acute myocardial infarction, coronary artery bypass graft, heart failure, community-acquired pneumonia, and hip and knee replacement. The project categorizes hospitals by clinical area. The top ten performing hospitals will realize an increase of 2% in their Medicare base rate in the targeted clinical area. Low-performing hospitals in the third year will realize a payment reduction of 1% or 2%. Benchmarks for low performance are results beyond a minimum threshold set during the first year (Centers for Medicare and Medicaid Services, 2004).

Statistical Process Control

Statistical process control (as discussed in Chapter Seven) deals with the analysis and interpretation of data. These activities help the quality improvement practitioner identify what changes are occurring in health care processes and how the changes are affecting outcomes. Statistical process control was developed to evaluate quality in manufacturing. Applications in health care are frequently performed in standardized processes, like surgical procedures to correct strabismus (Self and Enzenauer, 2004). When an indicator is repeatedly measured in time, the results often fluctuate around a mean or a center value. This observed variation is known as common-cause variation because the variability is the product of inherent factors.

Large fluctuations in variability are usually externally induced. This externally induced variability is known as special-cause variation. Special-cause variation is crucial to the understanding of changes brought about by quality improvement interventions. Control charts are tools used to depict variability in statistical process control. The control chart has two components: a series of quantified observations charted in time sequence and the control boundaries and center lines (Benneyan, Lloyd, and Plsek, 2003). These lines are usually labeled the upper control limit (UCL), the lower control limit (LCL), and the center line (usually a mean value). The UCL, LCL, and center line are data-driven, and repeated measures will produce a fluctuation of these control limits.

The control limits are statistically set to expand to 3 standard deviations above and below the center line. This is an example of 6-sigma variation. When observations vary within the control limits, we assume a common-cause variation; when observations vary beyond the control limits, we assume a special-cause variation.

Six-Sigma Technology

Six-sigma technologies refer to the use of tools to reduce process variation to statistically measurable processes. *Six-sigma* is a statistical term that refers to 3.4 defects per million opportunities (or 99.99966% accuracy); in control charts, 6 sigma is equivalent to 3 standard deviations above and below the center line value. A defect can be a faulty surgical implement, a wrong dose of a medication, or an incorrect patient bill. Six-sigma initiatives use detailed and rigorous data collection and statistical analysis to identify sources of errors and to find ways to eliminate them. The define-measure-analyze-improve-control methodology provides a road map to reduce variation to a point where standardization aids in improving health outcomes and reducing waste (Goedert, 2004).

Six-sigma uses graphic data tools to represent and exemplify qualitative and quantitative data collection efforts with the intent of solving a problem, learning from the experience, and standardizing the process. The most common graphic data tools are checklists, flowcharts, cause-and-effect diagrams, histograms, Pareto charts, scatter diagrams, and control charts (Torpy, 2002).

Checklists, or affinity diagrams, are products of quality improvement team brainstorming efforts. They offer an organized and thematic representation of important information to standardize a process (see Figure 8.2).

Flowcharts are pictorial representations that describe a process. They are used to plan stages of a project and provide people with a common language and reference point for a project or process. Figure 8.3 shows some common elements used in flowcharts. Analysis of actual-process and best-process flowcharts allows the discovery of areas where there is variation. It is the identification and management of variation that leads to correction of defects and standardization of processes.

Cause-and-effect diagrams depict factors leading to an outcome in an inverted event tree format. These inverted event trees are also called fishbone diagrams. The effect node is the primary concern for improvement, and the cause nodes are the branches affecting the effect node. Consensus among quality improvement experts is sought to identify the causal factors for the selected outcome (see Figure 8.4).

FIGURE 8.2. A CHECKLIST.

	Develop marketing strategy		Implement Web portal		Develop customer-centered training
O	Task	O	Task	O	Task
O	Task	O	Task	O	Task
O	Task	O	Task	O	Task

FIGURE 8.3. A FLOWCHART.

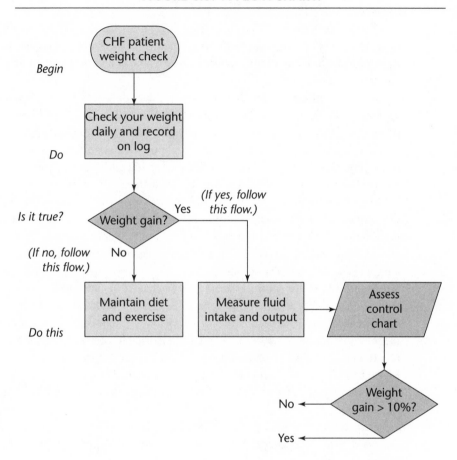

FIGURE 8.4. A CAUSE-AND-EFFECT OR FISHBONE DIAGRAM.

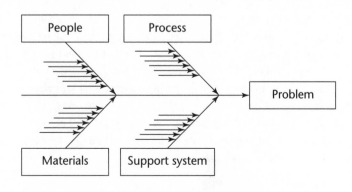

Histograms provide a graphic view of the accumulated data dispersion and central tendency (see Figure 8.5).

Pareto charts are specialized histograms; categories are ranked from most frequent to least frequent, making them useful for nonnumeric data. Pareto charts help the quality improvement team identify priority areas where action and process change are required (see Figure 8.6).

Scatter diagrams are graphic tools representing the relationship of one variable value to another variable value. For example, Figure 8.7 shows the distributions of physical and mental health summary scores in a south Texas population.

One illustration of the use of statistical process control involves a quality improvement program in a public health agency (Fos and others, 2005). Statistical process control was used as a tool to monitor improvement of latent tuberculosis infection (LTBI) control management efforts implemented statewide by the Mississippi State Department of Health quality improvement team. Quality improvement tools were used to measure LTBI medication completion rates before and after disease management intervention targeting statewide improvement by establishing an intermediate goal of a 95% completion rate.

Statistical process control was used to create control charts to depict spatial and temporal variability across health districts. Regression analysis was used to compare significance of pre- and postintervention LTBI medication completion rates. Resulting from this intervention was a mean LTBI medication currency rate for the twelve-month period of 89.5%, with a standard deviation of 4.2. A change from a rate of 84.1% to 95.0% was accomplished after the quality improvement team issued a memorandum establishing the goals and procedures to improve the LTBI medication currency rate. Further analysis revealed that the mean was significantly increased in all health districts except one. This effort appears to be a successful approach for managing a disease state using statistical process control as a quality improvement tool. Figure 8.8 depicts the quality control chart for the twelve-month study period.

The Malcolm Baldrige National Quality Program

The U.S. Department of Commerce established the Malcolm Baldrige National Quality Program in the 1990s to promote quality across all industries. The overall objective of the program is to improve the competitiveness of U.S. industries throughout the world. The specific objectives are to improve performance capabilities, to facilitate communication about best practices among and within U.S. industries, and to serve as a working model for understanding and managing performance, planning, and training (National Institute of Standards and Technology, 1999). Central to the concept of the Baldrige program is the relationship between the health care provider organization and the population.

FIGURE 8.5. A HISTOGRAM.

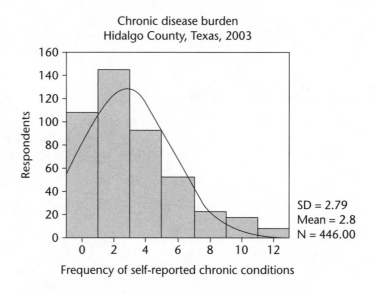

Chronic disease burden
Hidalgo County, Texas, 2003

SD = 2.79
Mean = 2.8
N = 446.00

Frequency of self-reported chronic conditions

FIGURE 8.6. A PARETO CHART.

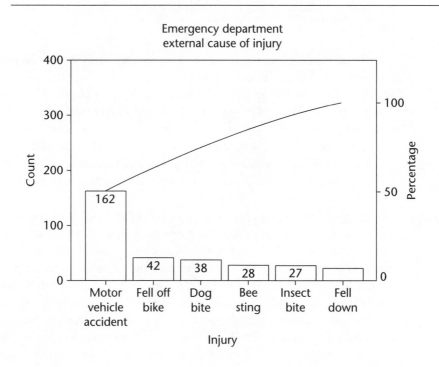

Emergency department
external cause of injury

Injury

FIGURE 8.7. A SCATTER DIAGRAM.

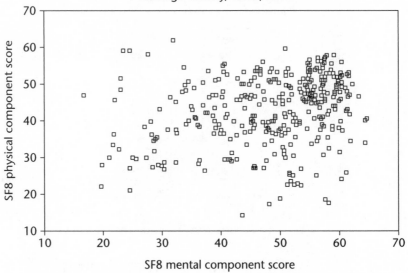

Adult physical and mental component scores
Hidalgo County, Texas, 2003

Source: Zúniga, Blakely, and Tromp, 2003.

The Baldrige program is based on core criteria, which are the foundation for the results-oriented quality improvement program. These criteria are customer-oriented quality, leadership, continuous improvement, valuing employees, rapid response, design quality and prevention, long-range view of the future, managing by facts, partnership development, community responsibility, and results focused (National Institute of Standards and Technology, 1999). The Malcolm Baldrige National Quality Award is presented to U.S. organizations that volunteer to undergo a self-assessment. Eligible for the award are business, education, health care, and not-for-profit organizations.

The Baldrige award, given to a maximum of three organizations a year, has seven categories of criteria: leadership, strategic planning, customer and market focus, information and analysis, human resource focus, process management, and business results. Leadership involves both organizational leadership and community responsibility. Strategic planning is focused on strategy development and deployment. Customer and market knowledge as well as customer satisfaction are evaluated. The processes of measurement and analysis of organizational performance are reviewed. The human resource focus is concerned with the structure of work systems, employee development, and employee satisfaction. Process management is associated with product and

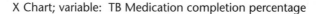

FIGURE 8.8. A QUALITY CONTROL CHART.

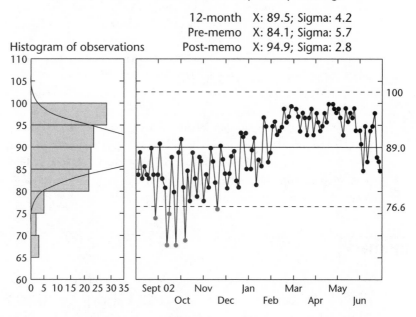

X Chart; variable: TB Medication completion percentage

	12-month	X: 89.5; Sigma: 4.2
	Pre-memo	X: 84.1; Sigma: 5.7
Histogram of observations	Post-memo	X: 94.9; Sigma: 2.8

service, support, supplier, and partnering processes. Business results are defined by customer-focused, financial and market, human resource, supplier and partner, and organizational effectiveness results.

Quality of Life and Global Burden of Disease

Quality-of-life outcomes measures incorporate individual perceptions of health care services into the assessment process. Psychometric multidimensional quality-of-life measures developed for the general population are called generic measures; multidimensional specific measures for selected populations are known as condition-specific measures. Measures represented by a single score or value include quality-adjusted life years (QALYs), quality-adjusted life expectancy (QALE), quality-adjusted healthy life years (QAHLYs), health-adjusted life years (HALYs), health-adjusted life expectancy (HALE), disability-adjusted life years (DALYs), and disability-adjusted life expectancy (DALE) (Drummond, Stoddart, and Torrance, 1994; Gold, Stevenson, and Fryback, 2002).

These measures of quality of life were developed in an attempt to express in one construct all health dimensions that are affected by health care services. The QALY quantifies a health outcome by assignment of a weight that represents the quality of life for a period of one year. Typically, a weight of 1 equals perfect health and 0 indicates death.

The weights are assigned by individual patients according to the foundations of utility theory and can be thought of as a measure of individual willingness to trade years of life in their present health state for a reduced number of years of perfect health. In this form, QALY represents an estimate of health-related utility for outcomes of specific health care interventions. QALE and QAHLY are modifications of this basic principle of health-related utility.

The World Health Organization sponsors an initiative called the Global Burden of Disease (GBD) (Murray and Lopez, 1996). This project uses available epidemiologic estimates of diseases, injuries, and risk factors to calculate GBD scores utilizing DALYs as a summary measure. The WHO *World Health Report, 2002* used epidemiologic data to rank all WHO members based on the GBD scores. This effort sought to develop a comparable, valid, and reliable epidemiologic information tool for a wide range of diseases, injuries, and risk factors.

Summary

Health outcomes have been increasingly important to managers in both fee-for-service and managed care environments. Epidemiology provides the methodologic framework needed to collect, analyze, and interpret data on health outcomes. Outcomes assessment focuses on both effectiveness and quality of health care.

Health outcomes are multidimensional, measuring physical, mental, and functional status. Functional status is further specified into health-related quality-of-life measures. Commonly used health-related quality-of-life measures include quality-adjusted life years.

Outcomes assessment is useful in cost analysis, cost-effectiveness analysis, establishment of clinical best practices through benchmarking, and quality-related reimbursement strategies. Outcomes are used for evaluation of performance of health care providers and can be expected to enjoy an increasingly important place in reimbursement mechanisms and provider panel selection processes.

With the advent of outcomes assessment, quality-of-care analysis has broadened its perspective. Patient satisfaction is a commonly used measure of the performance of health care providers. These measures are evaluated in conjunction with traditional medical record review.

Population health surveys have evolved over the past forty years. These surveys are in the form of indices and profiles. Such measures are important in assessing the health of a population, establishing baselines for future comparisons, evaluating health care policy, and making resource allocation decisions. Population health surveys have become specialized to address both general health and condition-specific health measurement.

Study Questions

1. The federal agency for Health Research and Quality produces a consumer-based checklist called "Your Guide to Choosing Quality Health Care" shown below. Using Donabedian's approach to quality-of-care measures, **S**tructure-**P**rocess-**O**utcome, mark with the letter S, P, or O each of the items on the checklist based on its role in quality-of-care measurement. Discuss the following question: Do a majority of indicators represent any of the quality measures or are the indicators evenly distributed between the measures?

Your Guide to Choosing Quality Health Care
Quick Checks for Quality

S/P/O

Look for a plan that

- ☐ Does a good job of helping people stay well and get better.
- ☐ Is accredited, if that is important to you.
- ☐ Has the doctors and hospitals you want or need.
- ☐ Provides the benefits you need.
- ☐ Provides services where and when you need them.
- ☐ Meets your budget.

Look for a doctor who

- ☐ Is rated to give quality care.
- ☐ Has the training and background that meet your needs.
- ☐ Takes steps to prevent illness (for example, talks to you about quitting smoking).
- ☐ Has privileges at the hospital of your choice.
- ☐ Is part of your health plan, unless you can afford to pay extra.
- ☐ Encourages you to ask questions.
- ☐ Listens to you.
- ☐ Explains things clearly.
- ☐ Treats you with respect.

Look for a hospital that

- ☐ Is accredited by the Joint Commission on Accreditation of Healthcare Organizations.
- ☐ Is rated highly by state or consumer or other groups.
- ☐ Is one where your doctor has privileges, if that is important to you
- ☐ Is covered by your health plan.
- ☐ Has experience with your condition.
- ☐ Has had success with your condition.
- ☐ Checks and works to improve its own quality of care.

2. Quality improvement organizations are focusing efforts on the health care delivery problems of underuse and overuse. How can clinical practice guidelines and treatment protocols aid in improving health outcomes and the quality of health care services? What is a practical source of evidence-based clinical practice guidelines?

3. What epidemiologic tools are used by quality improvement teams to enhance the quality of care and health outcomes using a six-sigma approach?

4. Describe current efforts to standardize the assessment of patient satisfaction and patient expectations. Use the CAHPS and HCAHPS initiatives for your discussion.

CHAPTER NINE

MARKETING HEALTH CARE FOR POPULATIONS

Chapter Outline

Introduction
Marketing and Population Health
Market Research
Summary
Study Questions

Learning Objectives

Upon completing this chapter, the reader will be able to do all of the following:

- Describe sampling techniques
- Discuss the role of epidemiology in marketing
- Discuss the new role of marketing in designing health care for populations
- Discuss the impact of epidemiology in market research

Introduction

Epidemiologic methods and data have been used for planning, developing, implementing, and evaluating health care services for many years. With respect to payment mechanisms, epidemiologic indicators of morbidity and mortality are of particular interest. For example, in fee-for-service and indemnity insurance methods of payment, these measures provide information necessary to measure organizational performance.

The advent of the Prospective Payment System (PPS) in 1982 and subsequent expansion of capitated methods of reimbursement have created opportunities to use additional epidemiologic information. PPS has increased the complexity of management in the health care industry, introducing an era in which health care managers must analyze and synthesize information with enhanced epidemiologic models in order to continue to plan, implement, and evaluate various programs and services. PPS has increased the impact of micro-level financial performance data that can be shared with physicians to illustrate the financial impact of their practice patterns.

This chapter will present the relationship of epidemiology to marketing and planning for health care services. The new role of health care marketing in designing and planning health care for populations will be outlined. In addition, sampling and marketing data and research will be discussed to highlight the role of formal analytic techniques.

Marketing and Population Health

Marketing is a management function that has not necessarily been performed with respect to population needs or population health. Traditional marketing is based on market surveys and focus groups, without a direct connection to population health information. Epidemiology is a natural bridge between traditional marketing practices and population health.

Marketing

Marketing can be defined as the art and science of understanding how people make choices and how they respond to their choices and of designing methods to influence their choice selection. The evolution to population-based health care has resulted in a change in the focus of marketing. Designing, planning, and financing health care for populations is changing decision making about the spending of health care dollars. Payers are evaluating the costs of health care and the associated benefits derived from the dollars spent.

Payers are exerting substantial pressure on the health care market, with cost containment as their goal. Payers are concentrating on negotiating discounted payment rates from providers of health care services and are increasingly entering into contract agreements with providers. These contracts describe discounted costs to payers and financial incentives to providers. A common theme in these contracts is capitation, a fixed payment per individual.

The focus on managing health care for populations has an effect on the manner in which health care marketing interacts and communicates with physicians, individual payers (for example, employers), and managed care entities. In the traditional role of health care management, individual users selected physicians, physicians selected hospitals to treat the individual users, and insurance programs financed the provision of health care services. Health care marketing concentrates on marketing physicians and hospitals to payers and individual users. This traditional perspective remains viable in markets dominated by fee-for-service reimbursement and low levels of managed care saturation.

In the evolving new role of health care management, which focuses on health care for populations, the traditional marketing activities may not be appropriate. In support of this new role, marketing attempts to market a comprehensive set of health care services as well as insurance. The payer is presented the planned health care services and insurance and then presents this plan to individual users, who make the final decision. This is a quite popular method for payers, because it allows the presentation of a series of options from which individual users may select their preferred choice.

The Role of Marketing

The traditional role of marketing has involved identifying product, price, promotion, and place aspects of a health care system's marketing plan. The product is the services that the health care system provides to its market, typically designed to meet its market's demands. The price is established to account for all costs associated with providing the product. Promotion encompasses activities that alert and educate the market about the product and its price. The place is where the product is offered to and used by the market and is identified on the basis of market demand (Berkowitz, 2004).

In designing health care for populations, objectives or marketing strategies are unchanged. Most traditional marketing activities are useful in this new role, particularly sound marketing research and public relations, but the focus of these objectives is modified. Traditionally, marketing efforts were directed at convincing individuals that a health care facility provided services that they should desire. To achieve objectives of health care for populations, marketing efforts must emphasize delivery of services that consumers need. This emphasis directly achieves the objectives of the traditional role of management and supports marketing to payers for health care services, including managed care organizations, traditional payers (third-party insurers), and out-of-pocket payers.

Marketing the Health Care System

In the traditional role of marketing, emphasis was placed on marketing the health care facility. The individual user was persuaded to think of physicians and hospitals. Marketing efforts were centered on distinguishing one hospital from another and one group of physicians from another. For example, typical marketing strategies centered around the notion that a facility possessed the best physicians and provided the best services. Individuals were encouraged to seek and purchase health care services at these facilities because of their superiority.

In marketing's new role, emphasis is placed on an integrated health care system that is designed to provide health care services for specific populations. Individual users choose between different delivery systems of health care services. Instead of attempting to convince individuals that a facility offers services that they should want to receive, marketing staff must research population needs as a basis for planning services.

Market Research

To successfully facilitate the shift in focus to designing health care for populations, the needs of the markets must be understood. This understanding requires information. One method for obtaining needed information is to translate epidemiologic and patient data into market research data. This information allows health care managers to shift to an external market-based (or population-based) focus.

Marketing involves establishing goals and objectives, estimating service demand, allocating available resources, and developing a method of monitoring and evaluation. Health care managers use internal information routinely, so acknowledging the need for information is not novel. But strategic market planning requires other data from external sources, due to the need to understand populations. Aggregating both internal and external data allows for the assessment of the current situation, as well as establishing future goals and objectives.

Sampling

Associated with selecting a study design is the principle of sampling. Data are collected by either random or systematic sampling. Sample data must reflect the characteristics of the population from which they are selected, in both the mean value and variability. Random samples possess this characteristic. Randomization is a notion that is important to ensure validity, because any attempt to influence the sample selection by human intervention is very likely to result in a study sample that is biased and does not accurately represent the total population. Random selection is the only method that can be used to ensure an unbiased study sample. The most common method of random selection is the use of a random number table that selects a sequence of numbers, or individuals, in the total study sample.

Systematic sampling involves the selection of a study sample that has the same unbiased characteristics as a random sample. To achieve this, a sampling fraction is used and a randomly preselected proportion of a population is included in the sample. For example, a sampling fraction of 1 in 50 would result in the selection of the first person and successive individuals at intervals of 50 (the 51st, 101st, 151st, and so on).

In addition to the specific study design, the sampling design is an important consideration. There are several commonly used sampling designs, including stratified, cluster, and multistage sampling. Stratified sampling is used when populations consist of a number of clearly defined subpopulations, known as strata. Using a process called stratification (see Chapter Five), data describing separate samples in each stratum are collected for analysis. Examples of population strata include age categories, males, females, whites, and African Americans.

Cluster sampling follows the concept that individuals in a population are found in natural groups, or clusters. Cluster sampling involves randomly selecting individuals from a cluster or grouping. For example, individuals are usually observed living in families, living in the same building, or living in the same subdivision of a city. Cluster sampling is advantageous due to decreased cost of sampling, the fact that data collection is concentrated in a relatively small number of locations, and the fact that it provides unbiased results.

Multistage sampling is used because individuals in a population can commonly be defined in a hierarchical manner. With respect to a hospital, there are employees and patients in a department, departments in the hospital, and hospitals in a network. Operationally, at each stage of the hierarchy, basic units are selected at random. Of the selected units, some corresponding subunits are selected at random. This specification continues until the study's needs are satisfied.

Market Research Data Analysis

Health care organizations have collected vast amounts of information for many years. But these data have not been fully employed to plan and design health care for populations. In fact, these data had little value in the traditional role of marketing. More recently, due to demands of payers and providers, health care data collection has improved significantly.

As discussed in Chapter Two, there are two basic types of data: primary and secondary. Primary data are collected to address a specific research concern or, as in this case, a specific market research concern. Primary data are frequently collected because needed information is not available. Primary data are characterized by high quality, but the collection process has some disadvantages. Collection is very costly and time-intensive, and designing and administering primary data collection surveys are difficult tasks with respect to validity and reliability, requiring a specific level of expertise.

Secondary data are routinely collected by others. The use of secondary data may not be directly correlated with those who collected it, but the data can be useful for other purposes. Health care marketing research makes frequent use of secondary data, which are readily available and typically inexpensive.

Marketing research data can be categorized as either internal or external. By definition, internal data are collected inside the organization, and external data are collected outside the organization, by others. Routinely collected epidemiologic data are an example of external data. These data indicate changes in populations served by health care systems that will affect the demand for health care services. Further, they help in identifying needed services and targeting segments of the population for outreach treatment and educational efforts.

Internal data illustrate the vast amount of information that has been collected over time by health care organizations as a result of providing health care services. All health care organizations have valuable information about their populations in their internal records. Internal data exist in the form of patient characteristics, financial information, health service use patterns and trends, and resource allocation and use.

One component of a hospital's internal data is known as case mix. Case mix can be defined as the measurement of the number of patients, types of patients, illnesses, and treated conditions. Patient data include information about age, sex, diagnosis, procedures, date of service, payer information, and physician. Case mix analysis is a process that relates patient demographics, clinical data, and financial data to hospital performance data.

Collection of external data is becoming increasingly important in the population-based environment of health care. Information about the characteristics of patients who receive health care services at a specific institution may not necessarily reflect the characteristics of the population. Demographic data are central to market research activities, and the characteristics of a target population and the health and disease status of this population are essential information for planning and market analysis.

Descriptive analysis identifies the characteristics of a population. This description can be accomplished using internal and external epidemiologic data. Case mix analysis is an excellent example of how epidemiologic data and methods can be used in marketing research. Data can be used in both a descriptive and comparative sense, with descriptive data allowing for interpretation of current status of the health care provider. These data can serve as baseline information for future study. For example, descriptive data can outline length-of-stay trends by service, disease or condition diagnosis, or treating physician.

Analytic analysis is accomplished using specific epidemiologic methods, including standardization of information and study designs (see Chapters Four and Five). Because the calculation of rates (see Chapter Three) is an important aspect of market research analysis, standardization of data is essential. Standardization allows for accounting for any potential confounding factors that may result in misinterpretation of market analysis.

Epidemiologic data that can prove useful are disease rates, mortality rates, and utilization rates. Important data include physician information, hospital-specific utilization rates, and hospital-specific disease rates. If specific demographic information is known, target areas can be identified for marketing activities. Population growth patterns, which may be a cause of an increase in utilization, can indicate a need for expansion of services and resources.

Associated with demographic information are other patient characteristics that are of interest for marketing of services. Patient payer classification proportions indicate potential revenue sources and estimates of expected revenue. Correlation of reimbursement rates by payer and payer proportions of patients can be used to determine expected revenue sources, expected revenue levels, and areas to target for increased revenue. For example, if a significant proportion of patients represent payers with a home health care benefit, a strategic marketing effort could be to develop or expand services in this area.

Epidemiologic data can be useful in identifying a market and the level of need for new service. This evaluation can be accomplished by reviewing historical internal data as well as external data. For example, if a health system plans to begin a neonatal intensive care service, the number of premature or low-birth-weight deliveries in the past must be identified for analysis. This information is used to identify characteristics of mothers who are at risk of having newborns in need of intensive care. In addition, population parameters such as infant mortality rate, neonatal mortality rate, low-birth-weight rate, fertility rate, percentage of pregnancies in teenage mothers, and proportion of mothers who receive adequate prenatal care should be reviewed to determine population need. Comparative data allow for contrasting and illustration of differences among areas of interest.

Patient Satisfaction

Satisfaction has become an important measure for outcomes assessment research. Satisfaction has always been a concern for health care marketing research efforts. In the new role of marketing, as is the case in outcomes assessment, patient satisfaction is used to assess the quality of care from the patients' perspective. For marketing and administrative purposes, satisfaction is useful for patient complaint management and as baseline data. For outcomes assessment purposes, satisfaction is becoming a measure of performance evaluation in the delivery of health care services. Satisfaction measurements can be used as goals for reimbursement and other reward incentives.

Patient satisfaction is the fundamental measure of how patients and payers feel about the interaction with the health care system. Satisfaction is measured on both the clinical and service aspects of this interaction. The actual measurement of satisfaction is quite difficult because of the problem of defining what is meant by satisfaction. This is due to the level of understanding of the health care delivery process by the population. In spite of this difficulty, understanding patient satisfaction is essential in developing approaches to improve the quality of care and health outcomes. Satisfaction with health care services received is a fundamental concern for managers.

Given this concern for patient satisfaction, a significant effort has occurred in the study of this area, focused on quality improvement. A study of office-based management of diabetes patients showed that psychological and economic concerns of patients must be considered to achieve optimal care (Goldsmith, Ward, and Howard, 2004). Radiation oncology patients who received a nutrition intervention demonstrated greater compliance and better outcomes than patients receiving the usual care regimen (Isenring, Capra, and Bauer, 2004). In addition, the patients who received a nutrition intervention reported higher overall satisfaction with the radiation oncology treatment. A study among elderly patients indicated that in situations in which the physician participated to a greater extent in the treatment, patient satisfaction was significantly higher (Xu, 2004).

To this end, a set of constructs of satisfaction has been identified that addresses the multiple issues, of differing importance, that determine satisfaction (Berkowitz, Pol, and Thomas, 1997). These constructs are accessibility and convenience, availability of resources, continuity of care, efficacy and outcomes of care, financial considerations, humaneness, information gathering, information distribution, pleasantness of surroundings, and quality and competence of health care personnel.

Demand Estimation

Forecasting demand for health care services in a population provides valuable information for management decision making. Staffing and physical resources allocation decisions are dependent on estimating the future demand in a population. One source of demand data is past utilization, but this information is often inadequate for accurate estimation of future demand because it describes only past demand for a subset of the entire population.

Given the absence of adequate or complete data, estimates, projections, and forecasts must be used for planning for future demand. Population estimates can originate from secondary sources, including the U.S. Census Bureau and other federal and state governmental agencies. It is often difficult to obtain estimates for a subpopulation or a small area because of the manner in which data are collected across the population. For example, U.S. Census Bureau data are specified to the block level, but for some subpopulations, this may not be adequate. This results in the need to use forecasting methods, including estimates and projections.

An estimate can be defined as a calculation for a current or past period (Berkowitz, Pol, and Thomas, 1997). Estimates usually are based on actual data from specified time periods. Prevalence measures are often estimates of the current disease distribution in a population.

Conversely, projections are estimates for some period of time in the future. Projection is based on past information but is a process of revising these data and projecting them into the future. Projections may be crude reflections of past trends or may be adjusted according to known or expected changes in the population. In practice, projections are presented as a series of data points, along with the assumptions used for the projected series.

Forecasts, like projections, reflect expectations in the future. Forecasts are characterized by their singular nature and are not reported as a series of data points. Forecasts are calculated statistically by applying either extrapolation or interpolation methods.

Demand estimation models allow for the development of estimates and projections of utilization of health care services within and across populations. For marketing research purposes, these methods can be used for estimating hospital admissions or outpatient utilization according to population strata. Demand estimation models can be classified as traditional utilization projections and population-based and econometric models.

Traditional utilization projections typically involve crude projections of utilization based on historical trends in the data. If past trends reflected increasing utilization, the projection would illustrate the same increase. These projections are not commonly used because the past is not a valid guide to future utilization of health care services.

Population-based models are characterized by population estimates and projections and valid utilization rates. One frequently used population-based model is to determine the product of the projected population and known utilization rates. Using the population numbers as a core component of the demand estimation, these models are becoming the most popular. This is due to the fact that the size of the population is the most significant factor in determining future utilization. Other factors influencing the popularity of these models are the availability of population data and the presentation of population information according to demographic characteristics.

Econometric models are used to project future situations under differing and complex conditions. Econometric models are a specialized type of time-series models that attempt to predict future trends through statistical manipulation of past information. Econometric models allow for forecasting in light of the effects of multiple factors over time. These models develop statistical equations that forecast utilization as a function of the relationship between the multiple factors.

Validity and Reliability of Market Research

Whenever information is collected by surveying a population, two concerns are important. The first is whether the survey measures what it is designed to measure; this is associated with the concept of validity. A second concern is whether the survey results can be replicated under similar situations; this is the concept of reliability. Both validity and reliability are multidimensional constructs.

Validity can be measured by face, content, construct, and criterion. Face validity is simple and straightforward: if the survey appears to be measuring what it is designed to measure, face validity is supported.

Content validity is concerned with whether the survey offers an adequate sample of what it is designed to measure. To support content validity, survey items should cover the range of dimensions of the phenomenon under study. For example, a survey on patient satisfaction with an outpatient dermatology clinic should address all points of contact a patient will experience during a clinic visit.

Content validity relies on judgments about whether the questions chosen are representative of the concepts they are intended to reflect. In other words, content validity refers to how good a sample of the empirical measures is of the theoretical domain they are presumed to represent. So it is important that there be some clear notion of the domain or universe of meaning implied in the concept being evaluated.

One way to ensure that a series of questions has a fair amount of content validity is to begin with questions and variables on the topic that have been used in other studies. In addition, expert consultants in the area may be asked whether in their judgment the questions being asked adequately represent the concept.

In the Medical Outcomes Study, researchers were interested in validating empirical measures of the dimensions of physical, mental, and social functioning and well-being, as well as general health perceptions and satisfaction. Content validity analysis involved thorough reviews of the literature on the concepts and measures within each dimension. The content of questions was then compared with the universe of items distilled from the literature review to evaluate whether at least one item was included to represent each of the major dimensions of health and certain concepts within each dimension (for example, depression and anxiety within the mental health dimension) and whether a sufficient number of items were included to represent adequately each dimension and concept (Stewart and Ware, 1992).

Construct validity evaluates both the survey and the underlying theory about what the survey is designed to measure. Convergent and discriminant validity are foundations of construct validity. Convergent validity is supported when different methods of measuring the same construct provide similar results. Discriminant validity is supported when different measures yield expected different results.

Criterion validity refers to the level of agreement between market research results and some external criterion. This demonstrates that survey results are systematically related to one or more external criteria. For example, criterion validity is supported if health status measured by survey in a population is negatively correlated with the population's resource use, the external criterion.

To evaluate the construct validity of a survey variable, it must be assumed that there are well-developed theories or hypotheses about the relationships of that variable to others being measured in the study. Construct validity examines whether and how many of the relationships predicted by these theories or hypotheses are empirically confirmed when the data are analyzed. The more often these hypothetical relationships are confirmed, the greater the construct validity.

Criterion validity refers to the extent to which the survey measure predicts or agrees with some criterion of the "true" value (or "gold standard") for the measure. The two major types of criterion-based validity are predictive and concurrent validity. Both types of criterion validity are generally quantified through correlation coefficients between the survey measure and the (future or concurrent) criterion source value. The higher the correlation, the greater the validity of the survey measure.

The predictive validity of a survey-based measure of functional status could be based on the correlation of this measure with the ability of the respondent to carry out certain physical tasks in the future. This form of validity analysis is used in designing tests to choose candidates for certain programs, such as health promotion programs, based on the correlation scores (of probable adherence) on screening tests with participants' later performance in the program (actual adherence).

Concurrent validity reflects the correspondence between survey measure and a criterion measure obtained at essentially the same point in time. Concurrent validity could be evaluated by correlating patient reports of the types of conditions for which they had seen three physicians during a year with the physicians' medical records for the same period of time.

In the Medical Outcomes Study, concurrent validity analysis included examining the correlation between a survey-based measure of depression and a gold standard measure derived from the *Diagnostic and Statistical Manual of Mental Disorders* (American Psychological Association, 1995). In addition, the correlation of a short-form measure of physical functioning with a validated longer-form measure of the same concept was examined (McHorney, Ware, and Raczek, 1993).

The distinction between criterion and construct validity analysis is primarily a function of the purpose of the analysis and the assumptions underlying it. Criterion validity examines primarily the strength of the association of the survey measure with what is deemed to be an accurate measure of the same concept. Construct validity tests whether a hypothesized association between the survey measure and a measure of the same concept, known as convergent validity, or a different concept, known as discriminant validity, is confirmed.

Correlational analysis is used to quantify construct validity. In the Medical Outcomes Study, it was hypothesized that different indicators of physical health (for example, physical functioning, mobility, and pain) would be correlated. Measures of physical health would not be highly correlated with measures of mental or social health. Measures of general health status and vitality would be correlated with the measures of physical health as well as with the mental and social health indicators. In the Medical Outcomes Study, construct validity analyses did confirm the hypothesized relationships for the health status variables (Stewart and Ware, 1992). The more that different measures meant to measure the same concept agree (in other words, the greater the convergence) and the more they differ from measures intended to measure other concepts, the greater the convergent and discriminant validity of the indicators.

Reliability of market research information can be measured by error, test-retest, and internal consistency. A market researcher must be able to identify reliability relative to absence of errors in the information. This is determined by error reliability. One way to think of this construct is to consider whether survey results obtained from a subset of the population are similar to what they would be if the entire population were surveyed.

If marketing surveys are repeated in the same population over time, test-retest reliability must be addressed. There is a chance that the Hawthorne effect, whereby the knowledge of being under study affects the behavior or responses of the subjects, may influence the results of repeated surveying (Last, 1995). Some stability of measures must be established to permit valid evaluation of the correlations between data collected at different points in time. Internal consistency is related to whether survey responses are consistent across data items. If three different survey questions are intended to measure health, all three responses must be similar, indicating the same level of health.

Internal consistency analysis is primarily used in constructing and evaluating summary scales. The sources of variation studied include the inconsistency or nonequivalence of different questions intended to measure the same concept. If the questions are not really equivalent, different conclusions about the concept will result, depending on which questions are used in constructing the summary scale to measure it.

The main procedures for estimating the internal consistency or intercorrelation among a number of different questions that are supposed to reflect the same concept are the correlated item–total correlation and the split-half and alpha reliability coefficients (Cronbach's alpha). Cronbach's alpha, or coefficient alpha, is the correlation coefficient used to estimate the degree of equivalence between answers to questions constructed in this fashion. The coefficient will be higher the greater the number of questions asked about the topic and the higher the average correlation between the scores for all possible combinations of the entire set of questions.

Summary

Planning of health care services involves collection, analysis, interpretation, and inferential application of information. Information is quantified as data that can be evaluated through statistical techniques. Statistical significance must be established before results of statistical analysis can be compared and interpreted for planning purposes. Central to statistical significance is adequate sample size.

Population-based health care requires a modification of traditional facility-based management strategic planning and marketing. Emphasis is placed on understanding which health care services a population needs and the dissemination of this information through health education and promotion. Health and disease trends and population sampling illustrate the health status of the population and its health care needs. This information supports short- and long-term planning within the health care system.

A benefit to managers is the use of this information in constructing relationships and negotiating contracts between providers of health care services and managed care entities. After identifying health status and disease trends in a population, a formal relationship can be established that is most beneficial to the population, the providers, and the managed care organization.

Study Questions

1. Stuart Pettingill, chief of the medical staff at East Bank Regional Hospital, has decided to recruit a neurologist to increase the staff of the hospital's existing cerebrovascular disease (CVD) clinical care center. This new physician will begin work on the first day of the following year. Pettingill needs to present a proposal to the hospital board for approval. To prepare, he asks Dana Lopez, who has recently been hired as vice president for clinical practice, to gather some information to "put some meat" into his planned presentation. Lopez reviews data from the CDC, the Census Bureau, and other sources for the defined population service area of East Bank Regional Hospital, which can be described as a moderate-sized metropolitan area. Partial results of this review are listed in Table 9.1.

TABLE 9.1. INCIDENCE OF CVD IN THE EAST BANK REGIONAL HOSPITAL SERVICE AREA.

Race	Number of newly diagnosed cases of CVD in the previous year	Midyear population	Incidence rate (per 1,000 population)
White	4,590	846,711	5.42
Black	2,470	425,064	5.81
Totals	7,060	1,271,775	5.55

Lopez knows that the prevalence of the disease in the East Bank Regional Hospital service area will be an important factor for determining the potential population with CVD in a given period in the targeted service area. She reviewed data from the CDC National Health Interview Survey, which showed that the prevalence rate for CVD is 10.7 per 1,000 population. In addition, she determined that the five-year annual mean incidence rate for CVD is 7.8 per 1,000.

Calculate the estimated number of persons with cerebrovascular disease in the targeted service area in the previous year.

2. There are at least ten other hospitals in East Bank Regional Hospital's service area. These hospitals (including East Bank Regional) treated 7,060 patients with a CVD diagnosis in the previous year. East Bank Regional Hospital's market share for the CVD product line is 6.66%.

   a. How many patients with CVD were treated at East Bank Regional Hospital the previous year?

   b. Assuming no changes in market share, estimate how many patients with CVD could potentially have been treated at East Bank Regional Hospital the previous year.

   c. Assuming no changes in market share, no deaths among the patients in the population with CVD, and static growth in the population of East Bank Regional Hospital's service area, estimate how many patients with CVD can be expected to be treated at East Bank Regional Hospital the following year.

   d. Should Pettingill hire a new physician? Why or why not?

CHAPTER TEN

ECONOMIC ANALYSIS OF HEALTH CARE FOR POPULATIONS

Chapter Outline

Introduction
Economic Evaluation
Cost Analysis
Cost-Benefit Analysis
Cost-Effectiveness Analysis
Discounting
Cost-Utility Analysis
Sensitivity Analysis
Burden-of-Disease Analysis
Example of Economic Analysis
Summary
Study Questions

Learning Objectives

Upon completion of this chapter, the reader will be able to do all of the following:

- Explain what is meant by economic evaluation
- Describe and perform cost analysis
- Describe cost-benefit analysis
- Describe and perform cost-effectiveness analysis

- Describe cost-utility analysis
- Describe and perform discounting of costs and benefits
- Explain the role of epidemiology in economic evaluation
- Explain the concept of burden of disease

Introduction

Planning for provision of health care services is a complex task with many explicit and implicit concerns. Inherent to such planning is policy analysis and economic evaluation. A selected course of action that affects large numbers of individuals is known as a policy. A policy typically involves some rule or agreed course of action that is applied in a significant number of cases. If this policy is selected or implemented by a governmental agency, it is known as public policy. An example of public policy that affects health is the Medicare drug benefit. This new policy is expected to offer greater choice to Medicare beneficiaries at lower cost. This will have far-reaching effects on planning and provision of health services and will result in an improved Medicare program and health care system in the United States (Gingrich, 2004).

A policy choice may involve setting administrative decisions, enacting a law, or establishing a treatment protocol. Before policy choices can be made, each choice must be analyzed. Policy analysis is the formal, systematic use of empiric information and subjective interpretation to select the best policy from a number of alternatives. A distinction must be made: policy analysis does not involve collecting data; rather it involves using secondary data, evaluating choices by relating concepts and outcomes.

An example of formulating health care policy to effect utilization of resources is the so-called rationing of medical care in Medicaid populations. This policy has been applied in two ways: prioritizing of health care services (as in the Oregon Medicaid proposal) and enrollment of Medicaid beneficiaries in managed care entities, especially HMOs (as in the Tenncare Model). Both approaches are intended to reduce program costs while maintaining access to and quality of care.

The state of Oregon attempted to apply a cost containment scheme to Medicaid expenditures. The Oregon legislature enacted the Basic Health Services Act, which established a commission to rank health service priorities based on comparative health benefits to the served population. A list was ranked to reflect each health service's priority with respect to its relative health benefit. This legislation was enacted in response to concerns over excessive Medicaid expenditures.

The Oregon Medicaid proposal represents one of the first attempts to apply economic evaluation to health resource allocation decision making. The priority list was based on the relative importance of each health service, determined by public preferences and values. The resultant list consisted of condition-treatment pairs, weighted according to the relationship among cost, health benefit, and preferences of the residents of Oregon.

The final recommendation of the Oregon commission established a priority cutoff point at the 587th ranked health service. This meant that of the 709 listed health services, the first 587 ranked services would be funded for the next fiscal year. If the Medicaid expenditures for that year are less than budgeted, the following year additional services on the list (ranked lower than 587) would be funded. Conversely, if Medicaid expenditures are more than budgeted, the following year fewer services on the list (ranked higher than 587) would be funded.

Fee-for-service payment systems have the potential to encourage greater than expected numbers of physician visits, which can increase costs. In contrast, prepaid health care may discourage delivery of necessary services, such as patient visits, that would lead to underprovision of needed care.

In many states, programs have been implemented to study the effects of Medicare and Medicaid managed care programs. Managed care programs in general are increasing in numbers of patients covered each year. One study focused on the actuarial split-sample method in assessment of the predictive accuracy of adjusted clinical groups (ACGs) for Medicaid enrollees in Georgia, Mississippi, and California (Adams, Bronstein, and Raskind-Hood, 2002). Georgia and Mississippi are states with low managed care penetration. The purpose of the study was to predict the occurrence of high-cost conditions in the sample states. The study used age, sex, poverty level, and disability as predictive variables. The results of the study indicated that ACGs are useful in identifying potential risky selection under managed care programs in all age groups. This predictive ability is less in areas with a high proportion of short-term enrollees, which is characteristic of Mississippi. Previous research has shown that it costs more per month in areas with short-term enrollees (Adams, Bronstein, Becker, and Raskind-Hood, 2001).

Another study investigated the relationship between supplemental benefits offered by Medicare + Choice plans and plan performance (Cox, Lanyi, and Strabic, 2002). Plan performance measurements included disenrollment rates and patient satisfaction. Results of the study indicated that varying supplemental benefits programs have no significant effect on patient satisfaction and that disenrollment rates were more sensitive to the alternative programs. Understanding whether these results indicate cost savings requires more analysis. This chapter presents economic analysis techniques useful for studying the relationship between costs and health outcomes.

Economic Evaluation

Economic evaluation can be thought of as efficiency evaluation. Two questions underlie economic evaluation: Is a planned or existing health care service worth providing, relative to other health care services, given the consumption of the same resources? Is the affected population satisfied with a planned or existing health care service (and its consumption of resources) compared to some other health care service that would consume the same resources?

Economic evaluation is important to health care managers because the supply of resources is finite and they must thus make choices about what resources to devote to health care services. Given changes in how health care is organized and financed, managers often seek formal methods of making resource allocation decisions so that they can evaluate health care outcomes associated with consumption of resources. Such systematic methods can identify possible and appropriate alternatives.

Economic analysis of health services focuses on costs and resulting consequences of providing services. This analysis can be thought of as identifying the inputs and outputs associated with health services. Economic evaluation determines the unit cost for the resulting unit of health benefit. Epidemiologic data are used to measure the relationship between health benefits and costs of providing a health service.

Four major types of economic evaluation are used in designing health care for populations: cost analysis, cost-benefit analysis, cost-effectiveness analysis, and cost-utility analysis. The remainder of this chapter will describe these different evaluation methods and their role in population health management.

Cost Analysis

Cost analysis is a formal technique that compares the costs of providing several different health services. It involves identifying the range of costs associated with a given health service. These costs are identified by direct measurement and estimation. A reasonable cost typology is as follows: total cost, which is the cost of providing a health service; fixed cost; variable cost, which varies with the level of output; cost function, the total cost expressed as a function of quantity; average cost per unit of output; and marginal cost, which is the additional unit of cost associated with producing an additional unit of output.

To determine the total cost of a particular health service delivered in an acute care hospital setting, several different costs must be considered. First, all costs directly attributable to a health service are determined. These are referred to as direct costs. Second, costs not associated with the health service must be quantified and deducted from the overall hospital costs. Then net hospital costs, adjusted by the total number of patient days, are added to the calculation. The formula to calculate total cost is as follows:

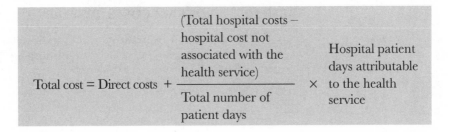

$$\text{Total cost} = \text{Direct costs} + \frac{(\text{Total hospital costs} - \text{hospital cost not associated with the health service})}{\text{Total number of patient days}} \times \begin{array}{l}\text{Hospital patient days attributable to the health service}\end{array}$$

Health economists make a distinction between marginal cost and average cost. Marginal and average costs are constructs related to quantity (McClellan and Newhouse, 1997). To understand this distinction, two questions are important: What are the costs of providing additional health care (marginal costs)? And does the average cost differ from the costs of changes in output?

Cost analysis can be illustrated in the following decision about program implementation. East Bank Regional Hospital's service area comprises a population with a high incidence and prevalence of lung cancer. Management and the board of directors must decide whether to conduct a community outreach program of screening and education over the next five-year period or to expand the in-hospital screening and educational activities for the same period of time. (These expanded activities would include in-service lung cancer awareness programs for hospital medical staff. Hospital staff would be encouraged to refer patients to the hospital's cancer center for screening and education.)

Table 10.1 presents the cost analysis for both programs for year 1. The community outreach program is more expensive in the first year because of the cost of developing the infrastructure for the program.

Table 10.2 presents the costs of both programs for the five-year period. The costs of the community outreach program decrease while the costs of the in-hospital program increase. Though the two programs appear to operate at the same five-year cost, the time value of money provides the analytic basis for establishing relative cost.

TABLE 10.1. COST ANALYSIS, YEAR 1

	Direct costs ($)	
	Outreach program	In-hospital program
Administration	2,000	500
Personnel (new)	15,000	0
Marketing	5,000	1,000
Miscellaneous	3,000	2,500
Totals	25,000	4,000

TABLE 10.2. PROGRAM COSTS, BY YEAR.

Year	Community outreach program ($)	In-hospital program ($)
1	25,000	4,500
2	20,000	9,000
3	12,000	13,500
4	8,000	18,000
5	4,000	24,000
Totals	69,000	69,000

Cost-Benefit Analysis

Many managers confuse cost-benefit and cost-effectiveness analysis, often failing to make a distinction between the two. Cost-benefit analysis evaluates programs with different objectives, while cost-effectiveness analysis compares different approaches to achieving the same objective. Cost-benefit analysis can also evaluate programs with similar objectives, but in practice it is not typically used for this purpose.

Both cost-benefit and cost-effectiveness analysis are useful tools for health care policy formulators. Both kinds of analysis involve information-gathering techniques, with the information structured and analyzed to guide policymakers and planners.

The distinction between the two types of analysis is in the method of valuing the desired outcomes, the health benefits. In cost-benefit analysis, all health benefits and costs are expressed in monetary terms. Health benefits (added years of life, number of lives saved, and so on) are converted to monetary terms, using valuations associated with work productivity. In cost-effectiveness analysis, only costs are expressed in monetary terms, with health benefits represented in natural units.

Because cost-benefit analysis is based on comparing the health benefits of programs in monetary terms, this monetary value is expressed in one of two ways: the cost per unit of health benefit or the health benefit per unit of cost. The intent of this analysis is to determine the best use of resources. Because all costs and health benefits are expressed in dollars, cost-benefit analysis has the ability to determine the "worth" of providing a health care service or program.

Cost-benefit analysis indicates the absolute benefit of health care services in dollars. It is typically employed when the health care service or program of interest is not being compared to other services or programs with the same managerial or clinical objective. For example, cost-benefit analysis is useful when evaluating the decision of whether to build a new hospital or to provide better roads to the hospital. In addition, cost-benefit analysis can evaluate the service or program of interest compared to "doing nothing."

The constraint of expressing health benefits in strictly monetary terms has made cost-benefit analysis in health care less popular than other comparative constructs. Those who propose not using cost-benefit analysis argue that expressing health benefits in monetary terms is unethical and immoral (Petitti, 1994). There are studies in health care that use cost-benefit analysis, but these focus on technical efficiency instead of economic efficiency. The perspective of these cost-benefit studies is of the health care entity of interest and not society. These studies use economic assumptions and principles that are relevant to a societal perspective; true cost-benefit ratios are not calculated because costs and benefits that may occur over time are neglected (Nas, 1996).

Cost-Effectiveness Analysis

Cost-effectiveness analysis is a method that compares the costs and outcomes associated with health services provided with the intent to improve health. Cost-effectiveness analysis, as with cost-benefit analysis, illustrates the cost of achieving one unit of health benefit by providing a health service. Cost-effectiveness analysis involves estimating incremental costs and health benefits of a particular health service compared with one or more alternative health services. This comparison is important when choosing between alternatives in resource allocation.

Cost-effectiveness analysis is based on the premise that "for any given level of resources available, society . . . wishes to maximize the total aggregate health benefits conferred" (Weinstein and Stason, 1977, p. 717). In contrast, cost-benefit analysis has been criticized because it fails to take into account the societal perspective.

Cost-effectiveness analysis can be thought of as a relative, comparative method. The results of cost-effectiveness analysis are meaningful only if the costs and benefits are compared with respect to the same time period. Managers benefit from the use of cost-effectiveness analysis because it allows comparison of the relative returns of decisions made at the same time.

Cost-effectiveness analysis focuses on the economic concept of opportunity cost. Opportunity cost evaluates the cost of a health service or program relative to use of the required resources in another health service or program. In other words, the opportunity cost of some resource is its value in some other use. The true cost of a resource, then, is not its market price but the lost opportunity for using it in some other way.

Cost-effectiveness analysis evaluates the comparative effects of using a given set of resources for the provision of different health care services. Central to this analysis is

Year	Community outreach program	In-hospital program
1	0	0
2	0	0
3	0	0
4	10	5
5	15	20
Total benefits	25	25

TABLE 10.3. BENEFITS OF COMMUNITY OUTREACH PROGRAM: REDUCTION IN INCIDENCE (CASES PER 100,000 POPULATION).

the cost-effectiveness ratio, which represents the difference between the costs of alternative health services divided by the difference in the health outcomes of these alternative health services. Health outcomes are a measure of effectiveness.

Table 10.3 presents information about the anticipated results of the lung cancer screening and educational programs discussed earlier in this chapter. The health effects of the programs are measured by a reduction in the incidence of lung cancer cases in East Bank Regional Hospital's service area.

Discounting

An important issue for managers involves costs of health care services or programs, the associated health benefits, and time. Costs and benefits may not occur at the same time, and the manager must account for this temporal disparity.

The process known as discounting can be used to solve this analytic dilemma. The value of money is dynamic over time, as is the value of a health benefit. For example, the value of $100 ten years from today will be less than it is now. Similarly, the value of one additional year of life is different ten years hence. Discounting makes it possible to work with current and future costs and health benefits by adjusting their value to form a summary measure.

In practice, discounting involves adjusting the value of money relative to time. For example, if money invested today is increasing in value at a rate of 5% each year, then $100 dollars invested today would have a value of $105 in one year. The following formula can be used to calculate the value of money over time:

$$I_n = I_o \times (1 + r)^n,$$

where I_n = value of invested money
       I_o = original amount invested
       r = growth rate
       n = number of years invested

If $100 is invested for ten years at a 5% growth rate, the value after ten years is

$$I_{10} = I_o \times (1 + 0.05)^{10}$$
$$I_{10} = \$100 \times (1 + 0.05)^{10}$$
$$I_{10} = \$162.89$$

Conversely, $100 spent today on a health service or program would have a value of $100 minus 5%, or $95, in one year. To determine the discounted value of money spent for a health service or program over time, the following formula may be used:

$$C_o = \frac{C_n}{(1+r)^n}$$

where C_o = present value of the money spent
C_n = total cost of the health service or program
n = number of years of the health service or program
r = discount rate
$(1 + r)^n$ = discount factor

If $100 were spent to establish a health service or program for a ten-year period, the discounted cost would be determined as follows:

$$C_o = \frac{\$100}{(1 + 0.05)^{10}}$$
$$C_o = \$61.39$$

If costs are to occur annually over a period of years, an alternative equation is used to discount the value of these costs. The calculation of the present value of costs is as follows:

$$PV = \Sigma\, C_n (1 + r)^{-n},$$

where C_n = future costs
r = discount rate
n = number of years

Before determining the marginal cost-effectiveness ratio, health benefits must be discounted, in the same manner as previously undertaken for costs. Using a 5%

discount rate, the calculation of the present value of the costs of the community outreach and in-hospital programs used earlier as examples is as follows:

Present value of the community outreach program

$$\text{Present value} = \frac{C_1}{1.05} + \frac{C_2}{(1.05)^2} + \frac{C_3}{(1.05)^3} + \frac{C_4}{(1.05)^4} + \frac{C_5}{(1.05)^5}$$

$$= \frac{25{,}000}{1.05} + \frac{20{,}000}{(1.05)^2} + \frac{12{,}000}{(1.05)^3} + \frac{8{,}000}{(1.05)^4} + \frac{4{,}000}{(1.05)^5}$$

$$= \$62{,}032$$

Present value of the in-hospital program

$$\text{Present value} = \frac{C_1}{1.05} + \frac{C_2}{(1.05)^2} + \frac{C_3}{(1.05)^3} + \frac{C_4}{(1.05)^4} + \frac{C_5}{(1.05)^5}$$

$$= \frac{45{,}000}{1.05} + \frac{9{,}000}{(1.05)^2} + \frac{13{,}500}{(1.05)^3} + \frac{18{,}000}{(1.05)^4} + \frac{24{,}000}{(1.05)^5}$$

$$= \$57{,}724$$

The following equations illustrate the calculation of the present value of the reduction in health benefits resulting from implementation of both programs, based on a 5% discount rate.

Discounted benefits of the community outreach program

$$\text{Present value} = \frac{O_1}{1.05} + \frac{O_2}{(1.05)^2} + \frac{O_3}{(1.05)^3} + \frac{O_4}{(1.05)^4} + \frac{O_5}{(1.05)^5}$$

$$= \frac{0}{1.05} + \frac{0}{(1.05)^2} + \frac{0}{(1.05)^3} + \frac{10}{(1.05)^4} + \frac{15}{(1.05)^5}$$

$$= 19.97 \text{ lung cancer cases per } 100{,}000$$

Discounted benefits of the in-hospital program

$$\text{Present value} = \frac{O_1}{1.05} + \frac{O_2}{(1.05)^2} + \frac{O_3}{(1.05)^3} + \frac{O_4}{(1.05)^4} + \frac{O_5}{(1.05)^5}$$

$$= \frac{0}{1.05} + \frac{0}{(1.05)^2} + \frac{0}{(1.05)^3} + \frac{5}{(1.05)^4} + \frac{20}{(1.05)^5}$$

$$= 19.78 \text{ lung cancer cases per } 100{,}000$$

The community outreach screening and educational program results in a slightly higher reduction in the incidence of lung cancer (19.97 lung cancer cases per 100,000, compared with 19.78 lung cancer cases per 100,000). The marginal cost-effectiveness ratio comparing these two programs is calculated as follows:

$$\text{Cost effectiveness ratio} = \frac{\text{differences in costs of the programs}}{\text{differences in health benefits of the program}}$$

$$= \frac{\$62,032}{19.97/100,000} - \frac{\$57,724}{19.78/100,000}$$

$$= \$22,678.88 \text{ per lung cancer case averted}$$

The analysis indicates that implementing the community outreach program, which has higher costs but a greater health benefit, will result in a cost of $22,678.68 for every lung cancer case averted.

Cost-Utility Analysis

Cost-utility analysis, a variation of cost-effectiveness analysis, is a form of economic evaluation that is concerned with the quality of health benefit resulting from a health care service or program. The distinction between cost-effectiveness and cost-utility analysis is in the method used to quantify the health benefit. In cost-effectiveness analysis, natural units are used to express the marginal health benefit (for example, number of inpatient admissions, number of inpatient days, number of cases of a disease diagnosed, number of outpatient visits, or number of lives saved). Cost-utility analysis uses the measure of quality-adjusted life years (QALYs). Table 10.4 presents the cost utility of selected medical procedures, which are designed to treat selected diseases or conditions.

Cost-effectiveness analysis is best used when comparing health services or programs with similar objectives. Cost-utility analysis, through the use of QALYs, allows for a broader application of cost-effectiveness analysis. QALY is a construct that incorporates many health dimensions into a single measure. QALY is a measure of health outcome weighted according to the quality of life at a given point in time or during a specific period of time. The number of QALYs represents the number of healthy years of life relative to actual health outcomes (Gold, Siegel, Russell, and Weinstein, 1996).

The QALY falls into the general category of health-related quality-of-life measurements. Health-related quality of life is a measurement that aggregates quality and quantity of life, as well as a function of the trade-off between quality and quantity. The QALY combines the benefit of reduced mortality and morbidity. It also adjusts the quality-of-life measure by weighting a year of life by a factor ranging from 1 to 0. A factor of 1 represents perfect health and 0 represents death.

QALY weights are obtained from one of several sources. The weights represent utility values (preferences) derived from individual judgment, judgment of groups of

TABLE 10.4. COST UTILITY OF SELECTED MEDICAL PROCEDURES.

Year performed	Disease and procedure	Cost per QALY (in 2002 U.S. dollars)
1999	*Anemias* Recombinant human erythropoietin versus blood transfusions	120,000–240,000
2000	*Cardiovascular diseases* Angioplasty with selective stent placement versus angioplasty alone in 60-year-old patients with intermittent claudication due to iliac artery stenosis	8,400
	Cardiac catheterization versus exercise echocardiogram in 55-year-old ambulatory women with definite angina	24,000
	Cardiac catheterization versus exercise echocardiogram in 55-year-old ambulatory women with probable angina	31,000
2001	*Cardiovascular diseases* Low-molecular-weight heparin versus warfarin in patients with an episode of venous thromboembolism	30,000
	Amiodarone therapy versus no anti-arrhythmic therapy in patients with past MI	47,000
	Drug treatment versus no drug treatment in stage I hypertensive patients: men age 80	4,800
	Drug treatment versus no drug treatment in stage I hypertensive patients: women age 80	4,900
	Drug treatment versus no drug treatment in stage I hypertensive patients: men age 70	7,100
	Drug treatment versus no drug treatment in stage I hypertensive patients: women age 70	8,300
	Drug treatment versus no drug treatment in stage I hypertensive patients: men age 60	12,000
	Drug treatment versus no drug treatment in stage I hypertensive patients: women age 60	14,000

individuals, and published literature (which is the most common source). Individual utility values are obtained through direct rating, standard reference gamble, and time trade-off methods.

Direct rating involves the assignment of linear utility values across two anchored scalar endpoints. Utility values are assigned in relation to a most preferred health state (usually assigned the value of 1) and a least preferred state (usually assigned a value of 0). The resulting utility values will range from 1 to 0.

The standard reference gamble is a traditional method based on cardinal utility theory (von Neumann and Morganstern, 1953). This method assesses preferences for health states relative to other states at various chances of being in a specific health state. Preferences are obtained for various health states in relation to a most preferred and least preferred state. This method has been used in many situations, including with cataract surgery patients (Lee and others, 2001, 2003).

Time trade-off is a method developed for health care decision making. This method measures the relative desirability of being in specific health states, as the time in each state is varied. Intermediate health states are compared to the best and worst health state (Shah and others, 2004).

Sensitivity Analysis

Economic evaluation is characterized by several uncertain components, including costs and benefits. The results of an economic evaluation may be affected by these uncertainties. In other words, the economic evaluation may be sensitive to the specific value of these uncertainties and the chance that these values will occur.

Sensitivity analysis studies the effect of the uncertain components of an economic evaluation. The objective of the analysis is to determine how the results of the economic evaluation depend on the data represented by the uncertain components. Specifically, the different uncertainties may have different effects on the validity, reliability, and robustness of the economic evaluation.

In addition to using sensitivity analysis to determine the impact of uncertainties incorporated in the analysis, it can be used to simulate the effect of the potential range of values. The range of values will depend on analysis assumptions and information, which are dynamic. In this sense, sensitivity analysis can be thought of as a form of uncertainty analysis. The greatest benefit of sensitivity analysis is that it confirms the results of the economic evaluation and increases the confidence in the results.

Burden-of-Disease Analysis

Epidemiologic trends indicate that in the next several decades, the distribution of health and disease will be very different from what it is in today's landscape. As during the early decades of the twentieth century in the industrialized world, the distribution of noncommunicable diseases in developing countries is beginning to overtake infectious diseases. Diseases such as heart disease and depression are replacing infectious diseases as leading causes of death and disability. In addition to noncommunicable diseases, unintentional and intentional injuries are becoming a global concern.

Around the world, the notion of burden of disease has become a focus of investigation, comparison, and intervention. Burden of disease is a useful measure of the level of mortality and morbidity in a population. Burden-of-disease analysis attempts to quantify health status using epidemiologic and demographic information.

The Harvard University School of Public Health, through support of the World Health Organization and the World Bank, established the Global Burden of Disease (GBD) study and released its first findings in 1993 (Murray and Lopez, 1996). In the GBD study, the impact of noncommunicable diseases is measured by the global burden of disease. This study required a new construct because traditional statistics of health and disease do not capture the impact of premature death and disability.

Given this need, disease burden is expressed using the measure called the disability-adjusted life year (DALY). The DALY combines the effect of premature death and disability into a single measure. It is the only quantitative construct of burden of disease that reflects the total amount of healthy life lost, caused by either premature death or disability during a specified period of time. It is important to note that disability can be caused by physical or mental problems. A DALY is equal to one year of healthy life that is lost due to death or disability.

The number of DALYs in a population indicates the amount of health care currently provided as well as whatever has been done to protect or damage the population's health. Interventions are introduced to prevent, cure, or provide palliative care, and their effectiveness is measured in DALYs as well. DALYs are compared across and among interventions.

DALYs incorporate the following values to measure the burden of disease: (1) duration of time lost to a death at each age (that is, potential years of life lost, PYLL), (2) disability weights, (3) age weights, and (4) time preference (discounting). The DALY is a measure of the time a person lives with a disability and the time lost due to premature mortality. The duration of time is determined using PYLL (Reidpath, Allotey, Koumane, and Cummins, 2003).

The burden of disease for a given population, in DALYs, is determined by the following equation:

$$\text{DALYs} = \text{YLLs} + \text{YLDs,}$$

where

YLLs = number of deaths $\times$ (life expectancy at age of death – age at death)
    = incidence of death $\times$ duration of premature death,

and

YLDs = number of years with a disability $\times$ disability weight.

EXHIBIT 10.1. LEADING CAUSES OF DEATH WORLDWIDE, 1990, RANKED BY DALYS.

1. Lower respiratory disease
2. Diarrheal diseases
3. Conditions during the perinatal period
4. Unipolar major depression
5. Ischemic heart disease
6. Cerebrovascular disease
7. Tuberculosis
8. Measles
9. Road traffic accidents
10. Congenital abnormalities

The number of years with a disability is determined by: incidence *times* duration or prevalence for one year (Hollinghurst, Bevan, and Bowie, 2000).

The DALY has been used to measure the burden of disease for many diseases. It is interesting to review the ten leading causes of death in DALYs for developed countries. Exhibit 10.1 presents the leading causes of death, ranked by the DALYs associated with each of these causes. The DALY measure indicates that communicable diseases were the most important cause of death in 1990, accounting for seven of the leading ten causes (Murray and Lopez, 1996).

Exhibit 10.2 presents the leading causes of death observed in 1990 and what is expected in the year 2020. As mentioned earlier, a new distribution of causes can be observed. Fewer infectious diseases are expected to be among the ten leading causes of death, with only four communicable diseases on the list. In addition, the percentage of deaths attributable to infectious diseases is also expected to decrease significantly.

EXHIBIT 10.2. LEADING CAUSES OF DEATH, WORLDWIDE, 1990 AND 2020.

1990	2020
1. Ischemic heart disease	1. Ischemic heart disease
2. Cerebrovascular disease	2. Cerebrovascular disease
3. Lower respiratory infections	3. Pulmonary diseases
4. Diarrheal diseases	4. Lower respiratory infections
5. Conditions during the perinatal period	5. Trachea, bronchus, and lung cancers
6. Pulmonary diseases	6. Road traffic accidents
7. Tuberculosis	7. Tuberculosis
8. Measles	8. Stomach cancer
9. Road traffic accidents	9. HIV
10. Trachea, bronchus, and lung cancers	10. Self-inflicted injuries

Source: World Health Organization, 2004.

Example of Economic Analysis

A specific application of epidemiology to economic evaluation focuses on the adjustment of Medicare capitation payments based on disease risk factors. Medicare capitation payments are routinely adjusted by the average adjusted per capita costs formula. Disease risk factors can be incorporated into this formula to more accurately adjust payments. Such factors include prior hospitalization, prior physician visits, number of cigarettes smoked per day, number of cigarette pack–years of smoking, systolic blood pressure, serum cholesterol level, blood sugar level, forced vital lung capacity, and two-year probability of cardiovascular disease.

In one study, these risk factors were added to the average adjusted per capita costs model, which consisted of age, sex, and institutional status. The study confirmed the expected relationships between Medicare payments and prior utilization and disability. Results also demonstrated an association of risk factors for chronic disease and Medicare payments. The contribution of this study includes the identification of epidemiologic risk factors, as well as utilization and disability level, as appropriate adjusters of Medicare capitation payments (Schauffler, Howland, and Cobb, 1992).

The clinical decision to employ prophylactic therapy is often associated with controversy. An example is misoprostol prophylaxis for the prevention of nonsteroidal anti-inflammatory drug–induced gastrointestinal complications. Treatment of nonsteroidal anti-inflammatory drug–induced gastroduodenal ulcers is not definitive and has several clinical options. If the nonsteroidal anti-inflammatory drug therapy can be terminated, most ulcers heal within four to eight weeks. However, in many cases suspension of drug therapy is not possible.

The cost-effectiveness of misoprostol prophylaxis is of interest to both clinicians and managers. Routinely coprescribing misoprostol to prevent nonsteroidal drug–induced gastrointestinal complications has clinical importance and profound cost implications. Consensus does not exist on whether the prophylactic use of misoprostol cotherapy is cost-effective.

A study used the marginal cost-effectiveness ratio to compare misoprostol prophylaxis with no prophylaxis in an attempt to determine if its additional cost was worthwhile (Loh, 1998). This study used a decision analytic model that incorporated costs, expected events, and the probability of these events. Effectiveness was defined as the number of episodes of clinically relevant gastrointestinal complications that were averted. The study population was divided into three groups: universal prescription program (misoprostol prophylaxis for all), targeted prescription program (misoprostol prophylaxis for high-risk group only), and no misoprostol prophylaxis.

The marginal cost-effectiveness ratio is defined as follows:

$$\text{Cost-effectiveness} = \frac{\text{Difference in costs}}{\text{Difference in effectiveness}}$$

where cost is quantified as the sum of the costs of misoprostol, ambulatory care, inpatient medical care, and inpatient surgical care. Effectiveness was measured as the number of gastrointestinal complications averted.

The study calculated both direct and overhead costs. Direct costs were those associated with misoprostol therapy. Estimating per-unit cost was accomplished by converting charge data to cost data, using the cost-to-charge ratio for the study institution. Overhead costs were determined according to the study institution's designated cost centers, which included ambulatory care, patient care services, institutional operations, and medical affairs.

Resource utilization and primary diagnosis were determined by medical record review. Study eligibility was based on the following criteria: primary diagnosis of gastrointestinal complications in arthritis patients (DRG 174–180) taking nonsteroidal anti-inflammatory drugs and patients receiving medical care from May 1994 to August 1996. The study evaluated the cost-effectiveness of using misoprostol universally and in a targeted high-risk population relative to not using misoprostol.

Study results indicated that not using misoprostol would result in 2 clinically relevant gastrointestinal complications, with an associated cost of $16,000. If misoprostol were used in all patients, 1.5 clinically relevant gastrointestinal complications would occur, with $9,400 in costs. In the targeted program, 1.6 clinically relevant complications would be experienced, with resulting costs of $11,400.

Further analysis reviewed the cost-effectiveness and determined that it would cost $15,000 to prevent one additional gastrointestinal complication. On average, the universal use of misoprostol in chronic nonsteroidal anti-inflammatory drug users is more cost-effective than either no use or the targeted prophylaxis program.

Summary

Economic evaluation is an important aspect of management because of the increasing emphasis on population-based health care. Public policy formulation typically requires choosing among several alternative programs to provide health care to populations. Strategic planning activities depend on economic evaluation.

The types of economic evaluation needed by managers include cost analysis, cost-benefit analysis, cost-effectiveness analysis, and cost-utility analysis. These analyses have a common goal to determine what is the best, or most efficient, use of resources to provide for the health needs of a population.

Discounting of both costs and health benefits is necessary to properly interpret the results of these analyses. In programs that will be in place for a period of time, the costs and health benefits will occur over time. When evaluating these, the present value of costs and health benefits can be determined by adjusting future costs and health benefits, using a discount rate.

Epidemiology has an important role in economic evaluation. The health benefits used in the analyses are either epidemiologic data or measures based on these data. In addition, epidemiologic data can be used to evaluate both costs and pricing of health care services. Such evaluation is especially important in managed care situations when capitation rates or exclusion provisions are negotiated.

Burden-of-disease analysis is a notion that relates epidemiology to economic evaluation. Not only is the effect of disease measured in health indicators, but the economic impact of disease is folded into the analysis to illustrate the effect on productivity. This analysis will continue to gain popularity in the future and will represent a new measure in public health, community health, and health care administration.

Study Questions

1. Placental examination has been controversial for many years. Differing views are held about the rationale and economic impact of such examination. On one hand, advocates argue that placental examinations are essential for clinical and medicolegal concerns. Others argue that these procedures waste resources and that inadequate empirical evidence exists to indicate whether they are cost-effective. They believe that placental examinations should be performed only on the basis of well-defined criteria.

    Clinical benefits of placental evaluation are twofold. First, information from this evaluation can improve management of subsequent pregnancies through diagnosis of pathology. Second, placental evaluation provides for assessing the risk of long-term neurological developmental conditions of the newborn.

    Several physicians at East Bank Regional Hospital began to perform routine placental cultures on all women at delivery. The hospital's Medical Care Review Committee has become concerned about overuse and associated increases in costs. The committee felt that the practice of routine placental cultures might be establishing different standards of care among the hospital medical staff. The underlying concern of the committee was the cost-effectiveness of this practice. In fact, the committee strongly suggested that the practice be discontinued.

    Before responding to the committee's recommendation, the group of physicians using the clinical protocol of routine placental cultures commissioned a formal cost-effectiveness analysis. The physicians in question had begun to perform routine placental cultures in 1999. Data were collected in two separate time periods: five years before 1999 (1994–1998) and five years since beginning the routine culture practice (1999–2003). The unit of analysis was each delivery, and the underlying study hypothesis was that fewer readmissions would be one outcome of performing routine placental cultures. If this hypothesis is supported, an associated study question will be what the cost is per unit health benefit (that is, decreased readmissions). In other words, is the cost of routine placental cultures worth the expense of resources?

Currently, the hospital charge for performing placental culture is $36.00. This charge has resulted from an annual increase of 9%, so the average charge since 1999 is $30.55. Medicaid has paid between 70% (in 1994) and 47.6% (in 2003) of these charges. According to information from the hospital's chief financial officer, the Medicaid payment has averaged 60% for the study period. This figure indicates that the average payment from Medicaid has been $18.33 per culture.

During the period from 1994 to 1998, the physicians in question did not perform routine placental cultures on all deliveries, and their patients experienced 25 readmissions in 1,070 deliveries, a rate of 23.36 readmissions per 1,000 deliveries. These readmissions resulted in total charges of $84,355.00, with an average charge of $3,374.20 (standard deviation of $1,862.74).

Beginning in 1999, the physicians in question began the practice of performing placental cultures on all deliveries. During this period, their patients experienced 10 readmissions in 2,605 deliveries, a rate of 3.83 readmissions per 1,000 deliveries. These readmissions resulted in total charges of $26,825.00, with an average charge of $2,682.50 (standard deviation of $1,212.69). The 2,605 cultures cost $79,582.75. Assuming that 100% of the cultures are charged to Medicaid, this would result in a payment of $47,749.65. Total charges associated with readmissions and cultures during 1999–2003 were $74,574.65.

a. What is the difference between the rate of readmission among the physicians in question from 1994 to 1998 and the readmission rate from 1999 to 2003?

b. What is the marginal cost-effectiveness ratio to determine the cost per health benefit associated with the additional charge of the placental cultures?

2. To extend the analysis, physicians who did not perform routine placental cultures were also evaluated. During 1999–2003, their patients experienced 21 readmissions in 2,135 deliveries, a readmission rate of 9.84 per 1,000 deliveries. These readmissions resulted in total charges of $62,685.00, with an average charge of $2,985.00 (standard deviation of $1,297.51).

a. What is the difference between the rates of readmission among the physicians in question and among other physicians from 1999 to 2003?

b. What is the marginal cost-effectiveness ratio to determine the cost per health benefit associated with the additional charge of the placental cultures during 1999–2003?

c. What would be your recommendation to the medical staff and board of directors?

CHAPTER ELEVEN

EXPANDING EMERGENCY HEALTH CARE SERVICES

Chapter Outline

Introduction
Emergency Department Use
Description of Hospitals
Time Analysis
Payment Sources
Patient Disposition
Reason for Visit
Risk of an Urgent Visit

Learning Objectives

Upon completing this chapter, the reader will be able to do all of the following:

- Evaluate and use a secondary database
- Explain the significance of demographic information
- Describe the planning process
- Explain the role of epidemiologic data in the planning process

Introduction

East Bank Regional Hospital System consists of four hospitals, with an average size of five hundred beds. This is a not-for-profit acute care hospital system serving an urban population and the surrounding suburbs. The total population served is approximately 2.5 million people. The hospital system has been profitable for many years but is currently experiencing a decrease in its operating margin. This decrease is caused, in part, by a reduction in Medicare reimbursements and the low Medicaid payment. Medicare is increasing its reimbursement at a rate that is about half the actual rate of increase in operating costs. The hospital system board has recommended that one area for evaluation is emergency health services. It is suspected that this may be a growth area for the hospital system and may reverse the trend in decreasing profits.

Understanding population characteristics is important because health and disease patterns are identified with respect to the "population at risk" or, in this case, the population to be served. Health and disease trends are expressed as epidemiologic measures, that is, rates and ratios, with geographic and demographic bounds. Table 11.1 presents information on the age and sex distribution of the population in the service area. Figure 11.1 presents a graphic representation of the population.

Overall, 21.4% of the population is under 15 years of age, and 12.5% is over age 65. These percentages are very similar to those for the United States as a whole. Of the population under age 15, 62% receive Medicaid and CHIP benefits. The mean age of the population is 42.89 years, with a median age of 38 years and a standard deviation of 19.76. The mean age of males is 44.04 years (standard deviation of 20.78 years), and the mean age of females is 41.59 years (standard deviation of 18.45 years). Whites are older than blacks, with a mean of 44.74 years for whites and 38.75 for blacks. With respect to payment source, Medicare patients have a mean age of 70.73, with patients from all other payment sources having means ranging between 35.33 and 43.80 years. Younger individuals in the population visit the emergency department because of injury (mean equal to 39 years), whereas individuals with a mean age of 45.32 do so because of illness. The service area population is predominantly white (69.3%). African Americans represent 27.5% of the population, with other races making up 3.2%. The ratio of whites to blacks is 2.5 to 1.

The hospital system board has tasked the administration to begin to include emergency health services reconfiguration and expansion in the strategic plan. The board's recommendations include the following:

- Identify growth areas for emergency health services.
- Identify areas for consolidation.
- Identify areas for expansion.

TABLE 11.1.　SERVICE AREA POPULATION, BY AGE AND SEX.

Age group	Distribution (%)
Overall population	100.0
Under 15 years	21.4
15–24 years	13.9
25–44 years	30.2
45–64 years	22.0
65–74 years	6.5
75 years and older	6.0
Males	49.1
Under 15 years	22.3
15–24 years	14.5
25–44 years	30.8
45–64 years	21.8
65–74 years	6.0
75 years and older	4.6
Females	50.9
Under 15 years	20.5
15–24 years	13.3
25–44 years	29.6
45–64 years	22.2
65-74 years	7.0
75 years and older	7.4

Note: Data used in this case study have been abstracted from the 2002 National Hospital Ambulatory Medical Care Survey conducted by the Centers for Disease Control and Prevention, with data compiled by the National Center for Health Statistics. Survey results are distributed through the CDC and are the source for all table and figure data in this chapter. Population numbers were abstracted from the 2000 U.S. census.

FIGURE 11.1.　SERVICE AREA POPULATION, PERCENTAGE DISTRIBUTION.

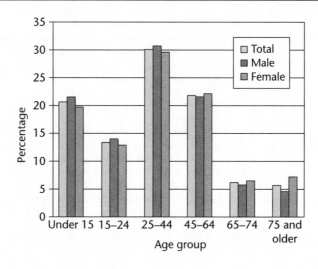

- Determine the level of profitability for the growth and reconfiguration areas.
- Develop a strategic plan with target objectives that are measurable.
- Create a timeline for activities.

The board has requested that a plan be submitted before its next quarterly meeting.

It is important to note that any expansion, consolidation, or other reconfiguration will require certificate of need (CON) approval from the state department of health. Depending on the specifics of the reconfiguration plan, CON approval may be problematic. Emergency health services CON regulations are presented in Exhibit 11.1.

The CEO of the hospital system has appointed an emergency health services strategic planning task force. Members of this task force include representatives from the hospital system board, medical staff, nursing staff, and administration. The hospital system planning department has been asked to gather information that may assist the task force.

1. Who, specifically, should be appointed to the strategic planning task force? Why?

2. What data and information should the hospital system planning department gather for the task force, and what insight would each data item provide to the strategic planning task force?

EXHIBIT 11.1. CERTIFICATE OF NEED REGULATIONS.

1. The applicant must demonstrate that the proposed emergency services facility will perform a minimum average of 10,000 emergency care services per year.
2. The applicant must demonstrate that the proposed emergency services facility has a population base of approximately 60,000 within 30 minutes travel time.
3. An applicant proposing to offer emergency services must document that the existing facilities in the area have been used for a minimum of 8,000 emergency services per year for the most recent twelve months.
4. The applicant must document that the proposed emergency facility will provide a full range of emergency care services.
5. The applicant must provide documentation that the proposed facility will be economically viable within two years.
6. The proposed facility must demonstrate support from the local physicians who will use the facility.
7. Medical staff for the facility must live within a 25-mile radius of the facility.
8. The proposed facility must have a formal relationship with a full-service hospital to provide services that are beyond the scope of the emergency services facility. The facility must have a formal process for providing follow-up services to patients through proper coordination mechanisms.
9. The applicant must affirm that it will provide a "reasonable amount" of indigent or charity care by stating the amount of indigent or charity care the applicant intends to provide.

Emergency Department Use

The planning department has provided data on patient characteristics (age, sex, and race), distribution of visits across the four system hospitals, duration of emergency department visits across the four system hospitals, distribution of time spent during emergency department visits, overall primary payment source, primary payment source across the four system hospitals, overall emergency department patient disposition, and emergency department patient disposition across the four system hospitals.

Table 11.2 presents the distribution of visits to the emergency departments of the hospital system, stratified by age. The total number of emergency department visits last year was 107,490. This is equal to a rate of 4.3 visits per 100 persons per year. In the under-15-years age group, there were 22,245 visits to the emergency departments of the hospital system, or 20.7%. The rate in the under-15 age group was equal to 3.7 visits per 100 persons per year.

The rate of visits to the emergency department in the 15–24 age group was 4.5 visits per 100 persons per year. The total number of visits in the 15–24 age group was 17,371, or 16.2%. The greatest number of visits, 32,732, was in the 25–44 age group. This also represents the greatest percentage of visits, 30.2%. The rate in this age group was 3.9 per 100 persons per year.

As the population increases in age, the trend in the number of visits decreases, except for the 75-years-and-older group. In the 45–64 age group, the total number of visits was 19,260, which represents 17.9% of all visits. The rate of visits in this age group was the lowest at 3.0 visits per 100 persons per year. In the 65–74 age group, the rate of visits was 3.6 visits per 100 persons per year. This rate was based on 6,551 total visits, or 6.1%. The highest rate of visits was in the 75-and-older age group, which had a rate of 5.9 visits per 100 persons per year. This represents 8.7% of all visits to the emergency department.

The distribution of emergency visits according to sex and age is presented in Table 11.3. As might be expected, more than half of the visits were by females (53.2%), who also had the highest rate of visits (4.0 visits per 100 persons per year). Among females, the greatest number of visits was observed in the 25–44 age group. This age group had the greatest proportion of visits of all age categories, across both sexes, with 16.2% of the total. The least number of visits to the emergency department was seen in the 65–74 age category. The highest rate of visits for the total population (6.1 emergency department visits per 100 persons per year) occurred among women 75 years and older.

A similar trend was observed in males. The greatest number of visits was observed in the 25–44 age group. This represented a proportion of 14.2%, the highest among males and second highest in the total population. The least number of visits to the emergency department was by males in the 65–74 category. The highest rate of visits by men (5.7 emergency department visits per 100 persons per year) occurred in the

TABLE 11.2. EMERGENCY DEPARTMENT VISITS, BY AGE.

Age group	Number of visits	Distribution (%)	Number of visits per 100 persons per year[a]
Total visits	107,490	100.00	4.3
Under 15 years	22,245	20.7	3.7
15–24 years	17,371	16.2	4.5
25–44 years	32,732	30.5	3.9
45–64 years	19,260	17.9	3.0
65–74 years	6,551	6.1	3.6
75 years and older	9,332	8.7	5.9

[a] The population used to calculate the rate of visits was the population of the service area of East Bank Regional Hospital (2.5 million) and an assumed age distribution of this population.

TABLE 11.3. EMERGENCY DEPARTMENT VISITS, BY AGE AND SEX.

Age group	Number of visits	Distribution (%)	Number of visits per 100 persons per year[a]
Females			
Total visits	57,169	53.2	4.0
Under 15 years	10,096	9.4	3.4
15–24 years	9,783	9.1	5.1
25–44 years	17,456	16.2	4.1
45–64 years	10,447	9.7	3.2
65–74 years	3,464	3.2	3.5
75 years and older	5,923	5.5	6.1
Males			
Total visits	50,321	46.8	3.7
Under 15 years	12,148	11.3	3.9
15–24 years	7,588	7.1	3.9
25–44 years	15,276	14.2	3.7
45–64 years	8,813	8.2	2.8
65–74 years	3,087	2.9	3.8
75 years and older	3,409	3.2	5.7

[a] The population used to calculate the rate of visits was the population of the service area of East Bank Regional Hospital (2.5 million) and an assumed age distribution of this population.

75-years-and-older age group, as it did for women. The lowest rate of visits to the emergency department for the total population was observed in the 45–64 age group.

Race is a significant factor in the utilization of hospital services, especially emergency departments. Table 11.4 presents the number and rate of visits in the East Bank Regional Hospital System service population according to age and race. Overall, the greatest number of visits was by whites. Among whites, the 25–44-year age group had the greatest number of visits and the highest proportion of visits (22.8%) across the total population. The least number of visits by whites occurred in the 65–74 age group, which was similar to what was observed earlier. The 75-years-and-older category had the highest rate of visits among whites, with the 45–64 category showing the lowest rate.

Using Table 11.2 as a reference, answer the following questions:

3. Did sex affect the distribution of visits to the emergency departments? What effect did sex have on the rate of visits overall and by age group? Explain your answers. 25-54
4. Did race affect the distribution of visits to the emergency departments? What effect did race have on the rate of visits overall and by age group? Explain your answers. T blurb

TABLE 11.4. EMERGENCY DEPARTMENT VISITS, BY AGE AND RACE.

Age group	Number of visits	Distribution (%)	Number of visits per 100 persons per year[a]
Whites			
Total visits	82,012	76.3	3.6
Under 15 years	16,071	15.0	3.5
15–24 years	13,166	12.2	4.3
25–44 years	24,526	22.8	3.7
45–64 years	14,942	13.9	2.8
65–74 years	5,216	4.9	3.3
75 years and older	8,092	7.5	5.8
Blacks			
Total visits	22,238	20.7	6.4
Under 15 years	5,354	5.0	5.6
15–24 years	3,672	3.4	6.6
25–44 years	7,241	6.7	7.0
45–64 years	3,778	3.5	5.6
65–74 years	1,148	1.1	7.1
75 years and older	1,045	1.0	9.1
Asian[b]	2,099	2.0	2.7
Native Hawaiian or other Pacific Islander[b]	391	0.4	8.4
American Indian or Alaska Native[b]	612	0.6	2.3
Multiple races[b]	138	0.1	0.4

[a] The population used to calculate the rate of visits was the population of the service area of East Bank Regional Hospital (2.5 million) and an assumed age distribution of this population.

[b] These numbers are too small for their validity or reliability to be certain.

Description of Hospitals

Four hospitals make up the East Bank Regional Hospital System. Two of them are located within the limits of the city of East Bank, and two are in the suburbs. Each of the four hospitals has a comprehensive emergency department. Mid-City Hospital and Uptown Medical Center are located in the city and are typical urban hospital facilities. Mid-City Hospital has 585 licensed beds, and Uptown Medical Center, which contains a children's hospital, has 885 total licensed beds. North Suburbia Hospital is located in the north suburbs and has 300 licensed beds. South Suburbia Hospital, located in the south suburbs, is the newest to the system and has 230 licensed beds.

Table 11.5 shows the distribution of emergency department visits across the system hospitals. Uptown Medical Center had the greatest number of visits last year but the lowest rate of visits (2.6 visits per 100 persons per year). North Suburbia Hospital had the highest rate of visits (3.4 visits per 100 persons per year). The least number of visits and lowest rate of visits were observed at South Suburbia Hospital.

5. Which factors might explain the distribution of the numbers of emergency department visits across the four hospitals?
6. Why doesn't the distribution of the rate of visits correspond to the distribution of the number of emergency department visits?

Time Analysis

The duration of an emergency department visit can provide interesting information. Table 11.6 shows the time spent in the East Bank Regional Hospital System emergency departments, in hour intervals. Almost 70% of visits to the emergency depart-

TABLE 11.5. EMERGENCY DEPARTMENT VISITS, BY HOSPITAL.

Hospital	Number of visits	Distribution (%)	Number of visits per 100 persons per year[a]
Total visits	57,169	53.2	4.0
Mid-City Hospital	20,802	19.4	2.9
North Suburbia Hospital	26,688	24.8	3.4
Uptown Medical Center	40,512	37.7	2.6
South Suburbia Hospital	19,489	18.1	2.6

[a] The population used to calculate the rate of visits was the population of the service area of East Bank Regional Hospital (2.5 million) and an assumed age distribution of this population.

TABLE 11.6. DURATION OF EMERGENCY DEPARTMENT VISITS.

Time spent	Number of visits	Distribution (%)
Total visits	107,490	100.0
Under 1 hour	17,805	16.6
1–2 hours	26,945	25.1
2–4 hours	30,611	28.5
4–6 hours	14,363	13.4
6–10 hours	9,761	9.1
10–14 hours	4,468	4.2
14–20 hours	1,575	1.5
21–23 hours	1,439	1.3
23–24 hours	131	0.1
24 hours or more	391	0.4

TABLE 11.7. DURATION OF EMERGENCY DEPARTMENT VISITS, BY HOSPITAL.

Hospital	Mean duration (hours)	Median duration (hours)
Mid-City Hospital	3.5	2.3
North Suburbia Hospital	2.6	1.8
Uptown Medical Center	2.9	2.1
South Suburbia Hospital	3.1	2.2

ments lasted less than four hours. More than half of the visits lasted between one and four hours (53.6%). The largest proportion of visits was in the two-to-four-hour range (28.5%). One visit in six (16.6%) lasted more than six hours.

Continuing the evaluation of time, Table 11.7 presents information on the duration of emergency department visits in each hospital in the system. Mid-City Hospital had the highest mean and median durations, 3.5 and 2.3 hours, respectively. North Suburbia Hospital had the lowest mean and median, 2.6 and 1.8 hours, respectively. Uptown Medical Center, which had the greatest number of visits, had a mean duration of 2.9 hours and a median duration of 2.1 hours. The hospital with the lowest number of visits, South Suburbia Hospital, had a mean duration of 3.1 hours and a median of 2.2.

7. What information does the time analysis provide with respect to efficient use of emergency department resources?
8. What impact, if any, does the duration of emergency department visits have on expansion and reconfiguration planning?

Payment Sources

The service area population has a varied distribution of payment sources, including private insurance, Medicaid or CHIP, Medicare, self-pay, and workers' compensation. As in all hospital systems, some emergency department services are provided that are not reimbursed (referred to as "no charge"). Table 11.8 shows the distribution of payment sources.

TABLE 11.8. PRIMARY PAYMENT SOURCE.

Payment source	Number of visits	Distribution (%)
Total visits	107,490	100.0
Private insurance	43,213	40.2
Medicaid or CHIP	18,789	17.5
Medicare	15,879	14.8
Self-pay	15,854	14.7
Workers' compensation	2,665	2.5
No charge	1,042	1.0
Other or unknown	10,048	9.4

The majority of emergency department services are paid for through private insurance (40.2%). Nearly one-third (32.3%) of services are covered by governmental payment sources. The ratio of individuals with nongovernmental payment sources to those with governmental payment sources is 2.1 to 1. A small portion of services is reimbursed by workers' compensation insurance (2.5%), and 10.4% of services are either charity care or funded by another payment source.

Understanding the primary payment source for each hospital will be valuable information for the strategic planning effort. Table 11.9 shows the distribution of primary payment sources for the four system hospitals. Private insurance is the major payment source for all hospitals. Medicaid or CHIP is the second most common primary payment source for Mid-City Hospital and Uptown Medical Center, the two urban facilities. Medicare is the second most common payment source for the two hospitals in the suburbs. Medicare and Medicaid or CHIP represents the primary payment source for 34.7% of the visits in Mid-City Hospital, 27.1% in North Suburbia Hospital, 39.3% in Uptown Medical Center, and 21.1% in South Suburbia Hospital.

9. How does the distribution of primary payment sources affect expansion and reconfiguration planning?

TABLE 11.9. PRIMARY PAYMENT SOURCE, BY HOSPITAL.

Payment source	Number of visits (percentage of visits)			
	Mid-City Hospital	North Suburbia Hospital	Uptown Medical Center	South Suburbia Hospital
Private insurance	9,803 (47.1)	14,285 (53.5)	17,778 (43.9)	10,346 (53.1)
Medicaid or CHIP	4,637 (22.3)	2,879 (10.8)	9,516 (23.5)	758 (3.9)
Medicare	2,588 (12.4)	4,352 (16.3)	6,382 (15.8)	3,358 (17.2)
Self-pay	1,711 (8.2)	2,459 (9.2)	4,750 (11.7)	2,078 (10.7)
Workers' compensation	533 (2.6)	600 (2.2)	933 (2.3)	400 (2.1)
No charge	698 (3.4)	931 (3.5)	465 (1.1)	233 (1.2)
Other or unknown	832 (4.0)	1,182 (4.4)	688 (1.7)	2,316 (11.9)

Patient Disposition

Table 11.10 presents information concerning the disposition of patients who visited the emergency department. Of the 107,490 visits to the emergency departments in the East Bank Regional Hospital System, over 40% were referred to another physician or a clinic within the hospital system. About 40% of the patients were advised to return to the emergency department if necessary. Slightly less than 20% of the patients were returned to the referring physician, inside or outside the hospital system. Some 11.7% of patients were admitted to the hospital. About 10% of patients were released from the emergency department without any further treatment planned.

Reason for Visit

Table 11.11 shows the breakdown of the major reasons for visiting the emergency department. Illness is the main reason for the first visit to the emergency department, accounting for more than half of all visits. Injury is the second most common reason for the first visit. Follow-up visits for illness and injury represent a small proportion of visits, a total of 7.1%.

It is important to understand whether visits to the emergency department are related to use of alcohol or drugs. Table 11.12 documents alcohol- and drug-related

TABLE 11.10. EMERGENCY DEPARTMENT DISPOSITION.

Disposition	Number of visits	Distribution (%)
All visits	107,490	100.0
Referred to other physician or clinic for follow-up	43,598	40.6
Told to return if needed	40,759	37.9
Returned to referring physician	19,842	18.5
Admitted to hospital	12,626	11.7
Left with no follow-up planned	10,299	9.6
Transferred to other system facility	1,967	1.8
Transferred to nonsystem facility	1,593	1.5
Admitted to intensive care unit	992	0.9
Returned to nonphysician treatment	924	0.9
Admitted for 23-hour observation	814	0.8
Left against medical advice	642	0.6
Referred to alcohol or drug treatment program	414	0.4
Referred out from triage, without treatment	344	0.3
Died before arriving or while in emergency department	254	0.2
Other	2,708	2.5

TABLE 11.11. MAJOR REASONS FOR EMERGENCY DEPARTMENT VISITS.

Major reason	Distribution (%)
Injury, first visit	27.6
Injury, follow-up visit	3.4
Illness, first visit	54.5
Illness, follow-up visit	3.7
Other	10.8

TABLE 11.12. ALCOHOL- AND DRUG-RELATED EMERGENCY DEPARTMENT VISITS.

Category	Distribution (%)
Alcohol-related	5.7
Drug-related	7.9
Both alcohol- and drug-related	5.6

visits to the emergency department. These reasons accounted for 19.2% of all visits, with more than half of them drug-related.

Risk of an Urgent Visit

Understanding the potential use of the emergency department is very important information for planning expansion and reconfiguration. People use the emergency department for many reasons, including access to primary care. Table 11.13 presents the risk of an urgent visit to the emergency departments for the service area population of the East Bank Regional Hospital System. This distribution of risk is determined using relative risk and is presented according to individual predictive factors. The greatest risk is observed in people under 65 years of age and those with Medicaid or CHIP as their primary payment source. The risk is higher among women compared to men and among whites compared to blacks.

Table 11.14 shows the risk of alcohol- and drug-related visits to the emergency department. In terms of gender, the greatest risk for all alcohol- and drug-related reasons is among females, especially with respect to alcohol-related visits. In terms of race, the greatest risk is observed in African Americans, especially with respect to drug-related visits. In terms of age, risk is significantly greater for persons under 65 (by a factor of more than 4 to 1 for all alcohol- and drug-related visits).

TABLE 11.13. RELATIVE RISK OF AN URGENT EMERGENCY DEPARTMENT VISIT.

Factor	Relative risk
Sex	
Males	0.78
Females	1.23
Race	
Whites	1.12
Blacks	0.95
Age	
Under 65 years	0.39
65 years and older	4.34
Payment source	
Medicare	0.67
Medicaid or CHIP	3.54
Private insurance	1.45
Self-pay	0.75
Other	1.19

TABLE 11.14. RELATIVE RISK OF AN ALCOHOL- OR DRUG-RELATED EMERGENCY DEPARTMENT VISIT.

Factor	*Relative risk*		
	Alcohol-related visit	Drug-related visit	Alcohol- and drug-related visit
Sex			
Male	0.45	0.87	0.32
Female	4.15	1.76	3.87
Race			
White	1.56	0.55	0.80
Black	0.82	1.85	1.65
Age			
Under 65 years	5.16	4.56	4.12
65 years and older	0.35	0.22	0.24
Payment source			
Medicare	0.51	0.40	0.88
Medicaid or CHIP	1.89	1.68	1.21
Private insurance	0.43	0.55	0.37
Self-pay	2.23	2.13	1.98
Other	1.61	1.55	1.52

10. How does the information on risk of an urgent emergency department visit guide expansion and reconfiguration planning?

11. In which hospital in the East Bank Regional Hospital System should an aggressive reconfiguration or expansion be initiated?

12. In a two- to three-page written report, present the strategic plan that will be given to the East Bank Regional Hospital System board. Emphasize the points that the board presented to the strategic planning task force:
    a. Identify growth areas for emergency health services.
    b. Identify areas for consolidation.
    c. Identify areas for expansion.
    d. Determine the level of profitability for the growth and reconfiguration areas.
    e. Target objectives that are measurable.
    f. Provide a timeline for activities.

    Indicate in this report the specific epidemiologic information you used to develop the recommendation.

CHAPTER TWELVE

QUALITY OF HOSPITAL CARE

Chapter Outline

Introduction
Population Characteristics
Age
Days of Care
Age and Sex
Primary Payment Source
Patient Satisfaction and Quality Improvement
Managed Care Contracting

Learning Objectives

Upon completing this chapter, the reader will be able to do all of the following:

- Explain the significance of demographic information
- Explain the role of epidemiologic information in the planning process
- Explain the role of epidemiologic information in managed care contracting
- Explain the role of epidemiologic information in evaluation of quality of care
- Explain the use of quality control charts

Introduction

Mid-City Hospital is one of four hospitals in the East Bank Regional Hospital System, located in the city of East Bank. The East Bank Regional Hospital System is a not-for-profit acute care hospital system that serves an urban population and its surrounding suburbs. The total population served is approximately 2.5 million people. Mid-City Hospital has 585 licensed beds and features a comprehensive hospital-based clinic system and an emergency department. The hospital personnel consist of 1,500 employees and a medical staff of 225 physicians.

In recent months, a quality-of-care improvement strategy was initiated in the hospital system. This initiative consisted of a quality improvement plan, the training of administrative and selected hospital staff in quality improvement methods and procedures, a focus on the use of data in decision making, and the establishment of quality improvement teams. Fundamental to quality improvement interventions are goal setting, establishment of a multidisciplinary team, commitment of visionary leadership, an ongoing improvement evaluation process, and a mechanism for feedback (Fos and others, 2005).

Quality improvement teams were formed, consisting of administrative, hospital, and medical staff members. Specific, clear, and achievable objectives were established, and an ongoing improvement evaluation process was planned, including concise and timely feedback. The CEO of the hospital system strongly supports this quality improvement initiative, which has been mandated by the hospital system board of directors.

1. Who should be selected from administration, hospital, and medical staff? Be specific with respect to general characteristics.
2. Identify the quality improvement objectives that should be included in the initial planning.

Mid-City Hospital has had an average daily patient population of 287 over the past eighteen months. The primary services provided at Mid-City Hospital are acute medical and surgical, with a significant amount of behavioral medical service, related to inner-city drug and alcohol use. Due to the demographics of the inner city, more than half of the hospital and clinic patients are recipients of Medicaid or CHIP and Medicare.

Two important dates loom in the future for Mid-City Hospital. By January 1 of next year (six months from now), Mid-City Hospital must present a detailed analysis of quality of care to the hospital system board of directors. This plan must be in a format that meets the quality-monitoring functions required by the Joint Commission on Accreditation of Healthcare Organizations. Two months later, Mid-City Hospital must finalize a managed care contract with a national managed care entity to serve a new, larger regional population.

Population Characteristics

The characteristics of the population that the hospital now serves and will serve under the future managed care contract constitute important strategic information that will be crucial during negotiation of the contract. Health and disease are not randomly distributed in the population. Understanding population characteristics is important because particular patterns of health and disease are associated with populations at risk. These patterns are expressed as epidemiologic measures, that is, rates and ratios, with geographic and demographic bounds.

Population information has been acquired by the East Bank Regional Hospital System planning office. The information that is presented here is important for the development of a quality improvement plan and evaluation, as well as for the preparation for managed care contracting.

Age

Information about demographics is important because different subgroups in the population experience differing levels of health and disease. This translates into different needs and demands for health care services across the population, resulting in an unequal distribution of types and levels of health care needs and uses by these various subgroups.

Table 12.1 presents the population distribution in Mid-City Hospital's service area. The age groups used are under 15 years, 15 to 44 years, 45 to 64 years, and 65 years and older. Three subgroups are shown for the 65-and-older group: 65 to 74 years, 75 to 84 years, and 85 years and older. These groups will be standard throughout this case study. The 15-to-44 age group contains the greatest proportion of the service area population (40%), followed by the 45-to-64 group (24%). The under-15 and over-65 groups are very similar in distribution, 18.2% and 16.2%, respectively. In the 65-and-older category, 63% are between 65 and 74 years of age.

Table 12.2 presents information on discharges over the past three years (2001–2003) according to age. The most discharges were seen in the 65-and-older age group every year except 2001. This represents approximately one-third of all discharges during the past three years. The lowest number of discharges occurred in the under-15 age group.

TABLE 12.1. AGE DISTRIBUTION IN MID-CITY HOSPITAL SERVICE AREA, 2003.

Age group	Distribution (%)
Under 15 years	18.2
15–44 years	40.7
45–64 years	24.9
65 years and older	16.2
65–74 years	10.2
75–84 years	4.8
85 years and older	1.2

TABLE 12.2. NUMBER OF DISCHARGES, 2001–2003, BY AGE.

Age group	2001	2002	2003
All ages	30,788	30,722	31,827
Under 15 years	2,412	2,405	2,299
15–44 years	11,799	10,593	10,376
45–64 years	6,244	6,168	6,696
65 years and older	10,333	11,556	12,456
65–74 years	4,689	4,832	4,876
75–84 years	3,949	4,590	5,099
85 years and older	1,694	2,134	2,481

3. Using Table 12.1 as a reference, discuss the trend in and the major reasons for the distribution of the discharges according to age.

4. Discuss the trend in and major reasons for the distribution of the discharges within the 65-years-and-older age group.

Table 12.3 shows the discharge rate (per 1,000 population) during the three-year period 2001–2003, broken down by age. The overall discharge rate decreased from 122.3 to 116.5 per 1,000 population during the study period. This same trend was observed in all age groups except the 65-years-and-older group, in which the discharge rate increased from 334.1 to 365.3 per 1,000 population. An increase was observed in all three age categories within the 65-and-older group.

5. The discharge rate decreased from 2001 to 2003, except in the 65-and-older age group. What are some possible reasons for this decrease in the younger categories?

6. What are some possible reasons for the discharge rate increase in the 65-and-older age group?

7. What effect, if any, do these discharge rate changes for different age groups have on the planning for managed care contracting?

Days of Care

The number of days of care from 2001 to 2003 is an important indicator. Table 12.4 shows the breakdown of days of care over the three-year period. In general, an overall decreasing trend was apparent in all age categories. The total number of days decreased from 197,422 in 2001 to 160,914 in 2003.

Table 12.5 presents the rate of days of care, by age. The rate decreased in all categories. The overall rate decreased from 784.0 to 589.2 per 1,000 population. In the 65-and-older category, the group with the highest rate during the three-year period, the rate decreased from 2,895.6 to 2,264.2 per 1,000 population. Another characteristic of

TABLE 12.3. DISCHARGE RATE PER 1,000 POPULATION, 2001–2003, BY AGE.

Age group	2001	2002	2003
All ages	122.3	115.7	116.5
Under 15 years	43.1	40.4	38.3
15–44 years	99.3	87.8	85.1
45–64 years	135.5	118.5	117.3
65 years and older	334.1	347.7	365.3
65–74 years	261.6	260.0	267.6
75–84 years	395.7	415.6	430.2
85 years and older	560.6	592.5	616.1

TABLE 12.4. NUMBER OF DAYS OF CARE, 2001–2003, BY AGE.

Age group	2001	2002	2003
All ages	197,422	164,627	160,914
Under 15 years	11,655	10,715	10,669
15–44 years	54,062	40,825	38,566
45–64 years	42,153	34,207	34,468
65 years and older	89,552	78,880	77,211
65–74 years	37,422	31,310	29,082
75–84 years	35,926	31,974	32,302
85 years and older	16,204	15,597	15,827

this trend is that as age increases, there is a positive correlation with the rate. The lowest rate is observed in the under-15 age group, and the highest is seen in the 65-and-older group. The same trend is apparent in the subgroups within the 65-and-older category.

8. What are the major reasons and factors for the decreasing trend in the rate of days of care over the period 2001–2003?

Hospital length of stay (in days) is the common measure used to evaluate system utilization. Table 12.6 shows the mean length of stay (referred to as the average length of stay, ALOS) in the service area population, according to age. As was seen with the number and rate of discharges and days of care, the average length of stay decreased over the three-year period. The overall ALOS decreased from 6.4 to 5.1 days. The 65-years-and-older age group had the highest ALOS (8.7 in 2001 and 6.2 in 2003), and the 15-to-44 age group had the lowest (4.6 in 2001 and 3.7 in 2003).

TABLE 12.5. RATE OF DAYS OF CARE PER 1,000 POPULATION, 2001–2003, BY AGE.

Age group	2001	2002	2003
All ages	784.0	620.2	589.2
Under 15 years	208.4	179.9	178.0
15–44 years	454.9	338.4	316.1
45–64 years	914.4	657.5	603.9
65 years and older	2,895.6	2,373.7	2,264.2
65–74 years	2,087.8	1,684.7	1,596.1
75–84 years	3,599.5	2,894.7	2,725.2
85 years and older	5,361.7	4,330.6	3,930.1

TABLE 12.6. AVERAGE LENGTH OF STAY, 2001–2003, BY AGE.

Age group	2001	2002	2003
All ages	6.4	5.4	5.1
Under 15 years	4.8	4.5	4.6
15–44 years	4.6	3.9	3.7
45–64 years	6.8	5.5	5.1
65 years and older	8.7	6.8	6.2
65–74 years	8.0	6.5	6.0
75–84 years	9.1	7.0	6.3
85 years and older	9.6	7.3	6.4

9. Discuss reasons that might explain the decreasing trend, according to age, in ALOS. In general, consider the effect of different methods of insurance and reimbursement, including private insurance, Medicare, Medicaid, and managed care plans.

Age and Sex

Table 12.7 presents the number of discharges, the discharge rate (per 1,000 population), and the ALOS for 2003 by age and sex. Over 60% of patients discharged were females. Among them, 39.5% of patients discharged were between the ages of 15 and 44, and 37.7% were 65 and older. Among women over 65, the majority of discharges (40.8%) were in the 75-to-84 age group. Among males, the majority of discharges occurred in the 65-and-older group (41.4%). The largest proportion of discharges among males older than 65 was seen in the 65-to-74 age group (44.2%). Figures 12.1, 12.2, and 12.3 depict these statistics graphically.

TABLE 12.7. NUMBER OF DISCHARGES, DISCHARGE RATE, AND AVERAGE LENGTH OF STAY, 2003, BY AGE AND SEX.

Age group	Number of discharges	Discharge rate (per 1,000 population)	Average length of stay (days)
All ages	31,827	116.5	5.1
Males	12,469	93.5	5.5
Under 15 years	1,303	42.5	4.7
15–44 years	2,718	44.6	5.1
45–64 years	3,286	118.8	5.3
65 years and older	5,162	365.4	5.5
65–74 years	2,284	278.5	6.1
75–84 years	2,118	446.4	6.4
85 years and older	761	642.6	6.4
Females	19,358	138.5	4.7
Under 15 years	996	34.0	4.5
15–44 years	7,659	125.4	3.2
45–64 years	3,410	115.9	5.0
65 years and older	7,293	365.2	6.2
65–74 years	2,592	258.6	6.1
75–84 years	2,982	419.4	6.3
85 years and older	1,720	605.1	6.3

FIGURE 12.1. DISCHARGE RATE, 2003, BY AGE AND SEX.

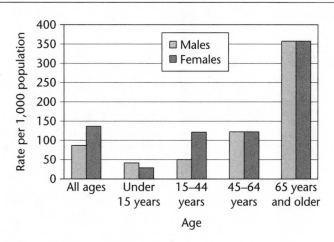

FIGURE 12.2. AVERAGE LENGTH OF STAY, 2003, BY AGE AND SEX.

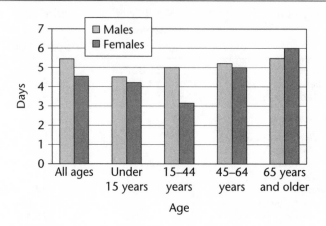

FIGURE 12.3. NUMBER OF DISCHARGES, 2003, BY AGE AND SEX.

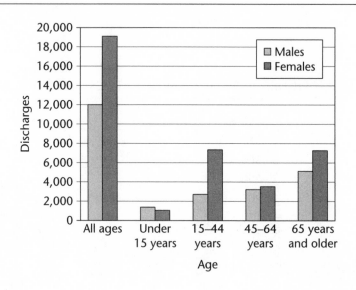

The discharge rate for females is 1.48 times greater than for males. The distribution across age among males and females is very interesting. The discharge rate consistently increases monotonically according to age in males, ranging from 42.5 to 365.4 per 1,000 population. In females, the discharge rate ranges from 34.0 to 365.2 per 1,000 population, but the rate for the 15-to-44 age group is higher than for the 44-to-64 age category, making it a nonmonotonic function. Another interesting fact is that the discharge rate for the 65-and-older age group is the same for males and females.

Reviewing ALOS by age and sex gives some interesting findings. The overall ALOS for males is higher than it is for females, 5.5 compared to 4.7 days. This comparison is true in all age categories up to age 65. But within the 65-and-older category, females had higher ALOS values. The 15-to-44 age group in females had the lowest ALOS, 3.2 days.

10. What new insights are provided by Table 12.7 for the discussion of the effect of decreasing discharge rates and ALOS on planning efforts?

11. Discuss the differences in the distribution of discharge rates across age for males and females. What could explain the nonmonotonicity of the female discharge rate distribution?

Primary Payment Source

Table 12.8 gives the breakdown of primary payment sources at Mid-City Hospital for 2003. Medicare beneficiaries represented the largest proportion of patients, closely followed by those covered by Medicaid or CHIP. This indicates that governmental sources paid for over half of the total costs of care during 2003 (51.2%). Private insurance accounted for slightly less than 20% of patients, with about 15% of patients paying their own way.

12. What, specifically, can be learned from the distribution of primary payment sources that can be translated to the planning efforts?

TABLE 12.8. PRIMARY PAYMENT SOURCE, 2003.

Payment source	Distribution (%)
Private insurance	18.2
Medicaid or CHIP	22.5
Medicare	28.7
Self-pay	14.7
Workers' compensation	3.5
No charge	8.0
Other or unknown	4.4

Patient Satisfaction and Quality Improvement

Excessive waiting is a major source of dissatisfaction for patients. Figure 12.4 is a graphic representation of the time patients spend waiting to be admitted. For thirty randomly selected patients, the average waiting time in the admissions office was 29.76 minutes, with a standard deviation of 10.25 minutes and a median waiting time of 30.50 minutes. This indicates that half of the patients waited 30 minutes or longer to be processed for admission into the hospital. The coefficient of variation is equal to 34.5%.

Figures 12.5, 12.6, and 12.7 are quality control charts of the distribution of the results from an inpatient satisfaction survey conducted at the time of discharge. These figures show the results of patient satisfaction surveys in three areas of Mid-City Hospital: admissions, medicine, and surgery. The survey responses were scored from 0 to 5, with 0 indicating not satisfied at all and 5 indicating complete satisfaction. The quality control charts present the mean and standard deviation values of twenty-five patients. The center line on the chart is the mean, and the hatched lines (known as control bounds) are ±3 standard deviations from the mean. Data points that are beyond the control bounds are referred to as being "out of quality control."

Figure 12.5 describes the patient satisfaction survey results for the admissions department. The mean value was 2.04, with a standard deviation of 1.22. The quality control chart indicates that all the survey responses were within the control bounds. Figure 12.6 presents the survey results for the patients in the medicine department. The mean was 3.40, with a standard deviation of 0.70. One patient's response was

FIGURE 12.4. ADMISSIONS DEPARTMENT WAITING TIME.

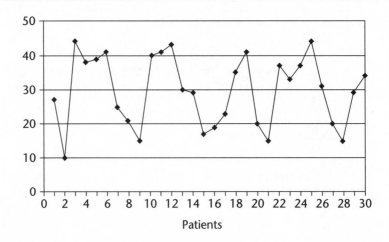

FIGURE 12.5. PATIENT SATISFACTION, ADMISSIONS DEPARTMENT.

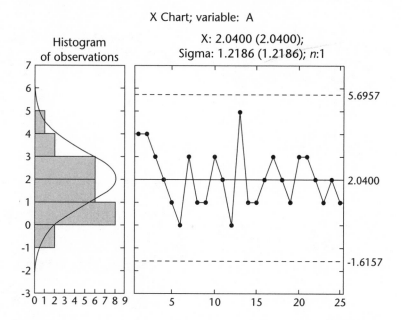

FIGURE 12.6. PATIENT SATISFACTION, MEDICINE DEPARTMENT.

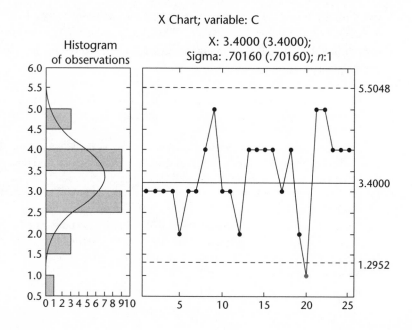

FIGURE 12.7. PATIENT SATISFACTION, SURGERY DEPARTMENT.

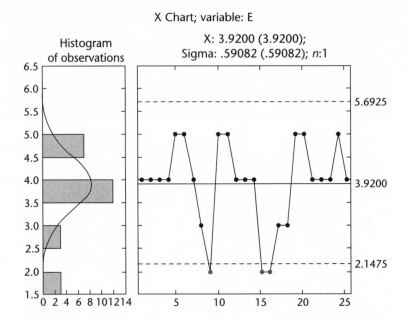

found to be out of quality control. Figure 12.7 shows the survey results from twenty-five patients in the surgery department. The mean satisfaction survey value was 3.92, with variation equal to 0.59. Among the surgery patients, three survey responses were out of quality control.

13. What are some possible causes of the variation in admissions department waiting times? Suggest a few potential remedies for the variation in and length of waiting time in the admissions department.

14. Using the quality control charts as a reference, answer the following questions:
    a. Is it better to have a high mean value of patient satisfaction and high variation or a moderate mean and low variation? Why?
    b. Which department would you target first, and what would you improve first, the mean or the variation?

15. Using patient satisfaction parameters, develop a brief report discussing areas for quality improvement and suggesting methods to achieve expected improvement.

16. What additional efforts should be undertaken to achieve the quality improvement objectives identified in question 2?

Managed Care Contracting

You must serve as the head of a team charged with negotiating a regional managed care contract for services provided by your health system. Assume that the entire Mid-City Hospital service area population will be included in this managed care contract. This contract will be negotiated with a national managed care entity. In preparation for the negotiation sessions, the team develops a list of questions that are assumed to be helpful. Answer the following questions.

17. What specific demographic considerations will become important when negotiating managed care reimbursement?
18. What special concessions might Mid-City Hospital have to include in the managed care contract, according to the characteristics of your population?
19. Which service area population subgroups cause the negotiating team the most concern with respect to the managed care contract?
20. In a two- to three-page written report, describe the negotiation strategy your negotiating team would recommend. Reference the specific epidemiologic information you used to develop your report.

CHAPTER THIRTEEN

PEDIATRIC INPATIENT SERVICES

Chapter Outline

Introduction
Population Characteristics
Westside Hospital Network
Historical Utilization Trends

Learning Objectives

Upon completion of this chapter, the reader will be able to do all of the following:

- Evaluate and use a secondary database
- Explain the significance of demographic information
- Explain the role of epidemiologic data in the planning process
- Explain the role of epidemiologic data in strategic planning

Introduction

Westside Hospital Network serves Westside City, East Coastal County, North Coastal County, and Southside County. Pediatric inpatient services have been targeted by the hospital network board as an area of excellence. The hospital network board has tasked the administration with developing a strategic plan to achieve recognition of excellence in pediatric inpatient services and an associated increase in market share. Current market share in Westside City is 16.6%, and an estimate of market share in the surrounding counties is 28.7%. The board's recommendations set out the following tasks:

- Identify growth areas for pediatric inpatient services.
- Identify existing areas of excellence.
- Identify existing areas for improvement.
- Determine the expected level of profitability as market share increases.
- Develop a strategic plan with target objectives that are measurable.
- Create a timeline for activities.

Population Characteristics

Westside City and the surrounding counties have a total population of 1,198,637. Westside City proper has a population of 484,674, with 46.9% male and 53.1% female. The median age is 33.1 years, with 7% of the population under the age of 5 years. The population under the age of 18 years equals 130,000. The racial distribution of Westside City is as follows: 135,956 white; 325,947 African American; 997 American Indian or Alaska Native; 10,972 Asian; 109 Native Hawaiian or other Pacific Islander; 10,699 other races or two or more races. Of the 484,674 in the population, 14,286 identify themselves as Hispanic or Latino of any race. Figure 13.1 presents a graphic representation of the population.

East Coastal County is a mixed urban-rural area with a total population of 455,466. The female-to-male ratio is 1.08. The median age is 35.9 years, with 30,226 people under the age of 5 years and 115,255 under the age of 18 years. The racial distribution is 318,002 white; 104,121 black; 2,032 American Indian or Alaska Native; 14,065 Asian; 154 Native Hawaiian or other Pacific Islander; 17,092 other races or two or more races. Of the 455,466 in the population, 32,418 are Hispanic or Latino of any race. Figure 13.2 presents a graphic representation of the population.

North Coastal County is a mixed residential-rural area with a total population of 191,268. There are 93,740 males (49%) and 97,528 females (51%) in the county. The

FIGURE 13.1. POPULATION OF WESTSIDE CITY, BY RACE.

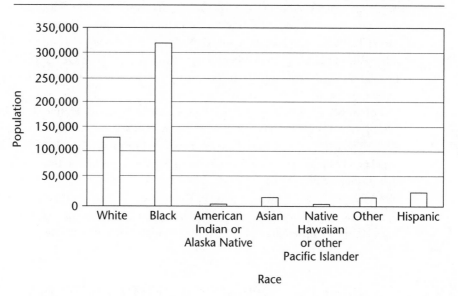

FIGURE 13.2. POPULATION OF EAST COASTAL COUNTY, BY RACE.

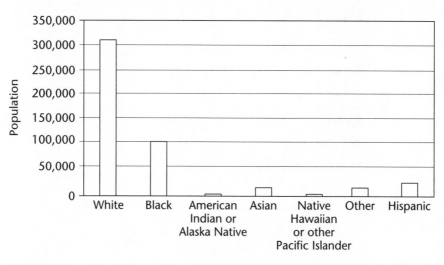

median age is 36.3 years, with 136,869 (71.6%) people over the age of 18 years. The pediatric population (under the age of 18 years) equals 54,399, with 13,556 people under the age of 5 years. The racial distribution is as follows: 166,458 white; 18,929 black; 825 American Indian or Alaska Native; 1,420 Asian; 57 Native Hawaiian or other Pacific Islander; 3,579 other races or two or more races. Of the 191,268 in the population, 4,737 are Hispanic or Latino of any race. Figure 13.3 presents a graphic representation of the population.

Southside County is similar to North Coastal County, given that it can be characterized as a mixed urban-rural area. Southside County has a total population of 67,229, with 32,495 males and 34,734 females. The median age is 36.6 years, with 4,242 people under the age of 5 years and 16,955 under the age of 18 years. The racial distribution is 59,356 white; 5,122 black; 329 American Indian or Alaska Native; 889 Asian; 14 Native Hawaiian or other Pacific Islander; and 1,519 other races or two or more races. Of the 67,229 in the population, 3,425 are Hispanic or Latino of any race. Figure 13.4 presents a graphic representation of the population.

FIGURE 13.3. POPULATION OF NORTH COASTAL COUNTY, BY RACE.

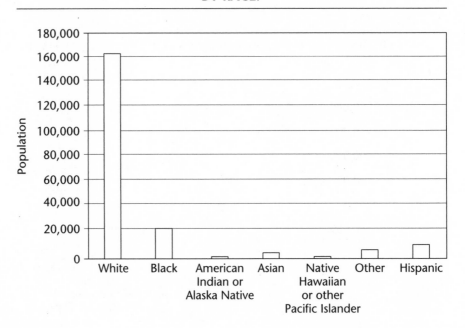

FIGURE 13.4. POPULATION OF SOUTHSIDE COUNTY, BY RACE.

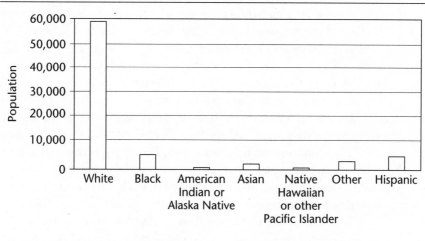

The total pediatric population for Westside City and the surrounding counties is 316,017. The total number of people employed in the labor force is 683,761 (57%); per capita income is $19,110, and median family income is $44,075. The number of individuals below the poverty level in each area is as follows: 130,896 in Westside City, 61,608 in East Coastal County, 18,336 in North Coastal County, and 8,687 in Southside County. The age distribution in the pediatric population in the entire service area is presented in Table 13.1. The majority of the pediatric population is under age 5 (51.83%), and over 25% is between the ages of 15 and 18 years.

TABLE 13.1. AGE DISTRIBUTION IN THE SERVICE AREA.

Age	Distribution (%)
Under 5 years	51.83
6–10 years	12.81
11–14 years	10.16
15–18 years	25.20

1. Discuss the differences in population in Westside City and the three surrounding counties. How would these differences affect planning?

2. Given the demographic information, which area of the Westside Hospital Network should be selected for expansion of pediatric services? Explain your selection.

Westside Hospital Network

The Westside Hospital Network is made up of three hospitals and six freestanding clinics. Two of the hospitals are located within the city limits of Westside City, with the remaining hospital in East Coastal County. Two clinics are in Westside City, two clinics are in East Coastal County, one clinic is in North Coastal County, and one clinic is in Southside County. Each of the three hospitals has a comprehensive emergency department, and the six clinics provide comprehensive ambulatory care services.

Westside Medical Center and Riverside Hospital are located in Westside City and are typical urban hospital facilities. Westside Medical Center has 645 beds, including a 200-bed children's pavilion. Riverside Hospital has 395 licensed beds and is a Level I trauma center. Westside Medical Center is a Level III trauma center and a Level II pediatric trauma center. Eastside Hospital is located in East Coastal County, has 200 licensed beds, and offers comprehensive services, including emergency medical services.

Table 13.2 presents information on the distribution of expected primary sources of payment for pediatric services in the Westside Hospital Network service area. The largest percentage of pediatric patients have private insurance coverage (52.79%), and more than 30% of the patients are Medicaid or CHIP recipients.

3. What information can you acquire from the distribution of primary payment sources? How will this distribution affect your plan?

Table 13.3 presents information on expected payment source by age of patient. As might be expected, the median age of patients covered by workers' compensation insurance is 17 years and the mean is 17.19 years, with a standard deviation of 0.83. The mean age for other primary payment sources ranges between 5.96 and 8.91 years. The median age for other payment sources ranges from 2 to 9 years.

4. What information can you acquire from the distribution of primary payment sources by age of patient? How will this affect your plan?

TABLE 13.2. EXPECTED PRIMARY PAYMENT SOURCES FOR PEDIATRIC SERVICES.

Primary payment source	Distribution (%)
Workers' compensation	0.18
Medicare	0.61
Medicaid or CHIP	31.13
Private insurance	52.79
Self-pay	8.49
Other	6.80

TABLE 13.3. EXPECTED PRIMARY PAYMENT SOURCES, BY AGE OF PATIENT.

Primary payment source	Mean age of patient	Median age of patient	Standard deviation
Workers' compensation	17.19	17.00	0.83
Medicare	5.96	2.00	6.95
Medicaid or CHIP	6.87	3.00	7.15
Private insurance	6.82	5.00	6.83
Self-pay	8.91	9.00	7.17
Other	7.24	6.00	6.40

Historical Utilization Trends

Historical inpatient utilization trends may be helpful in understanding the potential for increases in market share and profitability of future planning. Table 13.4 presents descriptive statistics on length of stay in the three hospitals in the Westside Hospital Network. The mean length of stay for the overall hospital network is 5.09 days (standard deviation of 6.17 days). Male patients have a longer length of stay than females do, and white patients have a shorter length of stay than patients of all other races do. Westside Medical Center has shorter stays than the other hospitals in the network. Medicare patients have longer stays, with private insurance patients demonstrating the shortest length of stay (mean of 4.92 days).

Table 13.5 presents information on length of stay, stratified into two categories (stays up to seven days and stays of more than seven days), from a sample of pediatric inpatients in the Westside Hospital Network. Overall, of slightly more than 9,000 inpatient stays, 7,854 (87%) were of seven days or less. This distribution remains constant regardless of population characteristics.

Figure 13.5 is a graphic representation of the distribution of short and long stays.

5. Assume that an LOS of up to seven days is classified as short, and an LOS greater than seven days is classified as long. Given this assumption, and using 2-by-2 contingency tables, determine the following ratios and risks:
   a. Risk of a long stay for whites as compared to African Americans
   b. Risk of a long stay for patients in Westside Medical Center as compared with patients in the other hospitals in the Westside Hospital Network
   c. Risk of a long stay for patients with private insurance as compared to patients with all other payment sources

6. Test the following hypotheses (see the Appendix):
   a. Patients in Westside Medical Center have shorter stays than patients in the other hospitals in the Westside Hospital Network.
   b. White patients have shorter stays than black patients.
   c. Male patients have shorter stays than female patients.

TABLE 13.4. LENGTH OF STAY, BY POPULATION CHARACTERISTICS.

Characteristic	Mean (days)	Median (days)	Standard deviation
Overall	5.09	3.00	6.17
Sex			
Male	6.49	4.00	8.77
Female	4.71	3.00	6.17
Race			
White	5.43	3.00	7.78
Black	6.72	4.00	7.10
Other	5.89	4.00	6.32
Hospital			
Eastside Hospital	7.23	5.00	8.51
Riverside Hospital	5.39	3.00	8.32
Westside Medical Center	5.31	3.00	7.14
Primary payment source			
Workers' compensation	4.98	3.00	6.44
Medicare	8.47	6.00	9.49
Medicaid or CHIP	5.51	3.00	6.23
Private insurance	4.92	3.00	6.57
Self-pay	5.80	3.00	7.39
Other	5.30	3.00	6.52

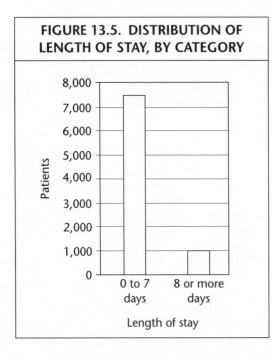

FIGURE 13.5. DISTRIBUTION OF LENGTH OF STAY, BY CATEGORY

d. Patients with private insurance have shorter stays than patients from all other payer sources.

7. The president of the hospital network wishes to seek regulatory approval to develop an innovative all-payer infant, child, and adolescent health care network. In a written report, design a program that will adopt a populationwide planning paradigm allowing such an initiative to work:

a. In the report, describe in detail the population according to the following characteristics: age, race, historical utilization, and primary payer.

b. Which subgroups of this population are at risk for a long stay? Why? Explain your answer.

8. In a written report, respond to the recommendations of the hospital network board:

TABLE 13.5. DISTRIBUTION OF SHORT AND LONG STAYS, BY POPULATION CHARACTERISTICS.

Characteristic	Number of short stays (up to 7 days)	Number of long stays (more than 7 days)
Overall	7,854	1,185
Age		
Under 5 years	3,995	690
6–10 years	1,023	135
11–14 years	780	138
15–18 years	2,056	222
Sex		
Male	3,774	649
Female	4,080	536
Race		
White	4,103	572
Black	1,651	283
Other	200	42
Hospital		
Eastside Hospital	981	74
Riverside Hospital	1,401	211
Westside Medical Center	5,472	900
Primary payment source		
Workers' compensation	15	1
Medicare	35	20
Medicaid or CHIP	2,209	363
Private insurance	4,175	596
Self-pay	690	77
Other	526	90

a. Identify growth areas for pediatric inpatient services.
b. Identify existing areas of excellence.
c. Identify existing areas for improvement.
d. Determine the expected level of profitability as market share increases.
e. Develop a strategic plan with target objectives that are measurable.
f. Create a timeline for activities.

CHAPTER FOURTEEN

COMMUNITY RELATIONS IN A HOSPITAL SERVICE AREA

Chapter Outline

Introduction
Population Characteristics
Pediatric Population
Adult Population
Population Health Characteristics
Resource Utilization
Health Status

Learning Objectives

Upon completing this chapter, the reader will be able to do all of the following:

- Evaluate and use a secondary database
- Explain the significance of demographic information
- Explain the role of epidemiologic data in the planning process
- Explain the role of epidemiologic data in strategic planning
- Explain the role of epidemiologic data in community outreach program planning

Introduction

Understanding all aspects of the population in a hospital's service area is a crucial aspect in managing the array of services offered. Specifically, evaluating past utilization, predicting future utilization, and understanding past and current health status, changes in health status, and the prevalence of diseases and conditions are necessary to plan for and provide health care services to the population in the service area. In addition to providing health services to meet medical needs, engaging in prevention and health promotion activities is an important concern.

The East Bank Regional Hospital System's board of directors has requested that the hospital system begin a formal program in community relations. This program will have the following objectives:

- To increase community awareness of services provided by the hospital system
- To identify target groups in the service area population for health education and promotion programs
- To determine the community's current and future trends in health status
- To design a plan for community outreach activities

Population Characteristics

The characteristics of the population of the service area are very important to the planning process for community-based activities. Knowledge of the distribution of population characteristics provides insight and may prove to be crucial information. To understand the characteristics of this population, the following information is needed: age, sex, race, payment source, health status, alcohol drinking status, smoking status, frequency of office visits to doctors, chronic disease prevalence, and body mass index. The information available is divided into two parts, data on the adult (18 years and older) and pediatric (under 18 years of age) segments of the population. The proportion of the population under age 18 is 21.4%.

Pediatric Population

Table 14.1 and Figure 14.1 present demographic information on the pediatric population in the service area. The greatest proportion (more than 50%) is children under 5 years of age. The mean age in the pediatric segment is 7.21 years, with a standard deviation of 6.83 years. The median age is 5 years. The mean age is 5.63 years for boys and 8.71 years for girls. Among whites, the mean age is 7.39 years, with a standard

TABLE 14.1. AGE INFORMATION FOR THE PEDIATRIC POPULATION.

Characteristic	Mean	Median	Standard deviation
All ages	7.21	5.00	6.83
Sex			
Male	5.63	3.00	6.07
Female	8.71	9.00	7.12
Race			
White	7.39	5.00	6.82
Black	7.10	4.00	6.99
Other	6.12	5.00	6.54
Payment source			
Private insurance	6.82	5.00	6.42
Medicaid	6.87	3.00	7.15
Medicare	5.96	2.00	6.95
Other	7.24	6.00	6.40
Uninsured	8.91	9.00	7.17

deviation of 6.82 years. Among African Americans, the mean age is 7.10 years, with a median age of 4 years. The mean age with respect to payment source is as follows: private insurance, 6.82 years; Medicaid, 6.87 years; Medicare, 5.96 years; other sources, 7.24 years; uninsured, 8.91 years.

Private insurance is the major primary payment source for the pediatric population in the East Bank Regional Hospital System's service area (see Table 14.2). Medicaid is the second most common payment source, covering 32.45% of all pediatric patients. Some 10.25% of the pediatric population is uninsured, and 12.26% of the patients are covered by some other payment source.

Table 14.3 presents hospital inpatient utilization information. The mean length of stay (LOS), in days, was 5.09, with a standard deviation of 6.17. For males, the LOS was 6.49, with a standard deviation of 8.77. For females, the mean (4.71) and the variation (standard deviation of 6.17) were both less than for males. African Americans had the highest mean LOS (6.72 days) compared to members of other races. The mean LOS for pediatric

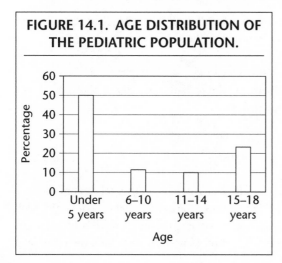

FIGURE 14.1. AGE DISTRIBUTION OF THE PEDIATRIC POPULATION.

TABLE 14.2. PAYMENT SOURCES FOR THE PEDIATRIC POPULATION.

Payment source	Distribution (%)
Private insurance	44.29
Medicaid	32.45
Medicare	0.75
Other	12.26
Uninsured	10.25

TABLE 14.3. LENGTH OF STAY FOR THE PEDIATRIC POPULATION.

Characteristic	Mean	Median	Standard deviation
Overall	5.09	3.00	6.17
Sex			
Male	6.49	4.00	8.77
Female	4.71	3.00	6.17
Race			
White	5.43	3.00	7.78
Black	6.72	4.00	7.10
Other	5.85	3.50	2.90
Payment source			
Private insurance	4.92	3.00	6.57
Medicaid	5.51	3.00	9.13
Medicare	8.47	6.00	9.49
Other	5.30	3.00	6.85
Uninsured	7.12	3.00	5.89

patients with private insurance was the lowest (4.92 days), and Medicare beneficiaries had the highest (8.47 days). The uninsured had the second highest mean LOS.

1. Discuss the pediatric population according to age, sex, and race.
2. Describe the utilization of services by the pediatric portion of the service area population.

Adult Population

Some 78.6% of the population in the East Bank Regional Hospital System's service area is 18 years of age and older. Table 14.4 shows the age distribution within the adult population. About half of the adults are between the ages of 18 and 44 years. Approximately a third are between the ages of 44 and 64 years, with the remaining fourth older than 65 years.

TABLE 14.4. AGE DISTRIBUTION OF THE ADULT POPULATION.

Age group	Distribution (%)
18–44 years	52.4
45–64 years	35.6
65–74 years	14.2
75 years and older	7.8

Risky lifestyle behaviors are important predictors of health and the use of health care services. In the East Bank Regional Hospital System's service area, alcohol consumption and smoking are two behaviors that have been of interest for some time. Table 14.5 presents information about alcohol drinking. The male-to-female ratio among current infrequent drinkers is 0.61 to 1. The ratio among current regular drinkers is 1.5 to 1. The 18-to-44 age group has the highest proportion of current regular drinkers, with more than half regularly consuming alcohol (55.2%). Almost half of the 45-to-64 age group are current regular alcohol drinkers (47.1%). Half of all whites are current regular alcohol drinkers, but only one-third of the members of other races. It is interesting to note that almost 56% of people with private insurance are current regular drinkers, the greatest proportion of all payment source categories.

Cigarette smoking status in the adult population is presented in Table 14.6. The male-to-female ratios are 1.21 to 1 for all current smokers, 1.20 to 1 for every day smokers, 1.37 to 1 for occasional smokers, 1.44 to 1 for former smokers, and 0.79 to

TABLE 14.5. ALCOHOL DRINKING STATUS.

Characteristic	Current infrequent drinkers	Current regular drinkers
Sex		
Male	10.4	58.9
Female	17.0	39.5
Age		
18–44 years	13.8	55.2
45–64 years	15.3	47.1
65 years and older	11.3	30.8
Race		
White	13.9	51.6
Black	13.7	34.7
American Indian or Alaska Native	16.1	37.6
Asian	11.6	34.4
Payment source		
Private insurance	14.4	55.8
Medicaid	15.1	30.3
Medicare	11.3	28.6
Other	14.7	41.0
Uninsured	13.7	46.5

TABLE 14.6. CIGARETTE SMOKING STATUS.

Characteristic	All current smokers	Every day smokers	Occasional smokers	Former smokers	Nonsmokers
Sex					
Male	24.9	20.4	4.8	26.4	48.5
Female	20.5	17.1	3.5	18.3	61.1
Age					
18–44 years	25.9	20.9	5.2	12.8	61.1
45–64 years	23.6	20.4	3.4	29.4	46.9
65 years and older	10.0	8.3	1.8	39.3	50.6
Race					
White	23.2	19.3	4.1	24.0	52.6
Black	22.0	17.4	4.9	14.4	63.4
American Indian or Alaska Native	31.5	25.6	5.8	21.0	47.5
Asian	12.5	10.7	1.9	9.6	77.7
Payment source					
Private insurance	21.5	17.4	4.2	20.5	57.8
Medicaid	37.9	32.9	5.3	14.1	47.8
Medicare	10.7	8.6	2.3	35.7	53.5
Other	35.6	31.9	4.1	24.3	39.6
Uninsured	34.4	28.8	5.9	12.5	52.8

1 for nonsmokers. The 18-to-44 age group had the largest proportion of current smokers (25.9%) and nonsmokers (61.1%).

American Indians and Alaska Natives represent the highest percentage of current smokers, with almost one-third of this subpopulation smoking cigarettes. The proportion of Asians who are current smokers is the lowest (12.5%), and the proportion who are nonsmokers is the greatest (77.7%).

Population Health Characteristics

The health of a population and its health risk can be evaluated in part by reviewing the prevalence of overweight and obesity. Overweight and obesity are caused by many factors, including behavioral, environmental, and socioeconomic issues. It has been suggested that as weight increases, the prevalence of health risks also increases. Overweight and obesity have been associated with high blood pressure, high blood cholesterol, heart disease, stroke, diabetes, and other conditions. As weight decreases, the effects of these diseases and conditions are reduced.

TABLE 14.7. BODY MASS INDEX (BMI) VALUES.

Weight category	BMI value	Approximate corresponding weight (pounds) for a person of average height	
		Men	Women
Healthy weight	18.5–24.9	121–163	108–144
Overweight	25.0–29.9	164–195	145–173
Obese	30 and above	196 and above	174 and above

Source: Centers for Disease Control and Prevention, 2001a.

A construct known as body mass index (BMI) is used to measure overweight and obesity. BMI is a function of weight and height, and its values are related to the categories of overweight ranges. Table 14.7 presents BMI values for healthy weight, overweight, and obesity. Studies have indicated that as BMI values increase, an individual's health risks increase.

Data on overweight and obesity originate from the National Health and Nutrition Examination Survey (NHANES), which is conducted by the Centers for Disease Control and Prevention's National Center for Health Statistics. Table 14.8 presents information from the 1998–1994 and 1999–2000 NHANES on the prevalence of overweight and obesity. The trend shows an increasing prevalence of overweight and obesity in the United States. In fact, after remaining constant over the two decades from 1960 to 1980, prevalence increased markedly over the next two decades, rising from 13% to 21% for men and from 17% to 26% for women.

Table 14.9 presents information on the distribution of BMI values in the East Bank Regional Hospital System's service area population. A total of 71.5% of the men and 50% of the women in the area are overweight or obese: 57.5% of whites and 67.2% of African Americans. The distribution of BMI values across age categories shows that the highest proportion of overweight and obesity is in the 45-to-64 age group (66.0%).

3. Discuss the adult portion of the population according to age. What insights can be gleaned from this information?

4. Describe the lifestyle behaviors in the adult population, including smoking and alcohol drinking. Which population groups should be targeted for an intervention?

5. What is the significance of the distribution of overweight and obese individuals in the adult population?

TABLE 14.8. TRENDS IN OVERWEIGHT AND OBESITY.

National Health and Nutrition Examination Survey	Overweight or obese (%)	Overweight (%)	Obese (%)
All adults			
1988–1994	56	33	23
1999–2000	64	34	30
Men, 1988–1994	60	40	20
Women, 1988–1994	51	26	25

TABLE 14.9. BODY MASS INDEX OF ADULTS IN THE SERVICE AREA POPULATION.

Characteristic	Underweight	Healthy weight	Overweight	Obese
Sex				
Male	0.8	32.7	43.8	22.7
Female	3.2	46.9	27.7	22.3
Age				
18–44 years	2.4	44.2	33.1	20.3
45–64 years	1.1	32.9	38.4	27.6
65 years and older	2.4	39.1	28.5	20.0
Race				
White	2.0	40.5	35.9	21.6
Black	1.4	31.5	34.9	32.3
American Indian or Alaska Native	4.5	33.5	34.5	27.5
Asian	6.1	61.3	26.3	6.3
Payment source				
Private insurance	1.7	40.4	35.7	22.2
Medicaid	3.2	35.0	26.8	35.1
Medicare	3.4	38.4	39.0	19.1
Other	2.2	35.4	35.6	26.9
Uninsured	2.8	41.0	34.7	21.5

Resource Utilization

Use of outpatient services is presented in Table 14.10 as office visits to doctors during the past twelve months. Females made more visits than males; 45.3% made four or more visits, compared to 29.1% of males. The largest proportion of the population making four or more visits occurred in the 75-years-and-older age group (64.6%), closely followed by the 65-to-74 age group (54.5%). Whites made more visits than blacks. Medicaid recipients had the highest proportion of four or more visits (57.4%) when compared to patients with all other primary payment sources.

TABLE 14.10. VISITS TO DOCTORS' OFFICES IN THE PAST TWELVE MONTHS.

Characteristic	Number of visits				
	None	One	Two or three	Four to nine	Ten or more
Sex					
Male	26.9	19.1	24.4	19.1	10.5
Female	12.7	14.7	27.3	28.1	17.2
Age					
18–44 years	25.0	19.5	26.0	18.6	10.9
45–64 years	16.4	15.7	27.1	25.8	15.0
65–74 years	8.5	11.9	25.2	33.9	20.6
75 years and older	6.2	8.2	21.0	40.7	23.9
Race					
White	18.7	16.4	26.3	24.3	14.4
Black	19.9	19.1	25.0	23.3	12.7
American Indian or Alaska Native	24.1	16.0	19.5	23.5	17.0
Asian	25.1	21.1	26.1	19.6	8.2
Payment source					
Private insurance	17.3	19.0	29.0	22.7	12.0
Medicaid	13.0	11.0	18.6	26.9	30.5
Medicare	11.3	12.2	20.9	36.7	18.9
Other	13.9	12.3	21.4	27.2	25.3
Uninsured	45.1	17.5	18.6	12.4	6.4

6. Discuss the distribution of office visits in the adult population. What insights or findings can be realized from this distribution that might be helpful in developing an initiative to increase community awareness of the East Bank Regional Hospital System?

Health Status

The self-assessed health status of the population in the service area is presented in Table 14.11. Overall, 38.4% of the members of this population rated their health status as excellent, 28.2% as very good, 20.5% as good, 9.5% as fair, and 3.4% as poor. Men rated personal health status higher than women did. As age increases, the proportion of the population with perceived excellent and very good health status decreases, and there is an accompanying increase in the proportion with perceived fair and poor health status. Asians have the highest proportion of excellent and very good health status self-ratings and the lowest proportion of fair and poor self-ratings.

TABLE 14.11. SELF-ASSESSED HEALTH STATUS.

Characteristic	Characterization of health status				
	Excellent	Very good	Good	Fair	Poor
All adults	38.4	28.2	20.5	9.5	3.4
Sex					
Male	39.5	23.6	21.4	12.3	3.2
Female	37.6	22.8	18.5	15.8	5.3
Age					
18–44 years	45.8	24.5	20.5	6.6	2.6
45–64 years	35.5	27.1	17.5	13.5	6.4
65–74 years	25.9	29.5	20.1	15.2	9.3
75 years and older	18.9	22.5	25.4	20.4	12.8
Race					
White	38.9	25.1	19.9	9.4	6.7
Black	33.6	22.5	19.5	11.5	12.9
American Indian or Alaska Native	34.5	23.2	18.2	10.5	13.6
Asian	43.8	25.8	20.8	6.8	2.8
Payment source					
Private insurance	42.5	25.9	20.2	8.4	3.0
Medicaid	25.8	28.4	25.2	12.8	7.8
Medicare	24.9	29.4	24.1	14.5	7.1
Other	33.8	24.5	22.1	11.5	8.1
Uninsured	38.5	26.2	19.4	10.2	6.7

It is interesting to evaluate change in self-assessed health status over time. Table 14.12 presents reports of changes in health status over the past year. A total of 18.3% of the members of the service area population reported that their health was better than it had been the year before. Only 4% reported that their health status had worsened over the past twelve months. More women reported better health status than men, and the same proportion stated that their health had worsened. As would be expected, as age increases, the proportion of the population reporting improved health status decreased. Conversely, as age increases, the proportion of the population stating that their health has worsened increased.

The change in health status across races indicated interesting findings. The proportion of Asians reporting improved health status was the lowest (15.0%). In addition, the proportion of Asians who reported that their health had worsened was the highest. A higher percentage of African Americans reported improved health status than whites did, with a greater proportion of whites stating that their health worsened over the past twelve months. Medicaid recipients had the greatest percentage reporting that their health had changed for the better or for the worse during the past twelve months.

TABLE 14.12. REPORTED CHANGE IN HEALTH STATUS OVER THE PAST TWELVE MONTHS.

Characteristic	*Characterization of health status*		
	Better than last year	**About the same as last year**	**Worse than last year**
All adults	18.3	77.7	4.0
Sex			
Male	17.4	78.7	4.0
Female	19.2	76.8	4.0
Age			
18–44 years	19.6	76.6	3.5
45–64 years	17.6	78.7	3.7
65–74 years	13.3	81.9	4.8
75 years and older	11.6	81.4	7.1
Race			
White	18.0	77.8	4.0
Black	19.4	76.9	3.7
American Indian or Alaska Native	21.5	74.2	4.3
Asian	15.0	79.8	5.2
Payment source			
Private insurance	18.8	77.6	3.6
Medicaid	25.9	67.8	6.3
Medicare	14.9	79.4	5.7
Other	15.2	82.3	2.5
Uninsured	13.3	86.7	1.6

Cancer prevalence in the service area population is presented in Table 14.13. Almost 7% of the population has some form of cancer. Of three major cancers, breast, cervical, and prostate, the prevalence in the population is less than 2%. Women have a slightly higher prevalence than men, and whites demonstrated a greater prevalence than all other races. As age increases, the prevalence of cancer increases, with 21.7% of the population in the 75-years-and-older age group exhibiting some form of cancer. In this age group, the prevalence of prostate cancer is 11.1%.

7. Which population groups should be targeted for interventions to improve their health status?

8. Write a report that would order a plan to increase community awareness of services provided by the hospital system. Include methods or sources of information that should be used to identify target groups in the service area population for health education and promotion programs.

9. Design a plan for community outreach activities, with timelines and expected outcomes of activities.

TABLE 14.13. PREVALENCE OF CANCER (PERCENTAGE OF POPULATION).

Characteristic	Site of cancer			
	Any site	Breast	Cervix	Prostate
All adults	6.9	1.1	1.1	1.5
Sex				
Male	6.2	0.0	0.0	1.5
Female	7.5	2.1	1.1	0.0
Age				
18–44 years	2.2	0.2	1.1	0.0
45–64 years	8.3	1.6	1.3	0.7
65–74 years	18.1	2.9	1.2	7.7
75 years and older	21.7	3.8	0.4	11.1
Race				
White	7.9	1.2	1.3	1.7
Black	2.9	0.6	0.4	1.1
American Indian or Alaska Native	2.6	0.2	0.0	1.3
Asian	0.9	0.2	0.3	0.3
Socioeconomic status				
Poor	6.3	1.1	1.5	1.5
Near poor	6.8	1.3	1.5	2.1
Not poor	6.5	1.0	1.2	1.2

APPENDIX

STATISTICAL CONCEPTS

This appendix is intended to assist the reader in understanding statistical concepts presented in the text. It is not intended to be a comprehensive introduction to the subject. It closely follows the work of Wayne W. Daniel (1995); see his work for an in-depth discussion.

Overview of Hypothesis Testing

There are two commonly used types of statistical inference: *estimation* and *hypothesis testing.* Both have the same purpose: to help a researcher or other investigator reach a conclusion about a population by examining a sample drawn from that population (Daniel, 1995). A hypothesis may be defined (in the context of this book) as a statement about one or more populations. A statistical hypothesis is stated in such a manner that it may be evaluated by an appropriate statistical technique. A flowchart of hypothesis testing is illustrated in Figure A.1.

Testing a Single Population Mean

There are three different conditions under which testing of a hypothesis about a population mean occurs: sampling is from a normally distributed population of values with known variance, sampling is from a normally distributed population with unknown variance, or sampling is from a population that is not normally distributed.

FIGURE A.1. FLOWCHART OF HYPOTHESIS TESTING.

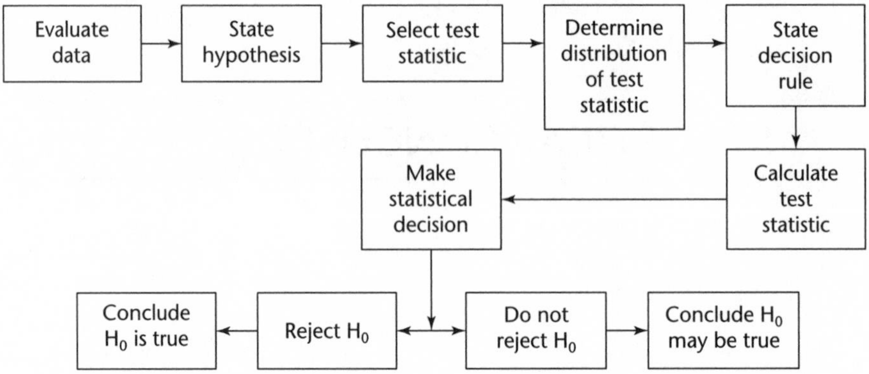

Example 1. The mean age of a population of registered nurses in a hospital department is of interest. Some observers have stated that the age of the population has changed over the past thirty years, when the mean was 30 years of age. The investigation of this statement consists of the following: $n = 10$ randomly selected individuals, sample mean = 27 years of age, and $\sigma^2 = 20$.

The null hypothesis is that the mean age of the registered nurse population is equal to 30 years of age; the alternative hypothesis is that it is not. The hypotheses are as follows:

$$H_0 : \mu = 30$$
$$H_A : \mu \neq 30$$

The population is assumed to be normally distributed and the population variance is known.

Choosing the decision rule concerns when to reject and when not to reject H_0. This depends on the significance level, α, which is the magnitude of the probability of the occurrence of a *Type I error.* Assume that $\alpha = 0.05$. The stated hypotheses do not indicate the direction of difference from the hypothesized mean (H_A: $\mu \neq 30$ indicates that the true μ may be greater or less than the hypothesized μ). Given this, α should be divided equally (to represent each direction), and $\alpha = 0.05/2$ or $\alpha/2 = 0.025$. This is an example of a two-sided (or two-tailed) test.

At an α of 0.025, the rejection or nonrejection areas of the normal distribution can be determined. The value of z to the right, which includes 0.025 of the area under the normal distribution, is 1.96. The value of z to the left, which also includes 0.025 of the area under the normal distribution, is -1.96. The rejection region is all values of z that are greater than 1.96 and less than -1.96. You should reject H_0 if $1.96 \leq z \leq -1.96$;

otherwise, you should not reject H_0. The values of the test statistic that separate the rejection and nonrejection regions are called the *critical values* of the test statistic, and the rejection region is called the *critical region* (in our example, 1.96 and −1.96 are the critical values).

p-Values

The *p*-value is the exact probability of getting a value as extreme as, or more extreme than, that observed if H_0 were true. A common and preferred practice is to state the computed value of the test statistic along with the *p*-value. The *p*-value is used instead of simply stating that the test statistic is significant or not. For example, assume that in Example 1, the test statistic is −2.12 and the *p*-value is 0.0340. The statement $p = 0.0340$ means that the probability of getting a value as extreme as 2.12 in either direction, when H_0 is true, is 0.0340. The *p*-value is found on the test statistic table, and it represents the probability of observing a $z \geq 2.12$ or a $z \leq -2.12$, when H_0 is true. That is, when H_0 is true, the probability of obtaining a value of z as large as or larger than 2.12 is 0.0170, and the probability of observing a z as small as or smaller than −2.12 is 0.0170. The probability of one or the other is the sum of the individual probabilities, or 0.0340.

By definition, the *p*-value for a hypothesis test is the probability of obtaining, when H_0 is true, a value of the test statistic as extreme as or more extreme (in the appropriate direction) than the value of the test statistic actually computed. The *p*-value can be alternatively defined as the smallest value of α for which H_0 can be rejected. In the preceding example, the *p*-value is 0.0340, so at $\alpha = 0.05$ you can reject H_0. At α less than 0.0340 (for example, 0.01 or 0.001), you could no longer reject H_0. If the *p*-value is greater than α, you do not reject H_0.

Stating *p*-values in the results of a study is more informative than stating that "the null hypothesis is rejected at the 0.05 level of significance" or "the results were not significant at the 0.05 level."

t-Distribution

The statistician William Gossett, who worked for the Guinness Brewery, solved the problem of whether a sample distribution is normally distributed. He called it the *Student's t-distribution* (Gossett's pseudonym was Student). He found that the shape of the distribution depended on the sample n. He realized that the *t*-distribution was a family of distributions indexed by a parameter known as degrees of freedom of the distribution. If $x_1, \ldots, x_n$ is normally distributed, then it is distributed as a *t*-distribution with $(n-1)$ degrees of freedom (df).

The notation of a *t*-distribution represents the level of significance and degrees of freedom. For example, the notation $t_{20,.95}$ represents the 95th percentile, or the upper 50th percentile of a t-distribution with 20 degrees of freedom. The t-distribution is always symmetrical around 0.

χ^2 (Chi-Square) Distribution

One problem facing data interpretation is the interval estimation of the mean of a normal distribution. Another problem of interest is obtaining interval estimates of the variance. These estimates will be valid only if the distribution is normally distributed. To obtain an interval estimate for s^2, the χ^2 distribution allows for the determination of s^2.

If $G = \Sigma x_i$, where $x_1, \ldots, x_n$ is normally distributed, G is said to follow a χ^2 distribution with n df.

The χ^2 distribution is not symmetrical around 0 for any number of degrees of freedom but only takes on positive values. In addition, the χ^2 distribution is usually skewed to the right. When $n > 100$, the distribution becomes more symmetrical.

The t-distribution and χ^2 distribution tables are constructed similarly. The major difference between the tables is that both lower ($p \leq 0.5$) and upper ($p > 0.5$) percentiles are listed for the χ^2 distribution. Only upper percentiles are listed for the t-distribution. This is due to the fact that the t-distribution is symmetric around 0, and the lower percentile can be obtained as the negative of the corresponding upper percentile. This cannot be done for the χ^2 distribution because it is usually a skewed distribution.

One-Sided Hypothesis Tests

In a two-sided (two-tailed) hypothesis test, the rejection region is divided between the two sides (tails) of the distribution of the test statistic. A hypothesis test may be one-sided (one-tailed), in which case the entire the rejection region is on one side of the distribution. Whether the hypothesis test is one-or two-sided depends on the study question.

Example 2. The mean age of a population of registered nurses in a hospital department is of interest. Some observers have stated that the age of the population has changed over the past thirty years, when the mean was 30 years of age. The investigation of this statement consists of the following: $n = 10$ randomly selected individuals, sample mean = 27 years of age, and $\sigma^2 = 20$. Can you conclude that $\mu < 30$?

The null hypothesis is that the mean age of the registered nurse population is greater than or equal to 30 years of age. The hypotheses are as follows:

$$H_o : \mu \geq 30$$

$$H_A : \mu < 30$$

The population is assumed to be normally distributed, and the population variance is known.

Choosing the decision rule concerns when to reject and when not to reject H_0. This depends on the significance level, α, which is the magnitude of the probability of the occurrence of a Type I error. Assume that $\alpha = 0.05$. The stated hypotheses indicate the direction of difference from the hypothesized mean (H_A: $\mu < 30$ indicates that the true μ may be less than the hypothesized μ). Because this is a one-sided test of the hypothesis, all the α values will go in one direction, and you want the rejection region to be where small values are, at the lower tail of the distribution. Using the normal distribution table, the value of z to the left of the distribution (which is the tail of interest), beyond which lies 0.05 of the area under the normal curve, is -1.65. You will reject H_0 if the calculated value of z is less than or equal to -1.65.

Statistical Power

In hypothesis testing, you define the null hypothesis (denoted H_0) as the hypothesis that is to be tested. In addition, you define the alternative hypothesis (denoted H_A or H_1) as the hypothesis that in some sense contradicts the null hypothesis (H_0). An objective of hypothesis testing is to compare the probabilities of the truth of these hypotheses.

By convention, the null hypothesis is typically expressed as an equality (for example, H_0: $\mu_1 = \mu_2$), and the alternative hypothesis is expressed as an inequality (for example, H_A: $\mu_1 \neq \mu_2$ or $\mu_1 > \mu_2$ or $\mu_1 < \mu_2$). In hypothesis testing, the possible decisions you can make are the following:

1. You decide that H_0 *is true* and state that you *accept* H_0, or
2. You decide that H_A *is true*, state that H_0 *is not true*, and you *reject* H_0.

The following possible events can occur:

1. You accept H_0 and H_0 is in fact true,
2. You accept H_0 and H_A is in fact true,
3. You reject H_0 and H_0 is in fact true, or
4. You reject H_0 and H_A is in fact true.

Error in hypothesis testing is classified as either *Type I* or *Type II error*. Type I error occurs when you reject H_0 and H_0 is in fact true. Type II error occurs when you accept H_0 and H^A is in fact true. Other important constructs are these:

1. α, which is referred to as the significance level of a test and is defined as the probability of a Type I error, and
2. β, which is defined as the probability of a Type II error (see Table A.1).

TABLE A.1. TYPE I AND TYPE II ERRORS.

	Actual truth	
Your decision	**H₀**	**Hₐ**
Accept H$_0$	H$_0$ is true and you accept H$_0$.	H$_A$ is true and you accept H$_0$ (Type II error) (β).
Reject H$_0$	H$_0$ is true and you reject H$_0$ (Type I error) (α).	H$_A$ is true and you reject H$_0$.

The power of a statistical test is defined as $1 - \beta$, or 1 minus the probability of a Type II error.

In general, you should endeavor to use statistical tests that make α and β as small as possible. The caveat to simply making these constructs arbitrarily very small is the following dilemma: making α small results in rejecting the null hypothesis (H$_0$) less often, and making β small results in accepting the null hypothesis (H$_0$) less often, which are contradictory actions. To mitigate this tension, the convention is to fix α at a specific level (for example, 0.10, 0.05, 0.01, and so on) and to use a test that minimizes β (that is, maximizes power).

The power of a statistical test can be defined, in words, as the ability of the test to detect true differences, that is, to find significant difference if H$_A$ is true. The power actually quantifies the probability that a test will detect true differences. If the power is low, then there is little chance of finding a significant difference even if there is a real difference (that is, if H$_A$ is true). One result of this is the acceptance of H$_0$. The most common cause of low power is inadequate sample size.

Example 3. This example illustrates the method to calculate the power of a test. The following data are from a study on low-birth-weight deliveries: number of full-term deliveries = 100 (n), sample mean birth weight = 115 oz. (μ_1), sample standard deviation = 24 oz. (s), U.S. mean birth weight = 120 oz. (μ_0), and U.S. standard deviation = 25 oz. (σ). Given these data, the power is defined by the following equation:

$$\text{Power} = \phi\left[\frac{z_\alpha\left(\left(\mu_o - \mu_1\right)n\right)}{\sigma}\right]$$

$$\text{Power} = \phi\left[\frac{z_{.05} + \left(\left(120 - 115\right)\left(10\right)\right)}{25}\right]$$

$$\text{Power} = \phi\left[\frac{-1.645 = 5\left(10\right)}{25}\right]$$

$$\text{Power} = \phi\left(0.355\right)$$

$$\text{Power} = 0.639$$

The symbol Φ denotes the normal distribution function (see the normal distribution function table in any standard statistics text), and z_α denotes the standardized normal variable. To calculate z, you must use the normal distribution function; for example, $\Phi(1.96) = 0.975$, $\Phi(1.645) = 0.95$, $\Phi(0) = 0.5$, $\Phi(-1.96) = 1 - \Phi(-1.96) = 1 - 0.975 = 0.025$; so $z_{0.975} = 1.96$, $z_{0.95} = 1.645$, $z_{0.5} = 0$, and $z_{0.025} = -1.96$.

This calculation indicates that there is a 63.9% chance of detecting a significant difference using a 5% significance level ($\alpha = 0.05$) with this sample size ($n = 100$).

Factors that affect the power include the following.

1. If the significance level is made smaller (α decreases), z_α decreases and power decreases.
2. If the standard deviation of an individual observation increases (σ increases), the power decreases.
3. If the sample size increases (n increases), the power increases.

Sample Size

Whenever studies are planned or designed, and when data are analyzed and interpreted, a major concern is the size of the study sample. The most common question is how large the sample should be to avoid erroneous interpretations. A simplistic approach would be to take as large a sample as possible, but this is a waste of valuable resources. Taking a conservative approach, which may result in a small sample, may lead to results that are meaningless due to the low power of the statistical test.

Sample Size for Estimating Means

Whenever you estimate an internal measure, you wish to obtain narrow intervals with high reliability (quantified by narrow *confidence intervals*). The components of a confidence interval are the *reliability coefficient* and the *standard error* (SE). The width of the confidence interval is the product of these two components: reliability coefficient x standard error. This construct is known as the margin of error.

Holding the standard error constant, if you increase reliability, the reliability coefficient increases, and a wider confidence interval results. If you hold the reliability coefficient constant, the width of the confidence interval is reduced by reducing the standard error. If σ is constant, the only method to reduce the SE is to increase the sample size (n). But how much should you increase n? The appropriate sample size depends on three things:

1. The size of σ
2. The desired degree of reliability
3. The desired confidence interval width

Assume that you desire a confidence interval to extend d units on either side of the estimator. Then d = reliability coefficient x standard error, and

$$n = \frac{z^2 \sigma^2}{d^2}.$$

The formula for sample size requires knowledge of the population variance (σ^2), which is usually unknown. So σ^2 must be estimated by one of the following methods:

1. A pilot sample may be drawn from a population, and the variance computed from this pilot sample is used as an estimate of σ^2. Observations used in the pilot sample may be included in the final sample.
2. Estimates of σ^2 may be available from previous or similar studies.
3. If the population from which the sample is drawn is thought to be approximately normally distributed, then you may assume that the range (R) is 6 standard deviations and that $\sigma = \frac{R}{6}$.

To use this method, you must know the smallest and largest value of the variable in the population.

Example 4. A national HMO wants to conduct a survey among a large population of physicians to determine their daily use of prescribed medications for HMO members (assume that this information is not routinely collected). How many physicians should be surveyed?

The HMO would like a confidence interval 10 prescriptions wide, which means that the estimate should be within about 5 prescriptions of the population mean in either direction (that is, a margin of error of 5 prescriptions). Assume that the HMO desires a confidence coefficient equal to 0.95 ($z = 1.96$), and the HMO (from previous surveys) feels that the population standard deviation is about 20. So if

z = 1.96 (0.95 confidence interval),
σ = 20 (from previous surveys), and
d = 5 (request of the HMO), then

$$n = \frac{z^2 \sigma^2}{d^2}$$

$$= \frac{(1.96)^2 (20)^2}{(5)^2}$$

$$= 61.47.$$

The HMO should take a sample of 62 physicians.

Sample Size for Estimating Proportions

The method is similar when determining the sample size for estimating means. Assuming random sampling and that conditions exist to assume approximate normality of the distribution of p, the sample size is determined as follows:

$$n = \frac{z^2 pq}{d^2}$$

where $q = 1 - p$.

This formula requires knowledge of p, which is the proportion of the population possessing the characteristic of interest. This is unknown, because it is the parameter that you are attempting to estimate. Methods to estimate p include the following:

1. A pilot sample may be drawn from a population, and the proportion of the pilot sample with the characteristic of interest is used as the population proportion, p.
2. Often an investigator has some idea of an upper bound of p (for example, you may know that less than 30% of a population can have the characteristic of interest, so 0.30 may be used as p).
3. If you have no idea, set p to 0.5. (Be aware, however, that this could lead to a larger sample than needed.)

Example 5. A hospital in the process of contracting with a local HMO in a large metropolitan area wants to conduct a survey to determine the proportion of people in the population at risk for a hospitalization in the next six months. The hospital CEO believes that the proportion cannot be greater than 0.35. A 95% confidence interval is desired (so $z = 1.96$), with $d = 0.05$. If $z = 1.96$ (0.95 confidence interval), $p = 0.35$ (from Fife), $q = 0.65$ ($q = 1 - p$), and $d = 0.05$ (request of the hospital), then

$$n = \frac{z^2 pq^2}{d^2}$$

$$= \frac{(1.96)^2 (.35)(.65)}{(.05)^2}$$

$$= 349.6.$$

The sample size should be 350 people.

Hypothesis Testing Using Categorical Data

Most of the data presented in the case studies in this book are in the form of categorical data. If the variable under study is not continuous and is classified into categories, then assumptions and inference procedures based on an underlying normal distribution are not applicable and alternative methods must be used.

Contingency Table Method

One alternative method employs 2-by-2 contingency tables. A 2-by-2 contingency table is a table composed of two rows and two columns. This provides a way to display data that can be classified by two different variables, each of which has two possible values; Table A.2 is an example of such a table. The cells of the table are referred to as O_{11}, O_{12}, O_{21}, and O_{22}. With a 2-by-2 contingency table, it is customary to make three sorts of tallies:

1. The number of units in each row, displayed in the right margins, called *row totals*
2. The number of units in each column, displayed in the bottom margins, called *column totals*
3. The total number of units in the table, displayed in the lower right-hand corner of the table, called the *grand total*

The principle used in hypothesis testing with the 2-by-2 contingency table method is to compare observed with "expected" contingency tables. After determining the expected values for the contingency table, a χ^2 test can be used to test a hypothesis. The following examples will illustrate the method.

Example 6. Assume the 2-by-2 contingency table in Table A.2 and Figure A.2 and the following hypotheses:

H_0: the proportion of males with a long stay is equal to the proportion of females with a long stay

H_A: the proportion of males with a long stay is not equal to the proportion of females with a long stay (two-tailed test)

or

H_A: the proportion of males with a long stay is greater than the proportion of females with a long stay (one-tailed test).

FIGURE A.2. A 2-BY-2 CONTINGENCY TABLE.

	Column 1	Column 2	Totals
Row 1	1, 1	1, 2	Row 1 total
Row 2	2, 1	2, 2	Row 2 total
Totals	Column 1 total	Column 2 total	Grand total

TABLE A.2. SAMPLE DATA.

	Long stay	Short stay	Total
Male	683	1,498	2,181
Female	2,537	8,747	11,284
Total	3,220	10,245	1,465

The expected values must be calculated. (These are the values that are expected if the null hypothesis is true.) If H_0 is true, this would indicate that there is no relationship between the dependent and independent variables. The method used to calculate the expected values is as follows:

E_{11}	E_{12}
E_{21}	E_{22}

1. Expected value for O_{11}

$$E_{11} = \frac{\left[(\text{row 1 total})(\text{column 1 total})\right]}{\text{grand total}}$$

2. Expected value for O_{12}

$$E_{12} = \frac{\left[(\text{row 1 total})(\text{column 2 total})\right]}{\text{grand total}}$$

3. Expected value for O_{21}

$$E_{21} = \frac{\left[(\text{row 2 total})(\text{column 1 total}) \right]}{\text{grand total}}$$

4. Expected value for O_{22}

$$E_{22} = \frac{\left[(\text{row 2 total})(\text{column 2 total}) \right]}{\text{grand total}}$$

Example 7. Calculation of expected values for Table A.3 would be as follows:

1. Expected value for O_{11}

$$E_{11} = \frac{\left[(2,181)(3,220) \right]}{13,465}$$
$$= 521.6$$

2. Expected value for O_{12}

$$E_{12} = \frac{\left[(2,181)(10,245) \right]}{13,465}$$
$$= 1659.4$$

3. Expected value for O_{21}

$$E_{21} = \frac{\left[(11,284)(3,220) \right]}{13,465}$$
$$= 2698.4$$

4. Expected value for O_{22}

$$E_{22} = \frac{\left[(11,284)(10,245) \right]}{13,465}$$
$$= 8585.6$$

The expected contingency table would be as shown in Table A.3.

After determining the expected values, the observed contingency table is compared with the expected contingency table. If the corresponding cells in the two tables are close in value, you would accept the null hypothesis. Conversely, if the corresponding cells in the two tables are far apart in value, you would reject the null hypothesis. How should you decide how far apart the cells must be to reject the null hypothesis?

Perhaps the best method is to compare the cells using the χ^2 statistic, which is

$$\frac{(O - E)^2}{E},$$

TABLE A.3. EXPECTED LENGTH OF STAY.

	Long stay	Short stay	Total
Male	521.6	1,659.4	2,181
Female	2,698.4	8,585.6	11,284
Total	3,220.0	10,245.0	13,465

where O = observed and E = expected number of units in a particular cell. In fact, under the null hypothesis, it can be shown that the sum of $(O - E)^2/E$ over the four cells in the table approximately follows a χ^2 distribution, with one degree of freedom. You reject the null hypothesis if this sum is large, and you accept the null hypothesis otherwise, because small sums correspond to good agreement between the two tables and large sums correspond to poor agreement. This test is used if no expected value in the table is less than 5.

Yates Corrected Chi-Square Test for a 2-by-2 Contingency Table

Under certain circumstances, a version of the χ^2 test statistic with a continuity correction yields more accurate p-values than the uncorrected version just discussed when approximated by a χ^2 distribution. This corrected statistic is

$$\frac{\left(|O - E| - \frac{1}{2}\right)^2}{E}$$

for each cell, rather than

$$\frac{(O - E)^2}{E}.$$

This test procedure is referred to as a χ^2 test using the Yates correction and is accomplished as follows:

1. The test statistic (T) is computed:

$$T = \left[\frac{\left(|O_{11} - E_{11}| - .5\right)}{E_{11}}\right] + \left[\frac{\left(|O_{12} - E_{12}| - .5\right)}{E_{12}}\right] + \left[\frac{\left(|O_{21} - E_{21}| - .5\right)}{E_{21}}\right] +$$

$$\left[\frac{\left(|O_{22} - E_{22}| - .5\right)}{E_{22}}\right]$$

which, under the null hypothesis, approximately follows a χ^2 distribution, with 1 df.

2. For a level α test, you reject H_0 if $T > \chi^2$ critical value (found in the χ^2 table) at 1 df (and $1 - \alpha/2$ for a two-tailed test and $1 - \alpha$ for a one-tailed test); and accept H_0 if $T \leq \chi^2$ critical value (found in the χ^2 table) at 1 df (and $1 - \alpha/2$ for a two-tailed test and $1 - \alpha$ for a one-tailed test).

3. This test is used if none of the four expected values is less than 5.

Example 8. To test the statistical significance of the data presented in Examples 6 and 7, we calculate the Yates corrected χ^2 statistic:

$$T = \left[\frac{\left(|638 - 521.6| - .5 \right)^2}{521.6} \right] + \left[\frac{\left(|1498 - 1,659.4| - .5 \right)^2}{1,659.4} \right] +$$

$$\left[\frac{\left(|2,537 - 2,698.4| - .5 \right)^2}{2,698.4} \right] + \left[\frac{\left(|8,747 - 8,585.6| - .5 \right)^2}{8,585.6} \right]$$

$$= \frac{(160.9)^2}{521.6} + \frac{(160.9)^2}{1,659.4} + \frac{(160.9)^2}{2,698.4} + \frac{(160.9)^2}{8,585.6}$$

$$= 49.63 + 15.60 + 9.59 + 3.02$$

$$= 77.84$$

The critical value in the χ^2 distribution table at 1 df and $1 - \alpha$ is 10.83. Since $T = 77.84$ ($T > 10.83$) and $p < 1 - 0.999$ ($p = 0.001$), you must reject the null hypothesis and conclude that there is a significant difference between the proportion of males with a long hospital stay and the proportion of females with a long hospital stay.

Extreme Values: Outliers

The arithmetic mean is a natural measure of central location in a data set and is commonly used as a measure of central tendency. A major limitation of the arithmetic mean is that it is very sensitive to extreme values and, if affected by them, may not be representative of the location of the great majority of points in the data set. Extreme values can be thought of as values that deviate significantly from most of the measurements in the data set. These extreme values are often referred to as *outliers.*

Identification of Outliers

Outliers may be defined in several ways. One method is to assume that the data set is normally distributed, and a function of the standard deviation from the mean of the data set is used to identify outliers. Remember that if the data set is normally distributed,

5% of the data points will be ±1.96 standard deviations from the mean of the data set. Various thresholds are used, including ±2.5 and ±3.0 standard deviations from the mean, as the defining characteristic. That is, all data points that are greater than or less than the threshold value (for example, greater than 2.5 or less than –2.5) are outliers. The Centers for Medicare and Medicaid Services use this method.

A more complicated method is as follows. First, upper and lower bounds of the data set are identified. The upper bound (UB) is defined as

$$UB = mean + standard\ error.$$

The upper bound is analogous to the 75th percentile of the data set distribution. The lower bound (LB) is defined as

$$LB = mean - standard\ error,$$

which is analogous to the 25th percentile of the data set distribution.

A data point is considered an outlier if it satisfies the following conditions:

$$Data\ point > UB + outlier\ coefficient\ x\ (UB - LB)$$

or

$$Data\ point < LB - outlier\ coefficient\ x\ (UB - LB).$$

The outlier coefficient is analogous to the threshold of the standard deviation; commonly used outlier coefficients are 1.5 and 2.0. The determination of the outlier coefficient is dependent on the variability and range of the data set.

A third method is to compare the data set with known population parameters. For example, the population mean can be used as the population parameter that will determine outliers. To identify outliers, you must compute the range around each population mean, as well as a range around each data subgroup. Outliers will be defined as values that fall outside the range. Data points that are less than the least value and data points that are greater than the greatest value in the population range are considered outliers.

An example involves determining length-of-stay (LOS) outliers according to diagnosis codes across types of hospitals, based on the number of hospital beds. For each diagnosis code, the mean LOS and standard deviation are determined across the population and hospital category. To identify outliers, you must compute the range around each population mean, as well as a range around each hospital category mean, for the same diagnosis.

LOS outliers are identified if the maximum of the LOS range for a hospital category exceeds the maximum of the LOS range for the population in each specific diagnosis code. In theory, LOS outliers should include extremely low LOS (out of the population range) as well as extremely high LOS. If you assume that maximum reimbursement is fixed at the population range maximum, you should be more concerned with controlling high LOS. Some of the very low LOS values could be caused by upcoding or coding errors, but they are not the first priority, as their impact increases profitability. But these low LOS values would be the next target of analysis to ensure quality of care.

What to Do with Outliers

After you have identified outliers, what should you do? First, you must determine whether the outlier is due to inaccurate measurement or recording of data points.

Assume that you evaluate two data points and find that an observation of 40 days was incorrect but 30 days was accurate. You must correct the observation with 40 days if possible; otherwise, eliminate the point from the data set. The data point of 30 days may remain in the data set after you have determined the effect it may have on your analysis (and this may be desirable if you have statistical power concerns). To determine the effect of outliers, test the study hypothesis with the outliers included in the data set and again with the outliers excluded. If the outliers cause an erroneous interpretation of the hypothesis test, eliminate the outliers from the data set; otherwise, maintain all data points in the data set.

REFERENCES

Adams, E. K., Bronstein, J. M., Becker, E. R., and Raskind-Hood, C. "Payment levels, resource use, and insurance risk of Medicaid versus private insured in three states." *Journal
of Health Care Finance,* 2001, *28,* 1–21.

Adams, E. K., Bronstein, J. M., and Raskind-Hood, C. "Adjusted clinical groups: Predictive
accuracy for Medicaid enrollees in three states." *Health Care Financing Review,* 2002, *24,*
43–60.

Agency for Healthcare Research and Quality. *HCAHPS Three-State Pilot Study Analysis Results.*
Rockville, Md.: Agency for Healthcare Research and Quality, 2003.

American Medical Association. *CPT-96: Physicians' Current Procedural Terminology.* Chicago:
American Medical Association, 1997.

American Psychological Association. *Diagnostic and Statistical Manual of Mental Disorders.* (4th ed.)
Washington, D.C.: American Psychological Association, 1995.

American Society for Quality, *Glossary* [online]. 2004 (http://www.asq.org/info/glossary/
b.html).

Anzalone, D.A., Anzalone, F. L., and Fos, P. J. "High-density lipoprotein-cholesterol: Determining hygienic factors for intervention." *Journal of Occupational and Environmental Medicine,*
1995, *37,* 856–861.

Association of State and Territorial Health Officers. *2002 Salary Survey of State and Territorial
Health Officers.* Washington, D.C.: Association of State and Territorial Health Officers,
2002.

Austin, C. J., and Boxerman, S. B. *Information Systems for Hospital Administration.* (5th ed.). Ann
Arbor, Mich.: Health Administration Press, 1998.

Benneyan, J. C., Lloyd, R. C., and Plsek, P. E. "Statistical process control as a tool for research and healthcare improvement." *Quality and Safety in Health Care,* 2003, *12,* 458–464.

Bergner, M. "Development, testing, and use of the Sickness Impact Profile." In S. R. Walker and R. M. Rosser (eds.), *Quality of Life Assessment: Key Issues in the 1990s.* Boston: Kluwer, 1993.

Berkman, L. F., and Kawachi, I. *Social Epidemiology.* Oxford: Oxford University Press, 2001.

Berkowitz, E. N. *Essentials of Health Care Marketing.* New York: Aspen, 2004.

Berkowitz, E. N., Pol, L. G., and Thomas, R. K. *Healthcare Market Research: Tools and Techniques for Analyzing and Understanding Today's Healthcare Environment.* New York: McGraw-Hill, 1997.

Butcher, A. H., Fos, P. J., Zúniga, M. A., and Panne, G. "Racial variations in cesarean section rates: An analysis of Medicaid data in Louisiana." *Journal of Public Health Management and Practice,* 1997, *3*(2), 41–48.

CAHPS Consortium. *The CAHPS Improvement Guide.* Cambridge, Mass.: Department of Health Care Policy, Harvard Medical School, 2003.

Centers for Disease Control and Prevention. *Direct Adjustment: Statistical Notes, Number 6 (Revised).* Atlanta: Centers for Disease Control and Prevention, 1995.

Centers for Disease Control and Prevention. *National Hospital Discharge Survey.* Atlanta: Centers for Disease Control and Prevention, 1998.

Centers for Disease Control and Prevention. *Asthma Surveillance Survey.* Atlanta: Centers for Disease Control and Prevention, 2000a.

Centers for Disease Control and Prevention. *Measuring Healthy Days.* Atlanta: Centers for Disease Control and Prevention, 2000b.

Centers for Disease Control and Prevention. *National Hospital Ambulatory Medical Care Survey.* Atlanta: Centers for Disease Control and Prevention, 2000c.

Centers for Disease Control and Prevention. *National Home and Hospice Care Survey.* Atlanta: Centers for Disease Control and Prevention, 2000d.

Centers for Disease Control and Prevention. *National Hospital Discharge Survey.* Atlanta: Centers for Disease Control and Prevention, 2000e.

Centers for Disease Control and Prevention. *National Health and Nutrition Examination Survey.* Atlanta: Centers for Disease Control and Prevention, 2001a.

Centers for Disease Control and Prevention. *National Health Interview Survey.* Atlanta: Centers for Disease Control and Prevention, 2001b.

Centers for Disease Control and Prevention. *National Hospital Ambulatory Medical Care Survey.* Atlanta: Centers for Disease Control and Prevention, 2001c.

Centers for Disease Control and Prevention. *National Hospital Ambulatory Medical Care Survey: 2000 Outpatient Department Summary.* Atlanta: Centers for Disease Control and Prevention, 2001d.

Centers for Disease Control and Prevention. "Summary of notifiable diseases, United States, 2001." *Morbidity and Mortality Weekly Report,* 2001e, *50,* 1–108.

Centers for Disease Control and Prevention. "Behavioral risk factor surveillance system." *Morbidity and Mortality Weekly Report,* 2003a, *52,* SS-8.

Centers for Disease Control and Prevention. "Benchmarking for prevention: The Centers for Disease Control and Prevention's National Nosocomial Infections Surveillance (NNIS) system experience." *Infection,* 2003b, 31(suppl. 2), 44–48.

Centers for Disease Control and Prevention. *National Health Interview Survey.* Atlanta: Centers for Disease Control and Prevention, 2003c.

Centers for Disease Control and Prevention. *National Vital Statistics Report,* Vol. 52, no. 3. Atlanta: Centers for Disease Control and Prevention, 2003d.

Centers for Disease Control and Prevention. "Transmission of hepatitis B and C viruses in outpatient settings—New York, Oklahoma, and Nebraska, 2000–2002." *Morbidity and Mortality Weekly Report,* 2003e, *52,* 901–906.

Centers for Disease Control and Prevention. *National Notifiable Disease Surveillance System.* Atlanta: Centers for Disease Control and Prevention, 2004a.

Centers for Disease Control and Prevention. "Tuberculosis outbreak in a community hospital—District of Columbia, 2002." *Morbidity and Mortality Weekly Report,* 2004b, *53,* 214–216.

Centers for Disease Control and Prevention, National Center for HIV, STD, and TB Prevention, Divisions of HIV/AIDS Prevention [online], 2004 (http://www.cdc.gov/hiv/dhap.htm).

Centers for Medicare and Medicaid Services. *CMS: Medicare Quality Improvement Priorities.* Publication No. 11041. Baltimore, Md.: U.S. Department of Health and Human Services, 2003.

Centers for Medicare and Medicaid Services. *Hospital Quality Initiative: Overview.* Baltimore, Md.: U.S. Department of Health and Human Services, 2004.

Chang, S. Crothers, C., and Lamm, S. "Pediatric neurobehavioral deseases in Nevada counties with respect to perchlorate in drinking water: An ecological inquiry." *Birth Defects Research Part A: Clinical and Molecular Teratology,* 2003, *67,* 886–892.

Chassin, M. R. "Is health care ready for six sigma quality?" *Milbank Quarterly,* 1998, *76,* 565–591.

Cohen, J. "A coefficient of agreement for nominal scales." *Education and Psychological Measurement,* 1960, *20,* 37–46.

Collins C. H. "John Snow: 'On the mode of communication of cholera.'" *Medical Sciences History,* 2003, *19,* 12–13.

Cooper, J. K., and others. "Health outcomes. New quality measure for Medicare." *International Journal for Quality in Health Care,* 2001, *13,* 9–16.

Cox, D., Lanyi, B., and Strabic, A. "Medicare health maintenance organization benefits packages and plan performance measures." *Health Care Financing Review,* 2002, *24,* 133–144.

Crawford, E. D. "Epidemiology of prostate cancer." *Urology,* 2003, *62*(suppl. 1), 3–12.

Daniel, W. *Biostatistics: A Foundation for Analysis in the Health Sciences.* (6th ed.) New York: Wiley, 1995.

Davis, M., and others. "Prescription drug coverage, utilization, and spending among Medicare beneficiaries." *Health Affairs,* 1999, *18,* 231–243.

Doll, R., and Hill, A. B. "Smoking and carcinoma of the lung: Preliminary report." *British Medical Journal,* 1950, *ii,* 739–748.

Donabedian, A. "The quality of care: How can it be assessed?" *Journal of the American Medical Association,* 1988, *260,* 1743–1748.

Drummond, M. F., Stoddart, G. L., and Torrance, G. W. *Methods for the Economic Evaluation of Health Care Programmes.* Oxford: Oxford University Press, 1994.

Dupaquier, J., and Dupaquier, M., *Histoire de la demographie [History of demography].* Paris: Perrin, 1985.

Edwards, W. "How to use multiattribute utility measurement for social decision making." *IEEE Transactions on Systems, Man, and Cybernetics,* 1970, *7,* 326–340.

Ellerbeck, E. F., and others. "Quality improvement in critical care access hospitals: Addressing immunizations prior to discharge." *Journal of Rural Health,* 2003, *19,* 433–438.

Epstein, R. S., and Sherwood, L. M. "From outcomes research to disease management: A guide for the perplexed." *Annals of Internal Medicine,* 1996, *124,* 832–837.

Eyler, J. M. "The conceptual origins of William Farris epidemiology: Numerical methods and social thought in the 1930s." In A. M. Lilienfeld (ed.), *Time, Persons and Places.* Baltimore: Johns Hopkins University Press, 1980.

Farnum, N. *Modern Statistical Quality Control and Implementation.* Belmont, Calif.: Wadsworth, 1994.

Fletcher, R. H., Fletcher, S. W., and Wagner, E. H. *Clinical Epidemiology: The Essentials.* Baltimore: Williams & Wilkins, 1988.

Ford, E. S., and others. "Determinants of quality of life among people with asthma: Findings from the Behavioral Risk Factor Surveillance System." *Journal of Asthma*, 2004, *41*, 327–336.

Fos, P. J., Bowen, F. W., and Zúniga, M. A. "Assessing performance of neonatal intensive care systems." Working paper, Department of Health Systems Management, Tulane University Medical Center, 1999.

Fos, P. J., and others. "The role of quality improvement in disease management: A state-wide tuberculosis control success story." *Journal of Public Health Management and Practice*, 2005.

Frank, J. W., and others. "Socioeconomic gradients in health status over 29 years of follow-up after midlife: The Alameda County study." *Social Science and Medicine*, 2003, *57*, 2305–2323.

Friede, A., O'Carroll, P. W., Thralls, R. B., and Reid, J. A. "CDC WONDER on the Web." *Proceedings of the American Medical Informatics Association Annual Fall Symposium*, 1996, pp. 408–412.

Frumkin, H. "Healthy places: Exploring the evidence." *American Journal of Public Health*, 2003, *93*, 1451–1456.

Gaynes, R., and others. "Outbreak of *Clostridium difficile* infection in a long-term care facility: Association with gatifloxacin use." *Clinical Infectious Diseases*, 2004, *38*, 640–645.

Gingrich, N. "Medicare gets much-needed shot in the arm." *Healthcare Financial Management*, 2004, *58*, 58–63.

Giovannucci, E., and others. "A prospective study of dietary fat and risk of prostate cancer." *Journal of the National Cancer Institute*, 1993, *85*, 1538–1540.

Goedert, J. "Crunching data: The key to six sigma success." *Health Data Management*, 2004, *12*, 44–48.

Gold, M. R., Siegel, J. E., Russell, L. B., and Weinstein, M. C. *Cost-Effectiveness in Health and Medicine*. New York: Oxford University Press, 1996.

Gold, M. R., Stevenson, D., and Fryback, D. G. "HALYs and QALYs and DALYs, oh my: Similarities and differences in summary measures of population health." *Annual Review of Public Health*, 2002, *23*, 115–134.

Goldsmith, G., Ward, K., and Howard, J. "Office-based management of diabetes: A two-year trial of primary care quality improvement." *Journal of the Arkansas Medical Society*, 2004, *100*, 300–305.

Gordon, T., and others. "Diabetes, blood lipids, and the role of obesity in coronary heart disease risk for women: The Framingham Study." *Annuals of Internal Medicine*, 1977, *87*, 393–397.

Gray, R. "Marketing for success through product-line development." *Trends in Health Care Management*, 1988, *14*(3), 76–83.

Greenfield, S., and Nelson, E. C. "Recent developments and future issues in the use of health status assessment measures in clinical settings." *Medical Care*, 1992, *30*(suppl.), MS23–MS41.

Grunbaum, J. A., and others. "Youth risk behavior surveillance: United States, 2003." *Morbidity and Mortality Weekly Report*, 2004, *53*, 1–96.

Hancox, J. G., Sheridan, S. C., Feldman, S. R., and Fleischer, A. B. "Seasonal variation of dermatologic disease in the USA: A study of office visits from 1990 to 1998." *International Journal of Dermatology*, 2004, *43*, 6–11.

Hauri, A. M., Armstrong, G. L., and Hutin, Y. J. "The global burden of disease attributable to contaminated injections given in health care settings." *International Journal of STDs and AIDS*, 2004, *15*, 7–16.

Hiebler, R., Kelly, T., and Ketteman, C. *Best Practices: Building Your Business with Customer-Focused Solutions*. New York: Simon & Schuster, 1998.

Hlady, W. G., Hopkins, R. S., Ogilby, T. E., and Allen, S. T. "Patient-to-patient transmission of hepatitis B in a dermatology practice." *American Journal of Public Health*, 1993, *83*, 1689–1693.

Holland, B. K., Foster, J. D., and Louira, D. B. "Cervical cancer and health care resources in Newark, New Jersey, 1970 to 1988." *American Journal of Public Health*, 1993, *83*, 45–48.

Hollinghurst, S., Bevan, G., and Bowie, C. "Estimating the avoidable burden of disease by disability-adjusted life year (DALYs). *Health Care Management Science*, 2000, *3*, 9–21.

"How safe is your hospital?" *Consumer Reports*, January 2003, pp. 12–19.

Hunt, S. M., McEwen, J., and McKenna, P. "Measuring health status: A new tool for clinicians and epidemiologists." *Journal of the Royal College of General Practice*, 1985, *35*, 185–188.

Idler, E. L., and Benyamini, Y. "Self-reported health and mortality: A review of twenty-seven community studies." *Journal of Health and Social Behavior*, 1997, *38*, 21–37.

Iezzoni, L. I. "Dimensions of risk." In L. I. Iezzoni (ed.), *Risk Adjustment for Measuring Healthcare Outcomes*. (2nd ed.) Chicago: Health Administration Press, 1997.

Institute of Medicine. *Crossing the Quality Chasm: A New Health System for the 21st Century*. Washington, D.C.: Institute of Medicine, 2001.

Institute of Medicine. *The Future of the Public's Health in the 21st Century*. Washington, D.C.: Institute of Medicine, 2002.

Isenring, E., Capra, S., and Bauer, J. "Patient satisfaction is rated higher by radiation oncology outpatients receiving nutrition intervention compared with usual care." *Journal of Human Nutrition and Diet*, 2004, *17*, 145–152.

Jackson, M. E., Eichorn, A., and Blackman, D. "Efficacy of nursing home preadmission screening." *Gerontologist*, 1992, *32*, 51–57.

Jarvis, W. R. "Benchmarking for prevention: The Centers for Disease Control and Prevention's National Nosocomial Infections Surveillance (NNIS) system experience." *Infection*, 2003, *31*(Suppl. 2), 44–48.

Jassal, S. V., and others. "Clinical practice guidelines: Prevention of cytomegalovirus disease after renal transplantation." *Journal of the American Society of Nephrology*, 1998, *9*, 1697–1708.

Jette, A. M., and Cleary, P. D. "Functional disability assessment." *Physical Therapy*, 1987, *67*, 1854–1859.

Jha, A. K., and others. "Differences in medical care and disease outcomes among black and white women with heart disease." *Circulation*, 2003, *108*, 1089–1094.

Jollis, J. G., and others. "Discordance of databases designed for claims payment versus clinical information systems: Implications for outcomes research." *Annals of Internal Medicine*, 1993, *119*, 844–850.

Keeney, R. L., and Raiffa, H. *Decisions with Multiple Objectives: Preferences and Value Trade-Offs*. New York: Wiley, 1976.

Kindig, D. A. *Purchasing Population Health*. Ann Arbor: University of Michigan Press, 1997.

Koontz, H., O'Donnell, C., and Weihrich, H. *Essentials of Management*. (4th ed.) New York: McGraw-Hill, 1986.

Last, J. M. *A Dictionary of Epidemiology*. (3rd ed.) New York: Oxford University Press, 1995.

Lau, J.T.F., and others. "SARS transmission among hospital workers in Hong Kong." *Emerging Infectious Diseases* [online], Feb. 2003 (http://www.cdc.gov/ncidod/EID/vol10no2/03-0534.htm).

Lee, J. E., and others. "Assessing health-related quality of life in cataract patients: The relationship between utility and health-related quality of life measurement." *Quality of Life Research*, 2001, *9*, 1127–1135.

Lee, J. E., and others. "Health-related quality of life of cataract patients: Cross-cultural comparisons of utility and psychometric measures." *Ophthalmic Epidemiology*, 2003, *10*, 177–191.

Leventhal, T., and Brooks-Gunn, J. "Moving to opportunity: An experimental study of neighborhood effects on mental health." *American Journal of Public Health*, 2003, *93*, 1576–1582.

Levin, M. L., Goldstein, H., and Gerhardt, P. R. "Cancer and smoking: A preliminary report." *Journal of the American Medical Association*, 1950, *143*, 336–338.

Li, S., McAlpine, D. D., Liu, J., Li, S., and Collins, A. J. "Differences between blacks and whites in the incidence of end-stage renal disease and associated risk factors." *Advances in Renal Replacement Therapy*, 2004, *11*(1), 5–13.

Lilienfeld, D. E. "John Snow: The first hired gun?" *American Journal of Epidemiology*, 2000, *152*(1), 4–9.

Loh, C. H. "Cost effectiveness of misoprostol in arthritis patients using nonsteroidal anti-inflammatory drugs." Unpublished dissertation, Tulane University, 1998.

Marmagas, S. W., King, L. R., and Chuk, M. G. "Public health's response to a changed world: September 11, biological terrorism, and the development of an environmental health tracking network." *American Journal of Public Health*, 2003, *93*, 1226–1230.

Mausner, J. S., and Kramer, S. *Epidemiology: An Introductory Text.* (2nd ed.) Philadelphia: Saunders, 1985.

McClellan, M., and Newhouse, J. P. "The marginal costs and benefits of medical technology: A panel instrumental-variables approach." *Journal of Econometrics*, 1997, *77*, 39–64.

McDowell, I., and Newell, C. *Measuring Health: A Guide to Rating Scales and Questionnaires.* (2nd ed.) New York: Oxford University Press, 1996.

McHorney, C. A. "Health status assessment methods for adults: Past accomplishments and future challenges." *Annual Review of Public Health*, 1999, *20*, 309–335.

McHorney, C. A., Ware, J. E., Jr., and Raczek, A. E. "The MOS 36-item Short-Form Health Survey (SF-36): II. Psychometric and clinical tests of validity in measuring physical and mental health constructs." *Medical Care*, 1993, *31*, 247–318.

Meynell, G. G. "Materials for a biography of Thomas Sydenham (1624–1689): A new survey of public and private archives." Folkestone, England: Winterdown Books, 1988.

Mills, P. K., Beeson, W. L., Phillips, R. L., and Fraser, G. E. "Cancer incidence among California Seventh-Day Adventists, 1976–1982." *American Journal of Clinical Nutrition*, 1994, *59*(suppl.), S1136–S1142.

Mississippi State Department of Health, Office of Health Informatics, 2004 (http://www.msdh.state.ms.us).

Murray, C.J.L., and Evans, D. B. *Health systems performance assessment: Debates, methods and empiricism.* Geneva: World Health Organization, 2003.

Murray, C.J.L., and Lopez, A. D. (eds.). *The Global Burden of Disease: A Comprehensive Assessment of Mortality and Disability from Diseases, Injuries, and Risk Factors in 1990 and Projected to 2020.* Cambridge, Mass.: Harvard School of Public Health, 1996.

Nas, T. *Cost-Benefit Analysis.* Thousand Oaks, Calif.: Sage, 1996.

National CAHPS Benchmarking Database. *What Consumers Say About the Quality of Their Health Plans and Medical Care: 2003 Chartbook,* 2 vols. [online]. January 2004 (http://ncbd.cahps.org/Home/chartbook.asp).

National Cancer Institute. *SEER Registries* [online]. 2000. (http://www.cdc.gov/cancer/npcr/uscs/2000/cancer_incidence.htm).

National Institute of Occupational Safety and Health, National Occupational Mortality Surveillance System (http://www.cdc.gov/niosh).

National Institute of Standards and Technology. *Baldrige National Quality Program Criteria for Performance Excellence.* Washington, D.C.: National Institute of Standards and Technology, 1999.

Newcomb, R. D., and Marshall, E. C. *Public Health and Community Optometry.* (2nd ed.) Boston: Butterworth's, 1990.

New York State Department of Health. *Coronary Artery Bypass Surgery in New York State, 1997–1999.* Albany: New York State Department of Health, 2002.

Onwuyani, A. E., Clarke, A., and Vanderbush, E. "Cardiovascular disease mortality." *Journal of the National Medical Association,* 2003, *95,* 1146–1151.

Parkerson, G. R., Jr., Broadhead, W. E., and Tse, C.K.J. "The Duke Health Profile: A 17-item measure of health and dysfunction." *Medical Care,* 1990, *28,* 1056–1072.

Patrick, D. L., and Erickson, P. *Health Status and Health Policy: Quality of Life in Health Care Evaluation and Resource Allocation.* New York: Oxford University Press, 1993.

Patrick, D. L., and others. "Cost and outcomes of Medicare reimbursement for HMO preventive services." *Health Care Financing Review,* 1999, *20*(4), 25–43.

Petitti, D. R. *Meta-Analysis, Decision Analysis, and Cost-Effectiveness Analysis: Methods for Quantitative Synthesis in Medicine.* New York: Oxford University Press, 1994.

Piednoir, E., and others. "Direct costs associated with a nosocomial infection in a long-term care institution." *American Journal of Infection Control,* 2002, *30,* 407–410.

Reidpath, D. D., Allotey, P. A., Koumane, A., and Cummins, R. A. "Measuring health in a vacuum: Examining the disability weight in the DALY." *Health Policy Planning,* 2003, *18,* 351–356.

Reinke, W. A. "An overview of the planning process." In W. A. Reinke (ed.), *Health Planning for Effective Management.* New York: Oxford University Press, 1998.

Rich, M. W., and others. "A multidisciplinary intervention to prevent readmission of elderly patients with congestive heart failure." *New England Journal of Medicine,* 1995, *333,* 1190–1195.

Rothman, K. J. *Modern Epidemiology.* Boston: Little Brown, 1986.

Salive, M. E., Collins, K. S., Foley, D. J., and George, L. K. "Predictors of nursing home admission in a biracial population." *American Journal of Public Health,* 1993, *83,* 1765–1767.

Schauffler, H. H., Howland, J., and Cobb, J. "Using chronic disease risk factors to adjust Medicare capitation payments." *Health Care Financing Review,* 1992, *14,* 79–90.

Self, C. A., and Enzenauer, R. W. "The application of statistical process control to horizontal strabismus surgery." *Journal of the American Association for Pediatric Ophthalmology and Strabismus,* 2004, *8,* 165–170.

Shah, V. A., and others. "TTO utility scores measure quality of life in patients with visual morbidity due to diabetic retinopathy or ARMD." *Ophthalmic Epidemiology,* 2004, *11,* 43–51.

Shortell, S. M., and Kaluzny, A. D. (eds.). *Essentials of Health Care Management.* Albany, N.Y.: Delmar, 1997.

Singer, C., and Underwood, E. A. *A Short History of Medicine. (2nd ed.)* Oxford, England: Clarendon Press, 1962.

Spendolini, M. J. *The Benchmarking Book.* New York: American Management Association, 1992.

Spitzer, W. O. "Quality of life." In D. Burley and W.H.W. Inman (eds.), *Therapeutic Risk: Perception, Measurement, Management.* New York: Wiley, 1988.

Sriniasan, S., O'Fallon, L. R., and Dearry, A. "Creating healthy communities, healthy homes, healthy people: Initiating a research agenda on the built environment and public health." *American Journal of Public Health,* 2003, *93,* 1446–1450.

Stewart, A. L., and Ware, J. E., Jr. *Measuring Functioning and Well-Being: The Medical Outcomes Study Approach.* Durham, N.C.: Duke University Press, 1992.

Stokols, D. "Establishing and maintaining healthy environments: Toward a social ecology of health promotion." *American Psychologist,* 1992, *47,* 6–22.

Swanson, K. *International Classification of Diseases, 9th Revision, Clinical Modification 4* (ICD-9-CM-4). Los Angeles: Practice Management Information Corporation, 2003.

Torpy, J. M. "Raising health care quality: Process, measures, and system failure." *Journal of the American Medical Association,* 2002, *287,* 177–178.

Trust for America's Health. "Ready or not? Protecting the public's health in the age of bioterrorism" [online]. December 2003 (http://healthyamericans.org/state/bioterror).

Tsevat, J., Slozan, J. G., and Kuntz, K. M. "Health values of HIV-infected patients: Relationship to mental health and physical functioning." *Medical Care,* 1996, *34,* 44–48.

Verderber, S. and Fine, D. J. *Healthcare architecture in an era of radical transformation.* New Haven, Conn.: Yale University Press, 2000.

von Neumann, J., and Morganstern, O. *Theory of Games and Economic Behavior.* (3rd ed.) New York: Wiley, 1953.

Voors, A. W., and others. "Studies of blood pressure in children, ages 5–14, in a total biracial community: The Bogalusa Heart Study." *Circulation,* 1976, *54,* 319–327.

Walker, M. W., and others. "Clinical process improvement: Reduction of pneumothorax and mortality in high-risk preterm infants." *Journal of Periodontology,* 2002, *22,* 641–645.

Ware, J. E., Jr., and Sherbourne, C. D. "The MOS 36-item Short Form Health Survey: I. Conceptual framework and item selection." *Medical Care,* 1992, *30,* 473–478.

Wechsler, H., Lee, J. E., Kuo, M., and Lee, H. "College binge drinking in the 1990s: A continuing problem." *Journal of American College Health,* 2000, *48,* 199–210.

Wechsler, H., and others. "Trends in college binge drinking during a period of increased prevention efforts." *Journal of American College Health,* 2002, *50,* 203–217.

Weinstein, M. C., and Stason, W. B. "Foundations of cost-effectiveness analysis for health care and medical practices." *New England Journal of Medicine,* 1977, *321,* 716–721.

Winkelstein Jr., W. "A new perspective of John Snow's communicable disease theory." *American Journal of Epidemiology,* 1995, *142,* 53–59.

World Health Organization. Preamble to the constitution of the World Health Organization. *Official Records of the World Health Organization,* 1948, no. 2, p. 100.

World Health Organization. *Manual of the International Statistical Classification of Diseases, Injuries, and Causes of Death, Ninth Revision.* Geneva: World Health Organization, 1977.

World Health Organization. *World Health Report, 2002: Reducing Risks, Promoting Healthy Life.* Geneva: World Health Organization, 2002.

World Health Organization. "Cumulative Number of Reported Probable Cases of SARS" [online]. July 11, 2003 (http://www.who.int/csr/sars/country/2003_07_11/en/).

World Health Organization. Global Burden of Disease [online]. 2004 (http://www.who.int/en/).

Wynder, E. L., and Graham, E. A. "Tobacco smoking as a possible etiologic factor in bronchiogenic carcinoma: A study of 684 proved cases." *Journal of the American Medical Association,* 1950, *143,* 329–336.

Xu, K. T. "The combined effects of participatory styles of elderly patients and their physicians on satisfaction." *Health Services Research,* 2004, *39,* 377–391.

Zelman, W. N., and McLaughlin, C. P. "Product lines in a complex marketplace: Matching organizational strategy to buyer behavior." *Health Care Management Review,* 1990, *15*(2), 9–14.

Zhang, J., Meikle, S., and Trumble, A. "Severe maternal morbidity associated with hypertensive disorders in pregnancy in the United States." *Hypertensive Pregnancy,* 2003, *22,* 203–212.

Zúniga, M. A., Babo, D. L., and Fos, P. J. "Patient satisfaction surveys: A performance assessment of two ambulatory care survey instruments." Unpublished manuscript, Tulane University Medical Center, 1996.

Zúniga, M. A., Blakely, C., and Tromp, M. "Evaluation of health and healthiness in South Texas *colonia* residents." Report to the Robert Wood Johnson Foundation, Texas A&M University System, School of Rural Public Health, 2003.

Zúniga, M. A., and Frentz, G. D. *Ambulatory Care Visit Specific Satisfaction.* New Orleans: Tulane University Hospital and Clinic, 2001.

Zúniga, M. A., and others. "Evaluación del estado de salud con la Encuesta SF-36: Resultados preliminares de su uso en México." [Evaluation of health status with the SF-36 survey: Preliminary results of its use in Mexico.] *Salud Pública de México,* 1999, *14,* 110–118.

Index

A

ACGs (adjusted clinical groups), 215
Active surveillance, 151
Adams, E. K., 215
ADL (activities of daily living), 174
Admissions department: patient satisfaction, 257*fig*; waiting time in, 256*fig*
Affinity diagrams (or checklists), 190*fig*
Age differences: average length of stay by, 254*fig*; cancer death rates by, 20*t*; crude case-fatality rates by, 106*t*; emergency department service area by, 235*t*; emergency department visits by, 49, 50*t*, 238*t*, 239*t*; expected cases by, 120*t*; expected cases using combined population by, 121*t*; frequency of cancer by, 25*t*; injury-related emergency department visits by, 19*t*, 22*t*, 23*t*; mortality rates for malignant neoplasm by, 63*t*; number of discharges by, 22*t*, 250*t*, 251*t*, 252–255; number of physician office visits by, 47–49*t*; outpatient department visits by, 99*t*, 110*t*; PMR for malignant neoplasms by, 68*t*; PMR for white male plant/system operators by, 68*t*; prevalence rate of women reporting pap test by, 58*t*; self-assessed health status and, 280*t*; tuberculosis cases by, 21*t*; uninsured by, 20*t*, 26*t*; as variable, 18–19

AIDS: case counts of, 44–46, 45*t*, 47*t*; rate of cases, 47, 48*t*
Alcohol use: community relations and population, 275*t*; lung cancer and, 101*t*
Allen, S. T., 144
Allocation, 81
Allotey, P. A., 226
ALOS (average length of stay), 252*t*, 253*t*, 254*fig*, 255. *See also* LOS (length of stay)
AMA (American Medical Association), 33–34
American Society for Quality, 182
Analytic study designs, 83
Anzalone, D. A., 84
Anzalone, F. L., 84
APC (ambulatory patient classification), 7